Penguin Education
Penguin Modern Psychology Texts

The Working Brain
An Introduction to Neuropsychology

A. R. Luria

Aleksandr Romanovich Luria is one of the most
distinguished Soviet psychologists of our time. For
forty years he has combined research on the meaning
for psychological functions of local brain lesions with
the meaning for the working of the brain of the
psychological functions – e.g. learning and
forgetting, perception and attention – that form the
central cluster of psychological concepts.

A. R. Luria is Professor of Psychology at the
University of Moscow and a member of the
Academy of Pedagogical Sciences. He is the author
of *The Nature of Human Conflicts, Traumatic Aphasia,
The Mentally Retarded Child, The Restoration of
Function After Brain Injury, Higher Cortical
Functions in Man, The Human Brain and Psychological
Processes, The Mind of a Mnemonist* and *The Man
with a Shattered World*. With F. Ia. Yudovich he is
the joint author of *Speech and the Development of
Mental Processes in the Child*, now available in
paperback from Penguin Education.

The Working Brain

An Introduction to Neuropsychology

A. R. Luria

Translated by Basil Haigh

Allen Lane The Penguin Press
Penguin Books

Penguin Education, Penguin Books Ltd, Harmondsworth,
Middlesex, England
Penguin Books, 625 Madison Avenue, New York,
New York 10022, U.S.A.
Penguin Books Australia Ltd,
Ringwood, Victoria, Australia
Penguin Books Canada Ltd, 41 Steelcase Road West,
Markham, Ontario, Canada
Penguin Books (N.Z.) Ltd, 182–190 Wairau Road,
Auckland 10, New Zealand

First published 1973
Reprinted 1976
Copyright © Penguin Books Ltd, 1973
Translation © Penguin Books Ltd, 1973
Allen Lane The Penguin Press ISBN 0 713 9 0532 8
Penguin Books ISBN 0 14 080654 7

Made and printed in Great Britain by
Hazell Watson & Viney Ltd,
Aylesbury, Bucks
Set in Monotype Times

Contents

Editorial Foreword

Over the past twenty-five years our knowledge of brain function has increased more than at any time in history except, perhaps, for the period of the last quarter of the nineteenth century. The current growth is based mainly on developments in the experimental analysis of animal behaviour, in electrophysiology and in neurochemistry, while the earlier period sought correlations between clinical observations and brain anatomy. My prediction is that the resulting bodies of evidence will soon engage and become married in a sophisticated science of human neuropsychology.

Aleksandr Romanovich Luria is uniquely fitted to herald this engagement. Early in his career he became an apostle of the great heritage of the previous century only to mould the then-current ideas into the images of the new. For the past fifty years he has refined clinical observation by devising bedside tests that could be administered to brain-damaged patients and correlated with surgical and pathological reports. Consistently he has shrewdly framed his interpretations of such correlations within the rapidly growing body of knowledge in the neurological and behavioural sciences.

The Working Brain summarizes these efforts and thus charts new horizons for us. The book serves two main purposes. As a Penguin it can reach that large readership which hungers to know the brain but finds brain facts simply presented hard to come by. As the most recent Luria pronouncement, it can serve brain scientists with what I believe to be the clearest statement available of his views, theoretical stance and some of the most important results of his researches. This clarity sharpens the issues and makes it possible to agree and disagree without ambiguity.

A case in point is Luria's Law of Diminishing Specificity of the central zones surrounding the sensory projection areas. The law either holds or it doesn't. My experience with non-human primate brains tells me that for the monkey, the law does not hold. My results therefore make me question whether the law does in fact apply to man's brain. If it does, we know at least one dimension of difference between the organization of human and non-human capacity; if it doesn't we search for other less sensory-specific integrating brain organizations. In the monkey these comprise the various 'motor' systems of the brain. The highly generative nature of man's behaviour, and especially his linguistic behaviour, suggest that in man also motor systems may be the roots of his unique capacities. Thus, experiments and observations need now to be done to test Luria's Law once again because by such tests we will come closer to an understanding of just what it is that makes man human.

There are, of course, chapters in *The Working Brain* which are less satisfactory than others. Neither Luria nor I are at all satisfied with the data on the mediobasal zones of the cortex and those on the right hemisphere. Observations on the mediobasal cortex are especially difficult to come by since restricted pathological lesions of these zones are rarely identified in the clinic. None the less, albeit too recent to include in the manuscript, major insights are currently being achieved in this area of investigation first by Oliver Zangwill, then by Brenda Milner and by Elizabeth Warrington and Lawrence Weiskrantz. These give promise of achieving as much understanding as have those regarding hemispheric specialization that were instigated by Colin Cherry and Donald Broadbent using the dichotic and dicoptic stimulation techniques and callosum sectioning developed by Roger Sperry.

The Working Brain must therefore be read as a carefully considered progress report on the current state of brain science constructed by one of its pioneers. As such it serves a new generation by clearly introducing data and ideas much as its author intends. As such it also serves Luria's peers as a provocative challenge to put up better fare or shut up shop. Can one ask more of a friend than this?

K. H. Pribram

Preface

Over the decades psychologists have studied the course of the mental processes: of perception and memory, of speech and thought, of the organization of movement and action. Hundreds of courses for university students have been prepared and thousands of books published during this period of intense activity to teach and describe the character of man's gnostic processes, speech and active behaviour. Their close study, in the context of the behavioural sciences, has yielded information of inestimable value and has given important clues to the nature of the scientific laws which govern these processes.

However, one very important aspect of this problem has remained unexplained: what are the brain mechanisms on which these processes are based? Are man's gnostic processes and motivated actions the result of the work of the whole brain as a single entity, or is the 'working brain' in fact a *complex functional system*, embracing different levels and different components each making its own contribution to the final structure of mental activity? What are the real brain mechanisms which lie at the basis of perception and memory, of speech and thought, of movement and action? What happens to these processes when individual parts of the brain cease to function normally or are destroyed by disease?

Not only would the answers to these questions be of great help to the analysis of the cerebral basis of human psychological activity, but they would also bring us much closer to the understanding of the *internal structure of mental activity*, assist with the study of the components of every mental act, and in this way enable a start to be made with the long but rewarding task of rebuilding psychological science on new and realistic foundations.

The purpose of this book is to bring this task to the reader's attention. It attempts to describe as succinctly as possible the results obtained by the author and his colleagues during almost forty years of research and to provide the student and graduate with an account of the basic facts of neuropsychology, this new branch of science.

The book begins with a brief analysis of the principal sources of the scientific facts used by the investigator when studying the brain, its structure and its functional organization, and with an account of the basic principles of neuropsychological research. The main part of the book describes what we know today about the individual systems which make up the human brain and about the role of the individual zones of the cerebral hemispheres in the task of providing the necessary conditions for higher forms of mental activity to take place. In the final part of the book the author analyses the cerebral organization of perception and action, of attention and memory, of speech and intellectual processes, and attempts to fit the facts obtained by neuropsychological studies of individual brain systems into their appropriate place in the grand design of psychological science.

Of course not all sections of neuropsychology receive equal treatment in this book, and some of them, such as the section dealing with medial parts of the cortex and with functions of the minor hemispheres (for which sufficient material has not yet been collected) can be dealt with only cursorily. Nevertheless the author hopes that in its present form the book will prove useful, in particular, to psychologists, neurologists and psychiatrists, to whom the study of the brain mechanisms of human complex activity is a matter of the greatest interest.

The author has the pleasant task of expressing his warm thanks to Professor Karl Pribram, who first suggested that he write this book, to Dr Basil Haigh who has translated it – excellently, as always – into English, and to the publishers – Penguin Education – for including it in their list.

Part One
Functional Organization and Mental Activity

Scientific interest in the study of the brain, as the organ of mental activity, has sharpened considerably in the past decades.

The human brain, this most sophisticated of instruments, capable of reflecting the complexities and intricacies of the surrounding world – how is it built and what is the nature of its functional organization? What structures or systems of the brain generate those complex needs and designs which distinguish man from animals? How are those nervous processes organized which enable information derived from the outside world to be received, analysed and stored, and how are those systems constructed which programme, regulate and then verify those complex forms of conscious activity which are directed towards the achievement of goals, the fulfilment of designs and the realization of plans?

The questions did not stand out so sharply a generation ago. At that time science was perfectly content to draw an analogy between the brain and a series of reactive systems and to direct the whole of its energies into representing the brain as a group of elementary schemes, embodying stimuli arriving from the outside world and the responses formed to these stimuli. This analogy of the brain with a series of passively responding devices, whose work was entirely determined by *past* experience, was regarded as adequate for the scientific explanation of its activity.

In the subsequent decades, the situation has changed radically. It has become abundantly clear that human behaviour is active in character, that it is determined not only by past experience, but also by plans and designs formulating the *future*, and that the human brain is a remarkable apparatus which cannot only create these models of the future, but also subordinate its behaviour to them. It has become evident at the same time that recognition of the decisive role played by such plans and designs, these schemes for the future and the programmes by which they are materialized, cannot be allowed to remain outside the sphere of scientific knowledge, and that the mechanisms on which they are based can and must be the subject of deterministic analysis and scientific explanation, like all other phenomena and associations in the objective world.

This tendency to create mechanisms whereby the future exerts its influence on current behaviour has led to the enunciation of some very important physiological hypotheses, and Anokhin's schemes of 'anticipatory excitation' or Bernstein's 'correlation between the motor task and its realization' as well as Pribram's ideas of T-O-T-E were signs of the radical shift of interest in the science of physiology, which began to recognize as its fundamental purpose the creation of a new 'physiology of activity'.

The theoretical basis of the science of the brain has also undergone a radical change. Although for many decades the theory of the brain was based on concepts likening its activity to that of certain well-known mechanical models and its purpose appeared to be to explain the work of the brain by analogy with a telephone exchange or control panel, the interests of science have now tended to move in the opposite direction.

The human brain has come to be regarded as a highly complex and uniquely constructed functional system, working on new principles. These principles can never be represented by mechanical analogues of such a sophisticated instrument, and knowledge of them must urge the investigator to draw up new mathematical schemes which really reflect the activity of the brain.

That is why the study of the intrinsic principles governing the work of the brain – however difficult their comprehension – has become the source for new constructions, and the new discipline of bionics has not merely prohibited the investigator from interpreting the work of the brain in the light of well-known mechanical schemes but, on the contrary, in order to understand the new principles, has compelled him when studying the brain to seek sources which would themselves influence the creative development of mathematics and technology.

The study of the laws governing the work of the brain as the organ of mental activity is a very difficult and complex problem and one which obviously will not be solved by the speculative invention of schemes which can only compromise this important branch of science and which, although apparently providing a solution to the highly difficult problems, in fact easily becomes an obstacle to further progress in this field. That is why the dozens of books dealing with 'models of the brain' or 'the brain as a computer' do not really help, but rather hinder, the advancement of truly scientific knowledge of the brain as the organ of the mind.

True progress in this important field naturally must not take place too quickly or otherwise real knowledge will be replaced by premature schemes which, although today they seem tempting, tomorrow will be baseless and forgotten. Progress must of course be based on real *facts*, on the achievement of real *knowledge*, on the result of scrupulously made observations in many difficult fields of science: morphology and physiology, psychology and clinical medicine. Such progress will naturally require time, and the ultimate goal will be reached by stages, each one making its own contribution to the solution of this most difficult problem.

It is now almost a quarter of a century since the appearance of Grey Walter's well-known book *The Living Brain*, in which, for the first time, an attempt was made to find an explanation of the intimate mechanisms of working of the human brain in terms of the facts of modern electrophysiology, and hypotheses (some of them confirmed, some of them still only the author's conjectures) concerning the basic forms of life of the brain and the basic principles governing its function were expressed.

A few years after this event, a second book appeared from the pen of the eminent anatomist and physiologist H. Magoun – *The Waking Brain*. This book records the first attempt to approach the brain, on the basis of the latest anatomical and neurophysiological data, as a system responsible for the waking, active state, the most important condition for all forms of behaviour of the living being. The importance of Magoun's book, which generalizes the achievements of a considerable group of brilliant investigators – Moruzzi, Jasper, Penfield and others – cannot be overestimated. With its appearance the brain of man and animals ceased to be regarded as a purely passively responding apparatus, and thus the first steps in its recognition as an active, waking system were taken.

Although this book described the mechanisms lying at the basis of waking, it did not attempt to analyse the fundamental forms of human concrete psychological activity. Questions of the fundamental mechanisms of activity (perception and thought), of speech and social communication, of the formation of plans and programmes of behaviour, and of the regulation and control of their active realization – none of this wide range of problems was discussed or considered in the numerous investigations on which the book was based.

However, facts which could permit an approach to the solution of these problems and lay the foundations of a science of the brain as the organ of concrete mental activity were gradually gathered in various fields of science.

An approach to the analysis of these facts has become possible through progress made in modern scientific *psychology*, a discipline whose purpose it is to describe the structure of human activity and to probe deeply into the functional structure of perception and memory, of intellectual activity and speech, of movement and action, and their formation in ontogenesis. A wealth of facts has been obtained in modern clinical *neurology* and *neurosurgery*. Advances in these fields have enabled the ways in which highly complex forms of behaviour are disturbed in local brain lesions to be studied in detail. A substantial contribution to success in the solution of these problems has been made by the creation of *neuropsychology*, a new branch of science with the specific and unique aim of investigating the role of individual brain systems in complex forms of mental activity.

As a result of these developments preparation of the present book, which its author has decided to call *The Working Brain*, has become possible. Its purpose is to generalize modern ideas regarding the cerebral basis of the complex working of the human mind and to discuss the systems of the brain which participate in the construction of perception and action, of speech and intelligence, of movement and goal-directed conscious activity.

This book is based on material collected by its author during his long period of work as a neuropyschologist, covering more than forty years and entirely devoted to the psychological study of patients with local brain lesions. This explains the fact that a large part of the book is concerned with the analysis of changes arising in human behaviour in the presence of local brain lesions. In the past decades neuropsychology has become an important field of practical medicine, with the consequent introduction of new methods to facilitate the early and more exact topical diagnosis of local brain lesions. At the same time, however, it has also become a powerful tool for the revision of our fundamental concepts of the internal structure of psychological processes, and a major factor leading to the creation of a theory of the cerebral basis of human mental activity.

The principal purpose of this book is to bring together the facts available at the present stage of our knowledge in the full understanding that this knowledge may be substantially changed in the stages which lie ahead.

Chapter 1
Local Brain Lesions and Localization of Functions

The neuropsychological study of local brain lesions can with every justification be regarded as the principal source of modern concepts of functional organization of the brain as the organ of mental activity. In this chapter we make a special examination of the knowledge that this study yields.

Early solutions

Attempts to examine complex mental processes as a function of local brain areas began in the very distant past. Even in the Middle Ages, philosophers and naturalists considered that mental 'faculties' could be localized in the 'three cerebral ventricles' (Figure 1), and at

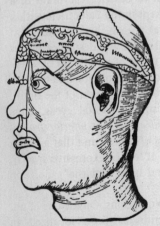

Figure 1 Diagram of the 'three cerebral ventricles'

the beginning of the nineteenth century the well-known anatomist, Gall, who first described the difference between the grey and white matter of the brain, confidently asserted that human 'faculties' are located in particular and strictly localized areas of the brain. If these areas are particularly well developed, this will lead to the formation of prominences in the corresponding parts of the skull, and observations on such prominences can therefore be used to determine individual differences in human faculties. Gall's 'phrenological' charts (Figure 2) were, however, attempts to project, without much factual basis, the 'psychology of faculties' in vogue at that time on to the brain, and they were therefore very quickly forgotten.

They were followed by attempts to distinguish functional zones of the cerebral cortex on the basis of positive observations on changes in human behaviour taking place after local brain lesions.

Clinical observations on the sequelae of local brain lesions began many years ago; even at an early stage it was discovered that a lesion of the motor cortex leads to paralysis of the opposite limbs, a lesion of the post-central region of the cortex leads to loss of sensation on the opposite side of the body, and a lesion of the occipital region of the brain leads to central blindness.

The true birth of scientific investigation of the disturbance of mental processes can rightly be taken as 1861, when the young French anatomist Paul Broca had the occasion to describe the brain of a patient who, for many years, had been kept in the Salpêtrière with a severe disturbance of motor (expressive) speech, and showed that the posterior third of the inferior frontal gyrus was destroyed in this patient's brain. Several years later, as a result of additional observations, Broca was able to obtain more precise information and to show that motor speech is associated with a localized region of the brain, namely the posterior third of the left inferior frontal gyrus. Thus Broca postulated that *the posterior third of the left inferior frontal gyrus is the 'centre for the motor images of words'* and that a lesion of this region leads to a distinctive type of loss of expressive speech, which he originally called 'aphemia' and later 'aphasia', the term still used today.

Broca's discovery was important for two reasons. On the one hand, for the first time a complex mental function had been 'localized' in a particular part of the cortex, and this 'localization' – unlike the

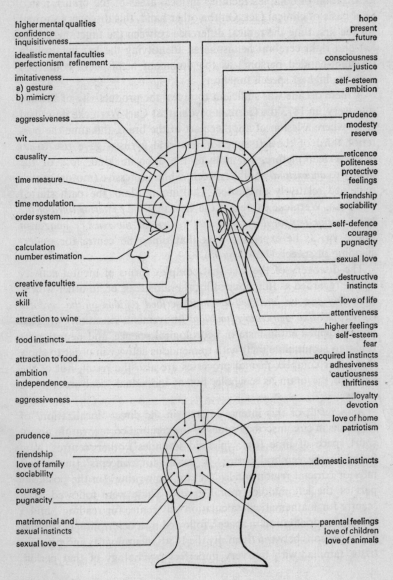

higher mental qualities
confidence
inquisitiveness

idealistic mental faculties
perfectionism   refinement

imitativeness
a) gesture
b) mimicry

aggressiveness

wit

causality

time measure

time modulation

order system

calculation
number estimation

creative faculties
wit
skill

attraction to wine

food instincts

attraction to food

ambition
independence

aggressiveness

prudence

friendship
love of family
sociability

courage
pugnacity

matrimonial and
sexual instincts

sexual love

hope
present
future

consciousness
justice

self-esteem
ambition

prudence
modesty
reserve

reticence
politeness
protective
feelings

friendship
sociability

self-defence
courage
pugnacity

sexual love

destructive
instincts

love of life

attentiveness

higher feelings
self-esteem
fear

acquired instincts
adhesiveness
cautiousness
thriftiness

loyalty
devotion

love of home
patriotism

domestic instincts

parental feelings
love of children
love of animals

Figure 2 Gall's phrenological chart

fantasies of Gall who, a generation before Broca, had tried to establish a scientific basis for his 'phrenology' (a doctrine of the localization of complex faculties in local areas of the brain), rested on a basis of clinical fact. On the other hand, this discovery showed for the first time the radical difference between the functions of the left and right cerebral hemispheres, identifying the left hemisphere (in right-handed persons) as the dominant hemisphere concerned with the highest speech functions.

A mere decade was sufficient to reveal the productivity of Broca's discovery: in 1873 the German psychiatrist Carl Wernicke described cases where a lesion of another part of the brain, this time the posterior third of the left superior temporal gyrus – gave rise to an equally clear picture, but now of the opposite kind, loss of the ability to *understand* audible speech, while expressive (motor) speech remained relatively unaffected. Continuing along the path started by Broca, Wernicke expressed the view that *the posterior third of the left superior temporal gyrus is the 'centre for the sensory images of words'* or, as he expressed it at that time, the centre for understanding of speech (*Wortbegriff*).

The discovery of the fact that complex forms of mental activity can be regarded as functions of local brain areas, or, in other words, that they can be *localized in circumscribed regions of the cerebral cortex, just like elementary functions* (movement, sensation), aroused unprecedented enthusiasm in neurological science, and neurologists began to accumulate facts with tremendous activity in order to show that other complex mental processes are also the result, not of the work of the brain as a whole, but of individual local areas of its cortex.

As a result of this intense interest in the direct 'localization' of functions in circumscribed zones of the cerebral cortex, within a very short space of time (the 'splendid seventies') other 'centres' were found in the cerebral cortex: a 'centre for concepts' (in the left inferior parietal region) and a 'centre for writing' (in the posterior part of the left middle frontal gyrus). These were followed by a 'centre for mathematical calculation', a 'centre for reading', and a 'centre for orientation in space', followed by a description of systems of connections between them. By the 1880s, neurologists and psychiatrists, familiar with the very imperfect psychology of that period, were thus able to draw 'functional maps' of the cerebral cortex which, as it seemed to them, finally settled the problem of the functional structure of the brain as the organ of mental activity once and for all. The accumulation of more material did not stop these attempts, and the tendency to localize complex psychological processes in local areas of the brain continued for more than half a century, with the addition of new facts from observations on patients with local brain lesions resulting from wounds or haemorrhage.

These attempts by the 'narrow localizationists', who observed how local lesions of the cerebral cortex led to the loss of recognition of numbers, disturbance of the understanding of words and phrases, inability to recognize objects, disturbances of motives or changes in personality, terminated in a fresh series of hypothetical maps of the 'localization of functions' in the cerebral cortex, totally unsupported by any detailed psychological analysis of the observed symptoms. The most clearly defined of these maps were suggested by the German psychiatrist Kleist (1934), who analysed a very large series of cases of gunshot wounds of the brain arising during the First World War, and, as a result, located in particular parts of the cortex functions such as 'the body scheme', 'the understanding of phrases', 'constructive actions', 'moods' and even 'the personal and social ego' (Figure 3), thereby producing maps which differed only very slightly, in principle, from Gall's phrenological maps.

These attempts to localize complex mental functions directly in local areas of the brain were so persistent that even in 1936 the well-known American neurologist Nielsen described localized areas, which in his opinion, were 'centres for the perception of living objects', distinguishing them from other areas where, in his opinion, the perception of 'non-living objects' was localized.

The crisis

It would be wrong, however, to suppose that the attempt to localize complex psychological processes directly in local brain lesions or, as it is generally called, 'narrow localizationism', remained the general line of development of neurological thought and that it encountered no natural opposition among influential neurologists. Even at the dawn of its development, in the 'splendid seventies', Broca and his

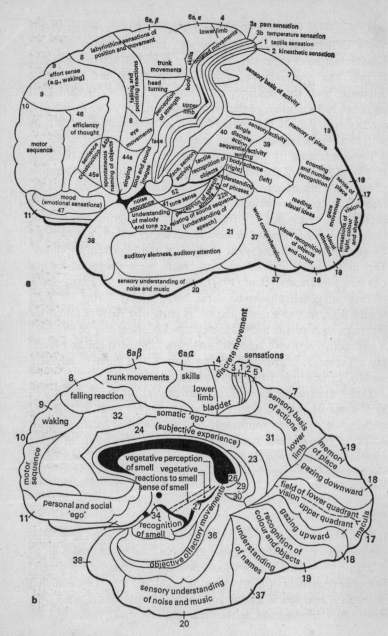

Figure 3 Kleist's localization chart (a) lateral surface; (b) medial surface

followers encountered a powerful opponent in the person of the famous English neurologist Hughlings Jackson, who put forward the hypothesis that the cerebral organization of complex mental processes must be approached from the standpoint of the *level* of their construction rather than that of their *localization* in particular areas of the brain.

Jackson's hypothesis, too complex for his time, was not taken up and developed until fifty years later, when it emerged once again in the writings of eminent neurologists in the first half of the twentieth century: Monakow (1914), Head (1926) and Goldstein (1927; 1944; 1948). Without denying the obvious fact that elementary physiological 'functions' (such as cutaneous sensation, vision, hearing, movement) are represented in clearly defined areas of the cortex, these investigators expressed valid doubts about the applicability of this principle of 'narrow localization' to the brain mechanisms of complex forms of mental activity.

These writers pointed with every justification to the complex character of human mental activity. They attempted to identify its specific features in the semantic character of behaviour (Monakow) or the 'abstract set' and 'categorial behaviour' (Goldstein), and were compelled to express their doubts that these 'functions' can be represented in circumscribed areas of the brain just like elementary functions of brain tissues. They therefore postulated that complex phenomena of 'semantics' or 'categorial behaviour' are the result of activity of the whole brain rather than the product of the work of local areas of the cerebral cortex. Doubts about the possibility of narrow localization of complex mental processes led these authors either to divorce mental processes from brain structures and to recognize their special 'spiritual nature', the position adopted towards the end of their lives by such eminent investigators as Monakow and Mourgue (1928) and Sherrington (1934; 1942), or to attempt to show that 'categorial behaviour' is the highest level of brain activity, dependent more on the *mass* of brain involved in the process than on the participation of specific zones of the cerebral cortex (Goldstein, 1944, 1948). The legitimate doubts regarding the validity of the mechanistic approach of the 'narrow localizationists' thus led either to the revival of realistic traditions of the acceptance of a 'spiritual' nature of mental processes or to the revival of other ideas of the brain as an undifferentiated entity, and of the decisive role of its mass in the performance of mental activity, which have repeatedly burst forth throughout the history of the study of the brain as the organ of the mind (Flourens, 1824; Goltz, 1876–1884; Lashley, 1929).

Whereas the mechanistic view of the direct localization of mental processes in local areas of the brain led the investigation of the cerebral basis of mental activity into a blind alley, the 'integral' (or, as they are sometimes called, 'noetic') ideas of mental processes clearly could not provide the necessary basis for further scientific research; they either preserved obsolete ideas of the separation of man's 'spiritual' life and of the impossibility, in principle, of discovering its material basis, or they revived equally obsolete ideas of the brain as a primitive, undifferentiated nervous mass.

Naturally this crisis compelled a search for new ways leading to the discovery of the true cerebral mechanisms of the highest forms of mental activity, retaining the same scientific principles of investigation for their examination as have proved themselves in the study of the elementary forms of physiological processes, but which would be adequate for the study of human conscious activity, with its social-historical origin, and its complex, hierarchical structure.

This task required the radical revision of the basic understanding of the term 'functions' on the one hand, and of the basic principles governing their 'localization' on the other.

A fresh look at the basic concepts

To approach the question of cerebral localization of human mental activity the first step must be a re-examination of the basic concepts, without which it would be impossible to solve this problem correctly. We shall re-examine first the concept of 'function', and follow this with a new look at the concept of 'localization', and finally, with a reassessment of what is called the 'symptom' or the 'loss of function' in local brain lesions.

Those investigators who have examined the problem of the cortical 'localization' of elementary functions by stimulating or excluding local brain areas have understood the term 'function' to mean the *function of a particular tissue*. Such an interpretation is unquestionably logical. It is perfectly natural to consider that the secretion of bile is a function of the liver, and the secretion of insulin is a function of the pancreas. It is equally logical to regard the perception of light as a function of the photosensitive elements of the retina and the highly specialized neurons of the visual cortex connected with them, and that the generation of motor impulses is a function of the giant pyramidal cells of Betz. However, this definition does not meet every use of the term 'function'.

When we speak of the 'function of digestion' or 'function of respiration' it is abundantly clear that this cannot be understood as a function of a particular tissue. The act of digestion requires transportation of food to the stomach, processing of the food under the influence of gastric juice, the participation of the secretions of the liver and pancreas in this processing, the act of contraction of the walls of the stomach and intestine, the propulsion of the material to be assimilated along the digestive tract and, finally, absorption of the processed components of the food by the walls of the small intestine.

It is exactly the same with the function of respiration. The ultimate object of respiration is the supplying of oxygen to the alveoli of the lungs and its diffusion through the walls of the alveoli into the blood. However, for this ultimate purpose to be achieved, a complex muscular apparatus incorporating the diaphragm and the intercostal muscles, capable of expanding and contracting the chest and controlled by a complex system of nervous structures in the brain stem and higher centres, is necessary.

It is obvious that the whole of this process is carried out, not as a simple 'function', but as a *complete functional system*, embodying many components belonging to different levels of the secretory, motor and nervous apparatus. Such a functional system (the term introduced and developed by Anokhin, 1935; 1940; 1949; 1963; 1968a; 1972), differs not only in the complexity of its structure, but also in the *mobility of its component parts*. The original task (restoration of the disturbed homeostasis) and the final result (the transportation of nutrients to the walls of the intestine or of oxygen to the alveoli of the lung, followed by their absorption into the blood stream) obviously remain unaltered in every case (or, as is sometimes said, they remain invariant). However, the way in which this task is performed may vary considerably. For instance, if the principal group of muscles working during respiration (the diaphragm) ceases to act, the intercostal muscles are brought into play, but if for some reason or other they are impaired, the muscles of the larynx are mobilized and the animal or person begins to swallow air, which thus reaches the alveoli of the lung by a completely different route. *The presence of a constant (invariant) task, performed by variable (variative) mechanisms, bringing the process to a constant (invariant) result*, is one of the basic features distinguishing the work of every 'functional system'. The second distinguishing feature is the *complex* composition of the '*functional system*', which always includes a series of afferent (adjusting) and efferent (effector) impulses.

This concept of a '*function*' as a whole *functional system* is a second definition, differing sharply from the definition of a function as the function of a particular tissue. Whereas the most complex autonomic and somatic processes are organized as 'functional systems' of this type, this concept can be applied on even stronger grounds to the complex 'functions' of behaviour.

This can be illustrated with reference to the function of movement (or locomotion), the detailed structure of which has been analysed by the Soviet physiologist Bernstein (1935; 1947; 1957; 1966; 1967). The movements of a person intending to change his position in space, to strike at a certain point, or to perform a certain action can never take place simply by means of efferent, motor impulses. Since the locomotor apparatus, with its movable joints, as a rule has a very large number of degrees of freedom, and this number is multiplied because groups of articulations participate in the movement, and every stage of the movement changes the initial tone of the muscles, movement is in principle uncontrollable simply by efferent impulses. For a movement to take place there must be constant correction of the initiated movement by afferent impulses giving information about the position of the moving limb in space and the change in tone of the muscles, so that any necessary correction in its course can take place. Only such a complex structure of the process of locomotion can satisfy the fundamental condition of the preservation of the invariant task, its performance by variative means, and the resulting attainment of an invariant result by these dynamically variative means. The fact that every movement has the character of a complex functional system and that the elements performing it may be interchangeable in character is clear because the same result can be achieved by totally different methods.

In Hunter's well-known experiments a mouse achieved its goal in a maze by running in a certain way, but when one element of the maze was replaced by a dish of water, it did so by swimming movements. In some of Lashley's observations a rat, trained to follow a certain pattern of movement, radically changed the structure of its movements after removal of the cerebellum or after division of its spinal cord by two opposite hemisections, so that no fibres were able to reach the periphery; in these cases, although unable to reproduce the movements learned through training, the rat was able to reach its goal by going head over heels, so that the original motor task was completed by achievement of the required result.

The same interchangeable character of movements necessary to achieve a required goal can also be clearly seen if any human locomotor act is carefully analysed: hitting a target (which is done with a different set of movements depending on the initial position of the body), manipulation of objects (which may be performed by different sets of motor impulses) or the process of writing, which can be performed either with pencil or pen, by the right or the left hand, or even by the foot, without thereby losing the meaning of what is written or even the characteristic handwriting of the person concerned (Bernstein, 1947).

Although this 'systemic' structure is characteristic of relatively simple behavioural acts, it is immeasurably more characteristic of more complex forms of mental activity. Naturally all mental processes such as perception and memorizing, gnosis and praxis, speech and thinking, writing, reading and arithmetic, cannot be regarded as isolated or even indivisible 'faculties', which can be presumed to be the direct 'function' of limited cell groups or to be 'localized' in particular areas of the brain.

The fact that they were all formed in the course of long historical development, that they are social in their origin and complex and hierarchical in their structure, and that they are all based on a complex system of methods and means, as the work of the eminent Soviet psychologist Vygotsky (1956; 1960) and his pupils (Leontev, 1959; Zaporozhets, 1960; Galperin, 1959; Elkonin, 1960) has shown, implies that the fundamental forms of conscious activity must be considered as complex functional systems; consequently, the basic approach to their 'localization' in the cerebral cortex must be radically altered.

Revision of the concept of 'localization'

Our examination of the structure of functional systems in general and of the higher psychological functions in particular has led us to take a completely fresh look at the classical ideas of localization of mental function in the human cortex. Whereas elementary functions of a tissue can, by definition, have a precise localization in particular cell groups, there can of course be no question of the localization of complex functional systems in limited areas of the brain or of its cortex.

We have already seen that a functional system such as respiration incorporates so complex and labile a system of components that Pavlov, when discussing the question of a 'respiratory centre', was compelled to recognize that, 'whereas at the beginning we thought that this was something the size of a pinhead in the medulla ... now it has proved to be extremely elusive, climbing up into the brain and down into the spinal cord, and at present nobody can draw its boundaries at all accurately' (1949a, vol. 3, p. 127). Naturally it is a far more complex matter with the localization of the higher forms of mental activity. The higher forms of mental processes have a particularly complex structure; they are laid down during ontogeny. Initially they consist of a complete, expanded series of manipulative movements which gradually have become condensed and have acquired the character of inner 'mental actions' (Vygotsky, 1956; 1960; Galperin, 1959). As a rule they are based on a series of external aids, such as language, the digital system of counting, formed in the process of social history, they are mediated by them, and cannot in general be conceived without their participation (Vygotsky, 1956; 1960); they are always connected with reflection of the outside world in full activity, and their conception loses all its meaning if it is considered apart from this fact. That is why mental functions, as complex functional systems, cannot be localized in narrow zones of the cortex or in isolated cell groups, but must be *organized in systems of concertedly working zones, each of which performs its role in complex functional system,* and which may be located in completely different and often far distant areas of the brain.

Two facts, which sharply distinguish this form of work of the human brain from the more elementary forms of work of the animal brain, are perhaps the most essential features of this 'systemic' concept of the localization of mental processes in the cortex. Whereas higher forms of conscious activity are always based on certain external mechanisms (good examples are the knot which we tie in our handkerchief so as to remember something essential, a combination of letters which we write so as not to forget an idea, or a multiplication table which we use for arithmetical operations) – it becomes perfectly clear that these external aids or historically formed devices are *essential elements in the establishment of functional connections between individual parts of the brain,* and that by their aid, areas of the brain which previously were independent become the *components of a single functional system.* This can be expressed more vividly by saying that *historically formed measures for the organization of human behaviour tie new knots in the activity of man's brain,* and it is the presence of these functional knots, or, as some people call them, 'new functional organs' (Leontiev, 1959), that is one of the most important features distinguishing the functional organization of the human brain from an animal's brain. It is this principle of construction of functional systems of the human brain that Vygotsky (1960) called the principle of 'extracortical organization of complex mental functions', implying by this somewhat unusual term that all types of human conscious activity are always formed with the support of external auxiliary tools or aids.

The second distinguishing feature of the 'localization' of higher mental processes in the human cortex is that it is never static or constant, but *moves about essentially during development of the child and at subsequent stages of training.* This proposition, which at first glance may appear strange, is in fact quite natural. The development of any type of complex conscious activity at first is expanded in character and requires a number of external aids for its performance, and not until later does it gradually become condensed and converted into an automatic motor skill.

In the initial stages, for example, *writing* depends on memorizing the graphic form of every letter. It takes place through a chain of isolated motor impulses, each of which is responsible for the performance of only one element of the graphic structure; with practice, this structure of the process is radically altered and writing is converted into a single 'kinetic melody', no longer requiring the memorizing of the visual form of each isolated letter or individual motor impulses for making every stroke. The same situation applies to the process in which the change to writing a highly automatized engram (such as a signature) ceases to depend on analysis of the acoustic complex of the word or the visual form of its individual letters, but begins to be performed as a single 'kinetic melody'. Similar changes take place also during the development of other higher psychological processes.

In the course of such development it is not only the functional structure of the process which changes, but also, naturally, its cerebral 'organization'. The participation of the auditory and visual areas of the cortex, essential in the early stages of formation of the activity, no longer is necessary in its later stages, and *the activity starts to depend on a different system of concertedly working zones* (Luria, Simernitskaya and Tubylevich, 1970).

The development of higher mental functions in ontogeny has yet another feature of decisive importance for their functional organization in the cerebral cortex. As Vygotsky (1960) showed some time ago, during ontogeny it is not only the structure of higher mental processes which changes, but also their relationship with each other, or, in other words, their 'interfunctional organization'. Whereas in the first stages of development a complex mental activity rests on a more elementary basis and depends on a 'basal' function, in subsequent stages of development it not only acquires a more complex structure, but also starts to be performed with the close participation of structurally higher forms of activity.

For instance, the young child thinks in terms of visual forms of perception and memory or, in other words, he *thinks by recollecting*. At later stages of adolescence or in adult life, abstract thinking with the aid of the functions of abstraction and generalization is so highly developed that even relatively simple processes such as perception and memory are converted into complex forms of logical analysis and synthesis, and the person actually begins to *perceive or recollect by reflection.*

This change in the relationship between the fundamental psychological processes is bound to lead to changes in the relationship between the fundamental systems of the cortex, on the basis of which these processes are carried out. Consequently, in the young child a lesion of a cortical zone responsible for a relatively elementary form of mental activity (for example, the visual cortex) invariably gives rise, as its secondary or 'systemic' effect, to the imperfect development of higher structures superposed on it, in the adult, in whom these complex systems have not only been formed but have come to exert a decisive influence over the organization of simple forms of activity, a lesion of the 'lower' areas is no longer so important as it was in the early stages of development. Conversely, a lesion of the 'higher' areas leads to disintegration of the more elementary functions, which now have acquired a complex structure and have begun to depend intimately on the most highly organized of activity.

This is one of the fundamental propositions introduced into the theory of the 'dynamic localization' of higher mental functions by Soviet psychological science. It was formulated by Vygotsky into a rule which states that a lesion of a particular part of the brain in early childhood had a systemic effect on the *higher* cortical areas superposed above it, whereas a lesion of the same region in adult life affects *lower* zones of the cortex, which now begin to depend on them. It can be illustrated by the fact that a lesion of the secondary areas of the visual cortex in early childhood may lead to systemic underdevelopment of the higher zones responsible for visual thinking, whereas a lesion of these same zones in the adult can cause only partial defects of visual analysis and synthesis, and leaves the more complex forms of thinking, formed at an earlier stage, unaffected.

All that has been said about the systemic structure of higher psychological processes compels the radical revision of the classical ideas on their 'localization' in the cerebral cortex. It is accordingly our fundamental task not to 'localize' higher human psychological processes in limited areas of the cortex, but to *ascertain by careful* analysis which groups of concertedly working zones of the brain are responsible for the performance of complex mental activity; what contribution is made by each of these zones to the complex functional system; and how the relationship between these concertedly working parts of the brain in the performance of complex mental activity changes in the various stages of its development.

Such an approach must radically modify the *practical mode of work* of the psychologist who is attempting to study the cerebral organization of mental activity. The attempt to determine the cerebral basis of a particular human mental process must be preceded by a *careful study of the structure of that psychological process* whose cerebral organization it is hoped to establish and by the identification of those of its components which can be classed to some extent among definite systems of the brain. Only by working in this way to clarify the precise functional structure of the psychological process to be studied, with the identification of its components and the further analysis of its 'location' among the systems of the brain, will a solution to the old problem of the 'localization' of mental processes in the cerebral cortex be found.

Revision of the concept of 'symptom'

Classical investigations into the localization of mental functions in the cortex, making use of observations on changes in behaviour after local brain lesions, started out from the simplified assumption that a disturbance of a particular mental function (speech, writing or reading, praxis or gnosis), arising as the result of destruction of a certain part of the brain, is direct proof that this 'function' is 'localized' in this (now destroyed) part of the brain. The facts examined above compel a radical re-examination of these over-simplified ideas.

A disturbance of general sensation must always indicate a lesion of the postcentral gyrus or of its tracts, just as the loss of part of the visual field must indicate a lesion of the retina, of the optic tracts, or of the visual cortex. In such cases to identify the *symptom* means to obtain definite information for the topical diagnosis of the lesion, and hence, for the localization of the function in the nervous system. It is a completely different matter in cases where higher mental processes are disturbed in patients with local brain lesions.

If mental activity is a complex functional system, involving the participation of a group of concertedly working areas of the cortex (and sometimes, widely distant areas of the brain), *a lesion of each of these zones or areas may lead to disintegration of the entire functional system,* and in this way the *symptom or 'loss' of a particular function tells us nothing about its 'localization'.*

In order to progress from establishment of the *symptom* (loss of a given function) to the *localization* of the corresponding mental activity, a long road has to be travelled. Its most important section is the *detailed psychological analysis of the structure of the disturbance and the elucidation of the immediate causes of collapse of the functional system* or, in other words, a *detailed qualification of the symptom observed.*

I shall clarify this with an example. In the clinical picture of local brain lesions a very frequently observed symptom is *apraxia*, when the patient is unable to manipulate objects in certain ways. In classical neurology it was sufficient to conclude that the lesion is located in the inferior parietal region, regarded as the 'centre for complex praxis' or, if the apraxia took the form of difficulty in carrying out a clearly represented movement scheme, it was a lesion localized in areas of the cortex lying anteriorly to this region. Nothing can be more mistaken than such an idea and such an attempt to 'localize' the symptom of apraxia (and, consequently, the function of 'praxis') in a narrow area of the cortex.

After the investigations of physiologists (notably the Soviet physiologist Bernstein), it became abundantly clear that any voluntary movement and, still more, any manipulative movement, must be a *complex functional system* incorporating a number of conditions, in the absence of which the movement cannot be carried out. In order to perform such movements, the first essential is its *kinaesthetic afferentation* or, in other words, the system of kinaesthetic impulses reaching the brain from the moving limb, indicating the degree of tone of the muscles, and giving information on the position of the joints. If these afferent impulses (the reception and integration of which are carried out by the general sensory areas in the postcentral cortex) are missing, the movement loses its afferent basis and the effector impulses passing from the cortex to the muscles become virtually uncontrolled.

As a result of this fact, even relatively fine lesions of the postcentral cortex may lead to a distinctive form of *'kinaesthetic apraxia'*, based on differentiation of the moving limb. This condition consists of a disturbance of finely differentiated movements including inability to place the hand in the necessary *position* for the manipulative action which it is to perform. But the presence of the essential kinaesthetic afferentation, however important it may be, is not in itself sufficient for the performance of the corresponding action.

Any movement, whether it be a movement in space, hitting a target, or a manipulative operation, is always effected in a certain system of *spatial coordinates*. It always takes place in the sagittal, horizontal or vertical plane, and it always requires the *synthesis of these visuo-spatial afferentations* which, on this occasion, is carried out by the tertiary zones in the parieto-occipital region of the cortex, receiving impulses from the visual and vestibular systems and the system of cutaneous kinaesthetic sensation. If this region of the brain is affected by a lesion and spatial syntheses are disturbed, a disturbance of movements of such structural complexity must take place. However, the apraxia arising in these cases is completely different in character, and it is manifested primarily as inability to give the performing hand its necessary position in space; the patient begins to have difficulty in making the bed, and often instead of laying the blanket along the bed, places it crosswise; he cannot keep the fork which he holds in the right direction, but often moves it vertically instead of horizontally, he cannot strike a target correctly, and so on. *Spatial apraxia* of this type clearly differs vastly from the 'kinaesthetic apraxia' described above, not only in its action and structure, but also in its mechanisms and in the localization of the effects responsible for it.

These two conditions alone are insufficient for the perfect performance of a movement or action. Every action consists of a *chain of consecutive movements*, each element of which must be denervated after its completion so as to allow the next element to take its place. In the initial stages of formation, this chain of motor elements is discrete in character and every motor element requires its own special, isolated impulse. In the formation of a motor skill, this chain of isolated impulses is reduced and the complex movements begin to be performed as a single 'kinetic melody'.

Essentially the *kinetic organization of movements* is performed by completely different brain systems: by the basal ganglia in the early stages of phylogenesis (the stages of elementary 'motor synergism') and by the premotor areas of the cortex in the late stages of formation of complex motor skills. For this reason, when these areas of the cortex are affected by pathological lesions, apraxia also arises, but this time it is a '*kinetic apraxia*', manifested as inability to synthesize the motor elements into a single smooth, consecutive melody, as difficulty in denervating an element of the movement on its completion at the proper time, and in passing on smoothly from one motor element to the next. The structure of this 'kinetic apraxia' naturally differs significantly from the forms of apraxia described previously, and the local origin of these symptoms is quite different.

We must now consider the last condition for the correct performance of movement. Any movement is aimed at a certain goal and carries out a certain *motor task*. At the level of instinctive behaviour, with its elementary structure, these motor tasks are dictated by inborn programmes; at the level of a complex conscious action formed during life, they are dictated by *intentions* which are formed with the close participation of speech, regulating human behaviour (Luria, 1961). Special investigations (Luria, 1962; 1963; 1966a; 1966b; 1966c; Luria and Homskaya, 1966) have shown that such complex intentions regulated by means of speech, are formed with the close participation of the *frontal lobes* of the brain. Massive lesions of the frontal lobe can thus lead to apraxia, but this 'apraxia of goal-directed action' differs radically from the forms described previously. As a rule it consists of inability of the patient to subordinate his movements to the intention expressed in speech, the disintegration of organized programmes, and the replacement of a rational, goal-directed action by the echopraxic repetition of the patient's movements or by inert stereotypes which have lost their rational, goal-directed character. We shall not discuss this type of disturbance of praxis at this point, for I have described it elsewhere and it will be specially examined later in this book.

An important conclusion can be deduced from these facts described. The symptom of a disturbance of praxis (apraxia) is a sign of a local brain lesion; however, by itself this symptom tells nothing about any specific localization of the focus causing its appearance. Voluntary movement (praxis) constitutes a complex functional system incorporating a number of conditions or factors dependent upon the concerted working of a whole group of cortical zones and subcortical structures, *each of which makes its own contribution to the performance of the movement* and supplies *its own factor* to its structure. *Complex manipulation of objects can thus be disturbed by lesions of different cortical areas (or subcortical structures); however, in each case it is disturbed differently* and the structure of this disturbance differs on each occasion.

The investigator's immediate task is to study the *structure of the observed defects and to qualify the symptoms.* Only then, by work leading to the *identification of the basic factor lying behind the observed symptom,* is it possible to draw conclusions regarding the localization of the focus lying at the basis of the defect. The concept of 'localization of a focus' thus does not coincide with that of 'localization of a function' and before the method of local brain lesions can be used to draw conclusions regarding 'localization of a function' (or, more exactly, the cerebral organization of a functional system), the syndrome must be subjected to complex structural analysis, which is the basis of the neuropsychological method of investigation.

Syndrome analysis and the systemic organization of psychological processes

The qualification of the symptom is only the first step in the analysis of the cerebral organization of mental processes. So that the results of this analysis shall be reliable, and the data of local brain pathology can serve as the basis for reliable conclusions regarding both the structure of mental processes and their 'localization' in the human cerebral cortex, the next step must be from qualification of the single syndrome to description of the complete symptom-complex or, as it is generally called, to the *syndrome analysis* of changes in behaviour arising in local brain lesions.

As I have said already, any human mental activity is a complex functional system effected through a combination of concertedly working brain structures, each of which makes its own contribution to the functional system as a whole. This means, in practice, that the *functional system as a whole can be disturbed by a lesion of a very large number of zones, and also that it can be disturbed differently in lesions in different localizations.* This last statement, as will easily be understood, is connected with the fact that each area of the brain concerned in this functional system introduces *its own particular factor* essential to its performance, and removal of this factor makes the normal performance of this functional system impossible. The example of the construction of a voluntary movement and the types of its disturbance in local brain lesions given above shows this clearly enough. The rules governing the structure and destruction of functional systems which I have described are of decisive importance for the next step, which occupies a central place both in the structure of mental processes and in their cerebral organization.

The neuropsychologist who is confronted by these problems must first ascertain *what factors are actually involved in the particular mental activity and what structures of the brain constitute its neuronal basis.* These two problems can only be solved by *comparison of all the symptoms which arise in lesions of one strictly localized focus in the cortex* (or subcortex), on the one hand, and by a thorough analysis of the *character of a disturbance of this system by brain lesions in different locations* on the other hand. Let us consider one example to illustrate this basic principle.

As I have said, the successful performance of a complex movement requires its precise spatial organization or, in other words, the structure of the movement in a system of definite spatial coordinates. This condition is satisfied by the tertiary 'visuo-kinaesthetic-vestibular' portions of the parieto-occipital cortex, and the removal of this condition causes disintegration of the spatially organized movement. However, the question naturally arises: *what other types of mental activity are disturbed by lesions of these parieto-occipital regions of the brain which are responsible for spatial organization of movements?* If we can answer this question, and if we can distinguish one group of processes which is affected by a focus in this localization, and another group of processes which remains intact in the presence of this pathological focus, we shall have made an important step towards discovering *which types of mental activity include the particular spatial factor directly connected with these parieto-occipital regions of the cortex.*

Facts showing that any local pathological focus arising in the cerebral cortex in fact disturbs the successful performance of some psychological processes while leaving others intact or, in other words, that every local focus gives rise to what the American neuropsychologist Teuber called the '*principle of double dissociation of function*', are found in great abundance by careful neuropsychological investigation. For instance, a local focus in the parieto-occipital (or inferior parietal) region of the left hemisphere, disturbing the spatial organization of perception and movement, invariably gives rise to other symptoms also: these patients as a rule cannot interpret the position of the hands of a clock or find their bearings on a map; they cannot find their way around the ward where they are staying: they cannot solve even relatively simple arithmetical problems and they are confused when faced with the problem of subtracting from a number of two digits requiring carrying over from the tens column: when subtracting 7 from 31, for example, they do the first stage of this operation ($30 - 7 = 23$) but then they do not know whether the odd 1 should be added or subtracted, or whether their final result should be '22' or '24'. Finally they begin to have great difficulty in understanding grammatical structures incorporating logical relationships, such as 'the father's brother' and 'the brother's father'; 'spring after summer' 'summer after spring', whereas the understanding of simpler grammatical structures remains unimpaired.

However, such a focus produces no disturbances of processes such as fluent speech, the understanding or playing of musical melodies, the smooth succession of the elements of movement, and so on.

All this shows that the *first group of processes indicated above includes a 'spatial' factor, whereas the second group of processes does not incorporate such a factor* and therefore remains intact in a lesion of the parieto-occipital region of the cortex. Quite the opposite arises in local lesions of the temporal (auditory) cortex. Lesions in this situation, as we shall see, lead to a disturbance of the complex organization of auditory perception, so that the organization of acoustic stimuli into their proper successive structure becomes impossible. Accordingly, patients with lesions in this situation are unable to reproduce correctly what is said to them or to retain traces of it. Fluent discriminative speech, like audio-verbal memory, can be substantially impaired in these patients. However, spatial orientation, the spatial organization of movement, mathematical operations, and the comprehension of certain logico-grammatical relationships as a rule remain unimpaired.

These observations clearly show that a careful *neuropsychological analysis of the syndrome* and *observations of the 'double dissociation' which arises in local brain lesions* can make a major contribution to the *structural analysis of psychological processes themselves* and can pick out the factors involved in one group of mental processes but not in others. As we shall see, this is a great help to the solution of the problem of the *internal composition of psychological processes*, which could not be solved by ordinary psychological investigations, for by this means, *apparently identical psychological processes can be distinguished* and *apparently different forms of mental activity can be reconciled*. Two examples will serve to illustrate this.

To the unprejudiced observer, *musical hearing and speech hearing* may appear to be two versions of the same psychological process. However, observations on patients with local brain lesions show that destruction of certain parts of the left temporal region leads to a marked disturbance of speech hearing (discrimination between similar sounds of speech is completely impossible), while leaving musical hearing unimpaired. In the report of one of my cases there is a description of a famous composer who, after a haemorrhage into the left temporal region, was unable to distinguish between the sounds of speech or to understand words spoken to him, yet he continued to compose brilliant musical works (Luria, Tsvetkova and Futer, 1965). This means that such apparently similar mental processes as musical hearing and speech hearing not only incorporate different factors, but also depend on the working of quite different areas of the brain.

Other examples demonstrating the intrinsic similarities between apparently totally different psychological processes also are known in neuropsychology. Would anybody be prepared to accept at once that such differing psychological processes as spatial orientation, arithmetical calculations, and the understanding of complex logico-grammatical structures have important links in common, on the basis of which they can be united into a single group of psychological processes? As I have already mentioned, a lesion of the left parieto-occipital (or inferior parietal) region of the cortex almost invariably leads to a disturbance of all these processes, so that a patient with such a lesion not only finds it difficult to find his bearings in space but also makes mistakes in his simplest calculations and misunderstands complex logico-grammatical structures. This means that all these apparently so widely different functions incorporate a *common factor*, and it allows an approach to be made to the more intimate analysis of the structure of psychological processes.

It will easily be seen that syndrome analysis sheds considerable light on the *cerebral organization of mental processes* and also gives *considerable insight into their internal structure*, something which for many centuries psychologists have been unable to do. The other aspect of this problem cannot be dealt with in such detail at this point.

The fact that every complex mental activity is a functional system which can be disturbed in different components and which can be impaired by brain lesions in different situations (even though it is impaired differently) means that we can get closer to the description of the *factors* composing it and thereby discover new ways of neurophysiological analysis of the internal structure of mental processes.

A complete part of this book will be devoted to illustrations of this principle, the importance of which cannot be overestimated, and so we will leave it aside for the moment.

From all the foregoing remarks it will be clear that the use of observations on changes in mental processes arising in local brain lesions can be one of the most important sources of our knowledge of the cerebral organization of mental activity.

However, the correct use of this method is possible only if *the attempt is resisted to seek the direct localization of mental processes in the cortex*, and only if this classical task is replaced by another – *by analysis of how mental activity is altered in different local brain lesions and what factors are introduced into the structure and complex forms of mental activity by each brain system.* This fundamental task defines the general direction of neuropsychology, the science of the cerebral organization of human mental processes.

Chapter 2
The Three Principal Functional Units

I have said that human mental processes are complex functional systems and that they are not 'localized' in narrow, circumscribed areas of the brain, but take place through the participation of groups of concertedly working brain structures, each of which makes its own particular contribution to the organization of this functional system. Accordingly, the first essential must be to discover the basic functional units from which the human brain is composed, and the role played by each of them in complex forms of mental activity.

There are solid grounds for distinguishing *three principal functional units of the brain* whose participation is necessary for any type of mental activity. With some approximation to the truth they can be described as a unit for *regulating tone or waking*, a unit for *obtaining, processing and storing information* arriving from the outside world and a unit for *programming, regulating and verifying mental activity*. Man's mental processes in general, and his conscious activity in particular, always take place with the participation of all three units, each of which has its role to play in mental processes and makes its contribution to their performance.

Another important feature is that each of these basic units itself is *hierarchical in structure* and consists of at least three cortical zones built one above the other: the *primary* (projection) area, which receives impulses from or sends impulses to the periphery, the *secondary* (projection-association), where incoming information is processed or programmes are prepared, and finally, the *tertiary* (zones of overlapping), the latest systems of the cerebral hemispheres to develop and responsible in man for the most complex forms of mental activity requiring the concerted participation of many cortical areas. Let us examine the structure and functional properties of each unit separately.

The unit for regulating tone and waking and mental states

For human mental processes to follow their correct course, the waking state is essential. It is only under optimal waking conditions that man can receive and analyse information, that the necessary selective systems of connections can be called to mind, his activity programmed, and the course of his mental processes checked, his mistakes corrected, and his activity kept to the proper course.

It is well known that such precise regulation of mental processes is impossible during sleep; the course of reminiscences and associations which spring up is disorganized in character, and properly directed mental activity is impossible.

'Organized, goal-directed activity requires maintenance of an *optimal level of cortical tone*', Pavlov stated many years ago, asserting hypothetically that if it were possible to see the system of excitation spreading over the cortex of a waking animal (or man), we would observe a moving, concentrated 'spot of light', moving over the cortex with the change from one activity to another, and reflecting a point of optimal excitation, without which normal activity is impossible.

With the subsequent development of electrophysiological methods it became possible to *visualize* this 'point of optimal excitation'. By the use of a special instrument, the 'toposcope' invented by Livanov (1962), which enables between 60 and 150 points of cortical excitation to be recorded simultaneously and dynamics of these points to be presented by television, we can see the way in which the point of optimal excitation in fact arises in the cortex of a waking animal, the pattern of its movement over the cortex, and the way in which it loses its mobility, becomes inert, and, finally, is completely extinguished as the animal passes into a state of sleep or, even more obviously, in a dying animal.

The credit not only for indicating the need for such an optimal state of the cortex for any form of organized activity to take place, but also for establishing the fundamental neurodynamic laws characterizing such an optimal state of the cortex, is due to Pavlov. As many of his observations showed, processes of excitation taking place in the waking cortex obey a *law of strength*, according to which every strong (or biologically significant) stimulus evokes a strong response, while every weak stimulus evokes a weak response. It is characterized by a certain degree of *concentration* of nervous processes and a certain balance in the relationships between excitation and inhibition and, finally, by high *mobility* of the nervous processes, so that it is easy to change from one activity to another.

It is these fundamental features of optimal neurodynamics which disappear in sleep or in the state preceding it, when cortical tone diminishes. In these states of inhibition or, as Pavlov calls them, these 'phasic' states the law of strength is broken, and weak stimuli may either evoke equally strong responses as strong stimuli (the 'equalizing phase'), or may evoke stronger responses than strong stimuli (the 'paradoxical phase'), or they may even continue to evoke a response whereas strong stimuli altogether cease to do so (the 'ultraparadoxical phase'). It is also known that in a state of lowered cortical tone the normal relationship between excitation and inhibition is disturbed, and the mobility of the nervous system, so necessary for mental activity to pursue its normal course, is lost. These observations show that maintenance of the *optimal level of cortical tone is essential for the organized course of mental activity*. This raises the question of which brain structures are responsible for maintaining the optimal level of cortical tone we have just mentioned. What parts of the brain regulate and modify cortical tone, maintain it at the proper time and raise it should it become necessary to do so.

A most important discovery, made only thirty years ago, was that the *structures maintaining and regulating cortical tone do not lie in the cortex itself, but below it, in the subcortex and brain stem*; it was also discovered that these structures have a *double relationship with the cortex, both influencing its tone and themselves experiencing its regulatory influence.*

The year 1949 initiated a new period in our knowledge of the functional organization of the brain. In that year two outstanding investigators, Magoun and Moruzzi, showed that there is a special nervous formation in the brain stem which is specially adapted, both by its morphological structure and by its functional properties, to play the role of a mechanism regulating the *state of the cerebral cortex*, changing its tone and maintaining its waking state. Unlike the cortex, this formation does not consist of isolated neurons, capable of sending single impulses along their long processes (axons) and, operating according to an 'all or nothing', law, generating discharges and leading to the innervation of muscles. This formation has the structure of a *nerve net*, among which are scattered the bodies of nerve cells connected with each other by short processes. Excitation spreads over the net of this nervous structure, known as the *reticular formation*, not as single, isolated impulses and not in accordance with the 'all or nothing' law, but *gradually*, changing its level little by little and thus modulating the whole state of the nervous system.

Some of the fibres of this reticular formation run upwards to terminate in higher nervous structures such as the thalmus, caudate body, archicortex and, finally, the structures of the neocortex. These structures were called the *ascending reticular system*. As subsequent observations showed, it plays a decisive role in *activating the cortex and regulating the state of its activity*. Other fibres of the reticular formation run in the opposite direction: they begin in higher nervous structures of the neocortex and archicortex, caudate body, and thalamic nuclei and run to lower structures in the mesencephalon, hypothalamus and brain stem. These structures were called the *descending reticular system* and, as subsequent observations showed, they subordinate these lower structures to the control of programmes arising in the cortex and requiring modification and modulation of the state of waking for their performance.

These two sections of the reticular formation thus constitute a single vertically arranged functional system, a single self-regulating apparatus built on the 'reflex ring' principle, capable of changing the tone of the cortex, but itself also under cortical influence, being regulated and modified by changes taking place in the cortex and adapting itself readily to the environmental conditions and in the course of activity.

With the discovery of the reticular formation, a new principle was thus introduced: the *vertical organization of all structures of the brain*. This put an end to that long period during which the attention of scientists attempting to discover the nervous mechanisms of mental processes was concentrated entirely on the cortex, the work of whose systems was deemed to be independent of the lower or deeper structures. With the description of the reticular formation, the *first functional unit of the brain* was discovered – an apparatus

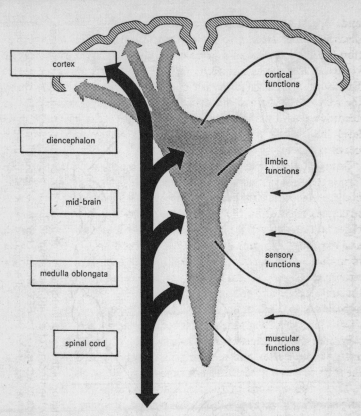

Figure 4 Scheme of the activating reticular formation

maintaining cortical tone and the waking state and regulating these states in accordance with the actual demands confronting the organism.

The function of the reticular formation in regulating the tone of the cortex and modulating its state was demonstrated by numerous experiments (Moruzzi and Magoun, 1949; Lindsley *et al.*, 1949; Lindsley, 1960; 1961; Bremer, 1954; 1957; Jasper, 1954; 1957; 1963; French *et al.*, 1955; Segundo *et al.*, 1955; Jouvet, 1956–1961; Nauta, 1964; 1968; Pribram, 1960; 1966b; 1967; 1971). These experiments formed the subject of a special survey by Magoun in his book *The*

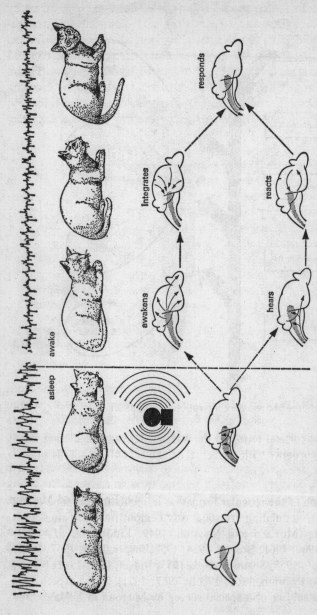

Figure 5 The activating effect of stimulation of the reticular formation on the cortex, evoking an arousal response (after French). The cat is awakened by the ringing of a bell; excitation arising in the reticular formation spreads to the auditory cortex and leads to arousal. The EEG waves change correspondingly. The reticular formation integrates brain activity and this results in a general organized response by the cat

Waking Brain (1958; second edition, 1963) and in publications by other workers (Hernández-Peón, 1969, etc.). This series of investigations showed that stimulation of the reticular formation (in the region of the mesencephalon, posterior part of the hypothalamus and adjacent subthalamic structures) evokes an arousal reaction (Figure 5) and increases excitability and sharpens sensitivity, by lowering both the absolute and differential thresholds of sensation (Lindsley, 1951; 1958; 1960) (Figure 6), thereby exerting a *general activating*

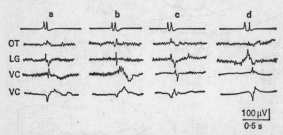

Figure 6 Activating effect of stimulation of the reticular formation, increasing sensitivity (discrimination of two flashes). Top line: flashes; line 2: optic tract; line 3: lateral geniculate body; lines 4 and 5: visual cortex (after Lindsley). (a) before stimulation of reticular formation; (b) during stimulation; (c) 0–10 sec, and (d) 10–12 sec after stimulation. The double response appearing in the visual cortex after stimulation will be noted

effect on the cortex. Excitation of the reticular formation of the brain stem results in a strengthening of the *motor* reactions to stimuli (Figure 7). The important fact was discovered that a lesion of these structures leads to a sharp decrease in cortical tone, to the appearance of a state of sleep associated with synchronization of the EEG (Figure 8) and, sometimes, to a state of coma. No arousal reaction is present in animals with such lesions, even in response to strong nociceptive stimulation (Lindsley *et al.*, 1949; French and Magoun, 1952; French, 1952; Narikashvili, 1961; 1962; 1968).

All this clearly showed that the reticular formation of the brain stem is a powerful mechanism for maintaining cortical tone and regulating the functional state of the brain, and that it is a factor determining the level of wakefulness.

Experiments by other workers (Jouvet, 1961; Hernández-Peón,

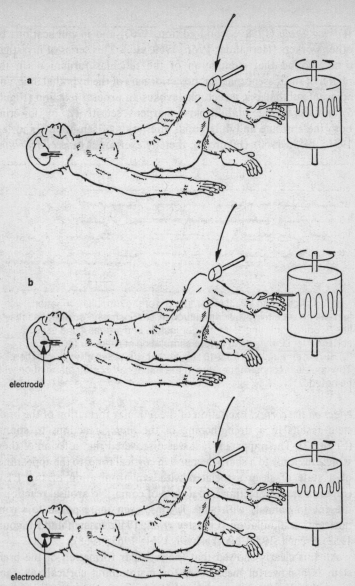

a

b

electrode

c

electrode

Figure 7 Activating role of stimulation of the reticular formation on the motor sphere (patellar reflex): (a) before stimulation of reticular formation; (b) during stimulation; (c) after stimulation of reticular formation (after French).

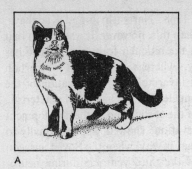 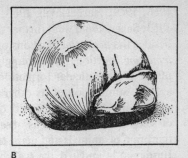

A B

a awake: midbrain lesion afferent paths

b asleep: lesion midbrain tegmentum

Figure 8 Development of sleep as a result of division of the tracts of the activating reticular formation: (A) Active state of the brain resulting from preservation of the activating influences of the reticular formation on the cortex; (a) the electroencephalogram awake. (B) State of sleep resulting from division of the higher levels of the brain-stem reticular formation and termination of the activating influences; (b) the electroencephalogram asleep (after Lindsley)

1966; 1969; Narikashvili, 1963; 1968; Narikashvili and Kadzhaya, 1963; Sager, 1968) went further than this, however. It was shown that besides the *activating* portions of the reticular formation, it also has *inhibiting* portions. Accordingly, whereas stimulation of certain nuclei of the reticular formation invariably led to activation of the animal, stimulation of its other nuclei led to changes characteristic of sleep in the electrical activity of the cortex, and to the development of sleep itself. This fact, as observations showed, applies equally to the brain of animals and man; that is why, when the Soviet surgeon Burdenko stimulated the wall of the third ventricle during neurosurgical operations, a state of sleep was induced artificially in the patient on the operating table.

The influence of the higher level of the brain stem and of the reticular formation on regulation of the waking state is no longer in doubt, and this fact has resulted in the closest attention being paid to the structures of the first unit of the brain. There is further proof of this in the study of the disturbances arising in human mental processes when lesions are present in these parts of the brain.

The reticular activating formation, the most important part of the first functional unit of the brain, was from the very beginning described as *non-specific*; this distinguished it radically from the great majority of specific (sensory and motor) cortical systems. It is considered that its activating and inhibitory action affects all sensory and all motor functions of the body equally, and that its function is merely that of regulating states of sleep and waking – the non-specific background against which different forms of activity take place.

The basic assumptions of the pioneers in neurophysiology who first described the activating system of the brain cannot however be regarded as completely correct. Subsequent observations have shown that the reticular system of the brain has certain features of *differentiation* or *'specificity'* as regards both its anatomical characteristics (Brodal, 1957; Scheibel and Scheibel, 1958) and its *sources* and *manifestations*, although this differentiation and specificity have nothing in common with the 'modality' of the primary sense organs, and as Anokhin (1959, 1962, 1963) and Yoshii (Yoshii *et al.* 1969) have shown, they are unique in character.

Let us consider for a moment the character of differentiation of the primary *sources* of the activation which is the basic function of the reticular system, that is, its differential *topographic organization* and then go on to examine the basic *forms of activation* in which its action is manifested.

The nervous system, as we know, always exhibits a certain tone of activity, and the maintenance of this tone is an essential feature of all biological activity. However, situations exist in which this ordinary tone is insufficient, and must be raised. These situations are the primary sources of activation. At least *three principal sources* of this activation can be distinguished; the action of each one of them is transmitted through the activating reticular formation, and, more significantly, by means of its various parts. This is the essence of the differentiation or specificity of functional organization of this 'non-specific activating system'.

The *first* of these sources is the *metabolic* processes of the organism or, as they are sometimes called, its 'internal economy'. Metabolic processes leading to maintenance of the internal equilibrium of the organism (homeostasis) in their simplest forms are connected with respiratory and digestive processes, with sugar and protein metabolism, with internal secretion, and so on; they are all regulated principally by the hypothalamus. The reticular formation of the medulla (bulbar) and mesencephalon (mesencephalo-hypothalamic), closely connected with the hypothalamus, plays an important role in this simplest, 'vital' form of activation.

More complex forms of this type of activation are connected with metabolic processes organized in certain inborn behavioural systems; they are widely known as systems of instinctive (or unconditioned-reflex) food-getting and sexual behaviour. A common feature of these two subdivisions is that metabolic (and humoral) processes taking place in the body are the source of activation in these cases. Their difference lies in the unequal complexity of their level of organization and the fact that whereas the first, the more elementary, processes evoke only primitive, automatic responses connected with oxygen deficiency or the liberation of reserve substances from their organic depots in starvation, the second are organized into complex behavioural systems, as a result of whose action the appropriate needs are satified and the necessary balance of the 'internal economy of the organism' is restored.

Naturally, in order to evoke these complex, instinctive forms of behaviour, a highly selective, specific activation is necessary, and the biologically specific forms of this food-getting or sexual activation are the responsibility of the higher nuclei of the mesencephalic, diencephalic, and limbic reticular formation. Many recent experiments (Olds, 1958; MacLean, 1959; Miller, 1966; Bekhtereva, 1971) show conclusively that highly specific nuclei of the reticular formation, stimulation of which can lead either to activation or to blocking

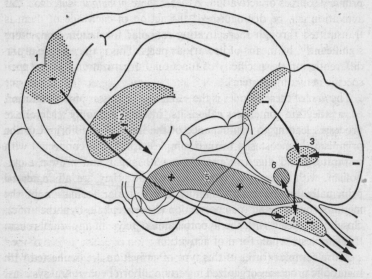

Figure 9 Excitatory and inhibitory influence of stimulation of the nuclei of the reticular formation; (5) facilitatory and (4) inhibitory zones of the brain-stem reticular formation and connections running to it from the cortex (1) and cerebellum (3)

of various complex forms of instinctive behaviour, are located in these structures of the brain stem and archicortex. A scheme showing the arrangement of these nuclei which activate or block food-getting, sexual and defensive behaviour is given in Figure 9.

The *second* source of activation is completely different in origin. It is connected with the *arrival of stimuli from the outside world* in the body and it leads to the production of completely different forms of activation, manifested as an *orienting reflex*.

Man lives in a world of constantly incoming information, and the need for this information is sometimes just as great as the need for organic metabolism. If a person is deprived of this constant inflow of information, as occurs in rare cases of exclusion of all receptor organs, he falls asleep and can be aroused only by a constant supply of information. A normal person tolerates restricted contact with the outside world with great difficulty, and as Hebb (1955) observed, if subjects are placed under the conditions of severe limitation of the inflow of excitation, their state becomes intolerable and they develop hallucinations which, to some extent, may compensate for this limited inflow of information.

It is therefore perfectly natural that special mechanisms providing for a *tonic form of activation* should exist in the brain and, in particular, in the structures of the reticular formation, using as their source the inflow of excitation from the sense organs and possessing comparable intensity with the source of activation just mentioned. However, this tonic form of activation, connected with the work of the sense organs, is only the most elementary source of activation of this type which will be described.

Man lives in a *constantly changing environment*, and these changes, which are sometimes unexpected by the individual, require a certain level of increased alertness. This increased alertness must accompany any change in the environmental conditions, any appearance of an unexpected (and sometimes, even an expected) change in those conditions. It must take the form of mobilization of the organism to meet possible surprises, and it is this aspect which lies at the basis of the special type of activity which Pavlov called the *orienting reflex* and which, although not necessarily connected with the primary biological forms of instinctive processes (food-getting, sexual, and so on), is an important basis of *investigative activity*.

One of the most important discoveries in recent times has been the demonstration that the link between the type of orienting reflex or activation and the mode of work of the reticular formation and limbic systems of the brain (Moruzzi and Magoun, 1949; Gershuni, 1949; Lindsley *et al.*, 1949; Sharples and Jasper, 1956; Gastaut, 1958; Sokolov, 1958; Sokolov *et al.*, 1964; Vinogradova, 1961) is not always identical in form. Tonic and generalized forms of the activation reaction, on the one hand, and phasic and local forms, on the other hand, have been described (Sharples and Jasper, 1956; Sokolov,

1958; Sokolov *et al.*, 1964; Lindsley *et al.*, 1949; 1960; Gastaut, 1958; Adey *et al.*, 1960; Vinogradova, 1961; Morrell, 1967). These forms of the activation reaction are linked with different structures of the reticular formation: the tonic and generalized forms with its lower regions, and the phasic and local forms with the higher regions of the brain stem and, in particular, with the non-specific thalamic region and limbic system.

Microelectrode studies have shown that the non-specific nuclei of the thalamus and also of the caudate nucleus and hippocampus are closely connected functionally with the system of the orienting reflex (Jasper, 1964; Vinogradova, 1969; 1970a; Danilova, 1967; 1970). Each response to a novel situation requires, first and foremost, the comparison of the new stimulus with the system of old, previously encountered stimuli. Such a comparison alone can show whether a given stimulus is in fact novel and whether it must give rise to an orienting reflex, or whether it is old and its appearance requires no special mobilization of the organism. This is the only type of mechanism which can permit a process of 'habituation', so that a repeatedly presented stimulus loses its novelty and special mobilization of the organism on its appearance is no longer necessary. In other words, this is the link by which the *mechanism of the orienting reflex is closely bound with the mechanisms of memory*, and by means of this link between the two processes the comparison of stimuli, one of the essential conditions of activation of this type, becomes possible.

Another important discovery in recent years has been that many neurons of the hippocampus and caudate nucleus, which have no modally specific functions, are in fact responsible for this function of 'comparing' stimuli, reacting to the appearance of novel stimuli, and blocking their activity with the development of habituation to repeated stimuli.

The activating and inhibiting or, in other words, the *modulating* function of neurons of the hippocampus and caudate nucleus, is thus, as recent work has shown, a vital source of regulation of tonic states of the cerebral cortex which are associated with the most complex forms of the orienting reflex, but on this occasion they are not instinctive but more complex, vital or conditioned-reflex in character. We shall see (part 3, ch. 10) the importance of a disturbance of the normal function of these regions of the brain in the production of changes in the course of human mental processes.

It now remains to examine, in the briefest outline, the *third* and perhaps the most interesting source of activation, in which the functional unit of the brain I have just described plays the most intimate part, although it is not the only brain structure concerned in its organization.

Metabolic processes or a direct inflow of information evoking an orienting reflex are not the only sources of human activity. Much human activity is evoked by intentions and plans, by forecasts and programmes which are formed during man's conscious life, which are social in their motivation and are effected with the close participation, initially of his external, and later of his internal, *speech*. Every intention formulated in speech defines a certain goal and evokes a programme of action leading to the attainment of that goal. Every time the goal is reached, the activity stops, but every time it is not reached, this leads to further mobilization of efforts.

It would be wrong, however, to regard the appearance of these intentions and the formulations of these goals as a purely intellectual act. The fulfilment of a plan or the achievement of a goal requires a certain amount of energy, and they are possible only if a certain level of activity can be maintained. The sources of this activity which are most important so far as the understanding of human conscious behaviour is concerned were for a long time unknown, and it is only recently that important progress had been made toward the elucidation of this problem.

The observations to which I refer have led to the overthrowing of the old hypothesis that the source of this activity must be sought entirely within cortical level. They show conclusively that in the search for mechanisms of these highest forms of organization of activity, the same *vertical principle* of construction of the functional systems of the brain must be retained and *connections existing between the higher levels of the cortex and the subjacent reticular formation* must be dealt with.

So far, when discussing the mechanisms of working of the first functional unit, we have considered the ascending connections of the activating reticular system. However, I mentioned that *descending connections* also exist between the cortex and the lower formations: it is these connections which transmit the *regulatory influence of the cortex on the lower structures of the brain stem* and which are the mechanism by means of which the functional patterns of excitation *arising in the cortex recruit the systems of the reticular formation of the 'old' brain and receive from them their charge of energy.*

The descending structures of the reticular formation have been investigated much less fully than its ascending connections. However, a series of studies (French *et al.*, 1955; Segundo *et al.*, 1955; Galambos and Morgan, 1960; Magoun, 1963; Narikashvili, 1962; 1963; 1968; Adrianov, 1963) has shown that through the intermediary of these cortico-reticular tracts stimulation of individual areas of the cortex can evoke a generalized arousal reaction (Brazier, 1960; Galambos and Morgan, 1960), facilitate spinal reflexes, modify the excitability of muscles through the system of γ-afferent fibres, increase the excitability of the cochlear apparatus (Hernández-Peón *et al.*, 1956; Narikashvili, 1963), and lower the thresholds of discriminatory sensation (Jouvet and Hernández-Peón,1957; Lindsley, 1951; 1958; 1960).

Both morphological and morphysiological investigations have thus reliably shown that, *besides the specific sensory and motor functions which we have already discussed, the cerebral cortex also performs non-specific activating functions*, that every specific afferent or efferent fibre is accompanied by a fibre of the non-specific activating system, and that *stimulation of individual areas of the cortex can evoke both activating and inhibitory influences on lower brain structures* (Jouvet, 1961; Buser *et al.*, 1961; Narikashvili, 1963; 1968; Sager, 1968; Hernández-Peón, 1966; 1969; Durinyan *et al.*, 1968). It has also been shown that the descending fibres of the activating (and also of the inhibitory) reticular system have a well-differentiated cortical organization. Whereas the most specific bundles of these fibres (raising or lowering the tone of the sensory or motor systems) arise from the primary (and, to some extent, the secondary) cortical zones, the more general activating influences on the reticular formation of the brain stem arise primarily from the frontal region of the cortex (French *et al.*, 1955; Segundo *et al.*, 1955; Nauta, 1964; 1968; Pribram, 1959b; 1960; 1966a; 1971; Homskaya, 1966b; 1969; 1972; Sager, 1968) (Figure 10). These descending fibres, running from the

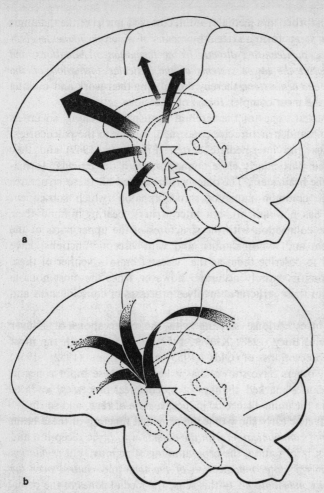

Figure 10 Diagram showing relations of cortical systems with brain-stem structures through the ascending reticular formation (after Magoun) (a) ascending, (b) descending tracts

prefrontal (orbial and medial frontal) cortex to nuclei of the thalamus and brain stems form a system by means of which *the higher levels of the cortex, participating directly in the formation of intentions and plans, recruit the lower systems of the reticular formation of the thalamus and brain stem*, thereby modulating their work and making possible the most complex forms of conscious activity.

The medial zones of the cerebral hemispheres belong, so far as their origin and structure are concerned, mainly to the paleocortex, archicortex and intermediate cortex (Filimonov, 1949) and they retain their particularly close connection with the reticular formations of the brain stem. The older writers united all these structures under the common name of rhinencephalon (which subsequent research has not upheld), but later writers, bearing in mind their very close connection with the structures of the upper parts of the brain stem and hypothalamus, and with visceral functions, have preferred to describe them as the 'visceral brain'. Neither of these appellations is entirely accurate, however, since the most notable function of these structures involves processes of consciousness and memory.

Early investigations, starting with the observations of Klüver (Klüver and Bucy, 1938; Klüver, 1952) and ending with the most recent observations of Olds (1955–9), MacLean (1952; 1958) and many others have shown that a lesion of these brain zones in animals causes marked changes in biochemical processes, leads to changes in the animal's needs, induces a state of rage, and so on.

These facts clearly show that the principal function of these brain zones is *not communication with the outside world* (the reception and analysis of information, the programming of actions), but *regulation of the general state, modification of the tone* and *control over the inclinations and emotions*. In this sense the medial zones of the hemispheres can be regarded as a system superposed above the structure of the upper part of the brain stem and reticular formation.

These views have been confirmed by morphological and physiological data. It has been shown, firstly, that the great majority of neurons in this part of the cortex do not possess any definite modal specificity, but respond actively to changes in the state of the organism. Secondly, it has been shown that stimulation of these zones does not lead to the appearance of differentiated discharges and, consequently, that it does not obey the 'all or nothing' rule but gives rise to gradual changes in states, and thus to a modification of the *general background* of behaviour. This description of the properties of the medial zones of the cortex will help to explain the type of disturbance of behaviour which arises as a result of a pathological lesion in them, for this type differs sharply from the disturbance of mental processes resulting from local lesions of the lateral cortical zones.

Lesions of the medial (and mediobasal) cortical zones *never cause disturbances of gnosis or praxis.* The visual, auditory and tactile perception of these patients remains intact, and they give no evidence of a disturbance of the reception of visual, auditory or kinaesthetic information. These patients can still perform any complex movement, their postural praxis remains intact, they easily reproduce positions of the hands in space in response to an instruction, they readily learn and reproduce rhythmic structures. Their speech, both phonetically and morphologically, remains unchanged, and were it not for its sluggishness and sometimes its monotony, and the quiet voice with which the patient responds to questions, and his general asthenia, it would show no perceptible abnormality. The writing of this group of patients likewise remains potentially intact, exhibiting only a tendency to fatigue and a rapid transition to micrographia, and it is difficult to detect any special peculiarities with respect to their reading. The cardinal features of all patients of this group are a definite *lowering of tone*, a tendency towards an *akinetic state*, and a tendency to become fatigued rapidly.

Although they begin to perform a task correctly, all their reactions very quickly become slow; this slowing of responses increases in severity, and often the patients cease to answer questions altogether although they continue to be clearly aware of their pathological state and of the inadequacy of their responses. Sometimes this state is accompanied by marked asthenia of movements, leading to manifestations of akinesia which may closely resemble stupor (Bragina, 1966). Sometimes these phenomena are manifested as changes in the voice, which may become sluggish and 'aphonic' and it is only by appropriate external stimulation that the tone can be temporarily increased. Against this background of a quantitative decrease in behavioural tone, these patients begin to show clearly defined affective changes.

Unlike patients with lesions of the frontal lobes and with a marked frontal syndrome, they never exhibit any features of emotional unconcern or euphoria. In some cases, their emotional tone is depressed and they begin to border on indifference; in other cases it assumes the character of anxiety or distress, accompanied by marked autonomic reactions, and sometimes it may be so acute that it has been described as a syndrome of 'catastrophic reactions' or 'experiences' or of 'breakdown of the world' (Baruk, 1926; Shmar'yan, 1949). This integrity, but sometimes distortion of affective experiences is a feature essentially distinguishing this group of patients from those with the frontal syndrome.

However, these facts constitute only the general background for the disturbances of mental activity observed in the patients of this group, which, although they varied in severity, formed the centre of the observed syndrome.

I refer, firstly, to *disturbances of consciousness*, and secondly, to *defects of memory*.

The patients of this group exhibited defects of orientation with respect to their surroundings far more frequently than patients with lesions in other situations. Frequently they could not be sure where they were, and either suggested that they were in hospital, or somewhere on active service, at the polyclinic, at home or staying with friends, that they were 'only lying down to rest' or, finally, that they were in some 'transitory' situation, such as at a railway station, at a place which they could not identify exactly. Often they were poorly oriented with respect to time, and even though they could tell approximately the period of the year or even the month, they made gross errors in telling the time of day; they either shrugged their shoulders helplessly when they were asked to state what time it was or even to name a time which differed sharply from the actual time.

They could not recognize the physician examining them and sometimes mistook him for an old friend, mentioning that they had met somewhere before.

They could not give a lucid account of their life history, mixed up the details of the history of their illness, and sometimes included in it confabulations, to which their attitude was by no means always sufficiently critical. For instance, some patients of this group declared that their relatives were waiting for them in the corridor, that they would leave the hospital in the morning and go back to work, or that they had only just returned from a mission, and so on (Luria, 1973).

Characteristically, these uncontrollable confabulations, of whose inaccuracy the patients themselves were not aware, were found particularly clearly only in patients with lesions of the *anterior zones* of the limbic region or with lesions of the *right hemisphere*. Patients with deep lesions of the posterior zones of the medial cortex exhibited confabulations much less frequently.

All these features, taken together, form a definite picture of disturbances of consciousness which, in the severest cases, closely resemble the typical phenomena of oneiroid states, the principal feature of which is loss of the selectivity of mental processes affecting all spheres of mental activity (Luria, Homskaya, Blinkov and Critchley, 1967).

Perhaps the most obvious symptom of patients with lesions of the medial zones of the hemispheres is a *defect of memory*, reflecting a general lowering of cortical tone, and *quite different in character from the modally-specific defect of mnestic processes* found in patients with local lesions of the lateral zones of the brain.

The disturbances of memory arising in lesions of the hippocampus and its connections, which have been described in the literature as the 'hippocampal ring' or 'Circle of Papez', comprising the thalamic nuclei, the fornix and the mamillary bodies (Figure 11) are well

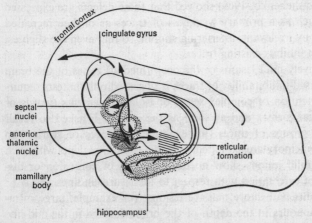

Figure 11 Diagram of the hippocampal circle (the circle of Papez)

known. It was Bekhterev who, in 1900, first pointed out that lesions of the medial zones of the temporal lobe can give rise to memory disturbances which sometimes resemble Korsakov's syndrome. Grünthal (1939) stated that memory defects of the same type can also arise as the result of a lesion of the mamillary bodies, the relay nuclei on to which fibres running from the hippocampus converge, and which receive fibres from other deep brain structures. Finally, investigations published more recently (Scoville, 1954; Scoville and Milner, 1957; Penfield and Milner, 1958; Milner, 1954; 1970; Popova, 1964) have shown that bilateral hippocampal lesions invariably lead to gross disturbances of memory. In other cases investigated by the author and his collaborators (Kiyashchenko, 1969; Luria, 1971; 1973; Luria, Konovalov and Podgornaya, 1970) the memory disturbances arising in deep brain lesions (especially in lesions of the medial zones of the hemispheres) were analysed in considerable detail.

These investigations showed that patients even with relatively silent lesions of the medial zones (for example, patients with pituitary tumours, spreading beyond the boundaries of the sella turcica and affecting the medial zones of the cortex), although they exhibited no defects of their higher mental processes, frequently complained of a defect of memory, which was not confined to any one particular (visual, auditory) sphere, but was modally non-specific in character. Tests (Kiyashchenko, 1969) showed that these defects are expressed not so much as a primary weakness of traces as of their increased inhibition by irrelevant, interfering stimuli, so that even the slightest distraction inhibits existing traces.

In relatively mild lesions of the deep (medial) zones of the brain this increased inhibitability of traces is observed only in tests requiring the retention of complex series of isolated elements (words or grammatical forms), and as soon as the patient is asked to recall organized groups of traces (for example, sentences or stories) no defects of memory are exhibited. For this reason, patients with such relatively mild lesions show no definite signs of confusion or disturbance of orientation with respect to their surroundings.

In patients with more massive lesions (for example, large intracerebral tumours in the depth of the brain, located in the mid-line and involving both hemispheres), the situation is very different, and the symptoms of a disturbance of memory, while still modally-non-specific in character, become more severe. Such patients can easily form the simplest type of sensorimotor structure (for example, it is easy to evoke in them a contrasting illusion of the inequality of two identical balls after being instructed to touch the larger one several times with one hand and the smaller with the other hand), but this contrasting illusion, which is the result of a 'fixed set' (Uznadze, 1966), disappears immediately if any interfering stimulus is brought to act on the patient (Kiyashchenko, 1969; Gorskaya, unpublished work).

These patients can readily grasp the similarity or difference between two geometrical figures presented one after the other at an interval of 1–1·5 minutes (Konorski's experiment); if, however, an irrelevant stimulus was introduced during this interval, the trace of the first shape disappeared to such an extent that it was impossible to compare the two shapes (Kiyashchenko, 1969). Similar phenomena, but in an even more conspicuous form, are found in tests of more complex types of memory; in such cases they affect not only the retention of isolated series of words (or series of visual elements), but also the retention of organized structures (sentences, anecdotes, thematic pictures). If, for example, the patient reads a relatively simple sentence, followed by another similar sentence, the traces of the first sentence are at once forgotten and it is impossible to recall it. The same result is found in tests on memorizing complete anecdotes. The patient can successfully repeat and retain a small fragment (such as Tolstoy's story *The Hen and the Golden Egg*), but if he is then asked to spend a minute solving arithmetical problems, or if immediately after the first story he is asked to read another similar one (such as Tolstoy's *The Jackdaw and the Pigeons*), the traces of the first story become so inhibited that it cannot be recalled. The fact that this disturbance of recollection is based, not on total obliteration of the traces, but on their excessive inhibition by the interfering stimuli, is clear because after a certain time has elapsed, the traces of the 'forgotten' story can suddenly and involuntarily reappear as a reminiscence (Kiyashchenko, 1969; Popova, 1964; Luria, 1971; 1973). In its most marked forms, this increased in-hibitability of traces is also manifested in the patient's actions. If, after he has carried out one action (for example, drawing a shape or placing a comb under the pillow), he is given another, distracting (interfering) task to do, his first action becomes 'forgotten' to such an extent that even if he is shown the drawing he made or asked how the comb came to be under the pillow he cannot recollect having done the action himself and he stubbornly denies ever having done so.

Such phenomena indicate very severe disturbances of memory in the patients of this group, and indeed they bear some resemblance to the picture of Korsakov's syndrome.

One of the most interesting observations is that if the lesion lies in the *posterior* parts of the medial zones of the cortex and results in bilateral involvement of the hippocampus, this increased inhibitability of traces may become complete and unaccompanied by any form of confabulation (Milner, 1954; 1966; 1968; 1969); conversely, if the lesion lies in the anterior parts of these zones, and involves the medial zones of the frontal lobes, the picture is substantially different and the patient will uncontrollably confuse two items given to him and exhibit signs of contamination (for example, when recalling the first sentence or the first anecdote, elements of the second will be interposed), and his attitude toward these phenomena will not be sufficiently critical. If the lesions of the frontal lobes are massive, and affect their medial zones also, any attempt to recollect previous traces will be disturbed by the pathological inertia of the last traces. Having repeated the last sentence (or anecdote) the patient exhibits perseveration and continues to reproduce it, thinking that he is giving the meaning of the first sentence (or the first story). If the pathological process takes place against the background of irritative phenomena, such as in massive mediobasal lesions (tumours, wounds, of the frontal region or haemorrhages and spasm of the anterior cerebral arteries accompanying rupture of an aneurysm) the picture of the disturbances of memory may become still more complex. When attempting to reproduce a short anecdote read to him, the patient will be unable to prevent the intrusion of irrelevant associations, and the selective reproduction of the anecdote becomes absolutely impossible (Luria, 1971; 1973; Luria, Konovalov and Podgornaya, 1970).

These disturbances constitute a link with some of the pathophysiological mechanisms of Korsakov's syndrome and they are thus of very great interest. At the same time they raise the question of the relations between disturbances of *memory* and disturbances of *consciousness*, a matter which has attracted the attention of psychiatrists for many decades but which has still found no precise neurophysiological or neuropsychological solution.

Thus the *systems of the first functional unit not only maintain cortical tone, but also themselves experience the differentiating influence of the cortex*, and *the first functional unit of the brain works in close cooperation with the higher levels of the cortex*, a matter which will be referred to again.

The unit for receiving, analysing and storing information

We have discussed the systems of the first functional unit of the brain which plays a role in the regulation of the state of cortical activity and the level of alertness. As we have seen, this unit has the structure of a 'non-specific' nerve net, which performs its function of modifying the state of brain activity gradually, step by step, without having any direct relationship either to the reception and processing of external information or to the formation of complex goal-directed intentions, plans and programmes of behaviour.

In all these considerations the first functional unit of the brain, located mainly in the brain stem, the diencephalon, and the medial regions of the cortex, differs essentially from the system of the *second functional unit of the brain*, whose primary function is the *reception, analysis and storage of information*.

This unit is located in the lateral regions of the neocortex *on the convex surface of the hemispheres*, of which it occupies the *posterior regions*, including the *visual (occipital)*, *auditory (temporal)* and *general sensory (parietal)* regions.

In its histological structure it consists, not of a continuous nerve net, but of *isolated neurons*, which lie in the parts of the cortex already described and which, unlike the systems of the first unit, do not work in accordance with the principle of gradual changes, but obey the 'all or nothing' rule, by receiving discrete impulses and relaying them to other groups of neurons.

In their functional properties, the systems of this unit are adapted to the reception of stimuli travelling to the brain the peripheral receptors, to their analysis into a very large number of very small component elements, and to their combination into the required dynamic functional structures (or in other words, their synthesis into whole functional systems).

Finally, it is clear from what has been said above that this functional unit of the brain consists of parts possessing *high modal specificity*, i.e. that its component parts are adapted to the reception of visual, auditory, vestibular or general sensory information. The systems of this unit also incorporate the central systems of gustatory and olfactory reception, although in man they are so overshadowed by the central representation of the higher exteroceptive systems, receiving stimuli from objects at a distance, that they occupy a predominantly minor place in the cortex.

The basis of this unit is formed by the *primary* or *projection* areas of the cortex, which consists mainly of neurons of afferent layer IV, many of which possess extremely high specificity, as was shown by Hubel and Wiesel, 1963. The neurons of the cortical visual systems, which respond *only* to the narrowly specialized properties of visual stimuli (shades of colour, the character of lines, the direction of movement).

Neurons which have undergone such a high degree of differentiation naturally preserve their strict modal specificity, and virtually no cells which respond only to sound can be found in the primary occipital cortex, just as no neurons responding only to visual stimuli can be found in the primary temporal cortex.

The primary zones of the individual cortical regions composing this unit also contain cells of a *multimodal* character, which respond to several types of stimuli, as well as cells which do not respond to any modally-specific type of stimuli, and which evidently retain the properties of non-specific maintenance of tone; however, these cells form only a very small proportion of the total neuronal composition of the primary cortical areas (according to some figures, not more than 4 per cent of the total number of cells present).

The primary or projection areas of the cortex of this second functional unit of the brain form the *basis* for this work, and as we have seen, they are surrounded by systems of *secondary* (*or gnostic*) *cortical zones* superposed above them, in which afferent layer IV yields its dominant position to layers II and III of cells, whose degree of modal specificity is much lower and whose composition includes many more associative neurons with short axons, enabling incoming excitation to be combined into the necessary functional patterns, and they thus subserve a *synthetic* function.

This hierarchical structure is equally characteristic of *all regions of the cortex constituting the second functional unit of the brain.* In the *visual (occipital) cortex,* above the primary visual area (Brodmann's area 17) there is a superstructure of secondary visual areas (Brodmann's areas 18 and 19), which convert the somatotopic projection of individual parts of the retina into its functional organization; they retain their modal (visual) specificity, but work as a system organizing visual stimuli reaching the primary visual area. Below we shall consider more fully the principles governing their work by analysing patterns of disturbances of visual perception observed in patients with local lesions of these cortical areas.

The *auditory (temporal) cortex* is constructed in accordance with the same principle. Its primary (projection) areas are concealed in the depth of the temporal cortex in the transverse gyri of Heschl (represented by Brodmann's area 41), the neurons of which possess high modal specificity and respond only to the highly differentiated properties of acoustic stimuli. Just like the primary visual area, these primary parts of the auditory cortex have a precise topographical structure. Many authorities consider that fibres carrying excitation from those parts of the organ of Corti which respond to high tones are located in the medial parts, while fibres from parts responding to low tones are located in the lateral portions of Heschl's gyrus. The only difference between the structure of the primary (projection) areas of the auditory cortex is that the right fields of vision of both eyes are represented in the projection zones of the visual cortex only in these zones of the left hemisphere, while the left fields of vision of both eyes are represented in the same zones of the right hemisphere, the corresponding systems of the organ of Corti are represented in the projection zones of the auditory cortex of both hemispheres, although (as we shall see below) the principally contralateral character of this representation is preserved.

Above the systems of the primary auditory cortex are superposed those of the *secondary auditory cortex,* located in the outer parts of the temporal region on the convex surface of the hemisphere (Brodmann's area 22 and part of area 21), and which also consists pre-

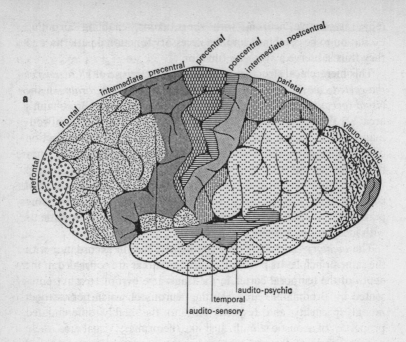

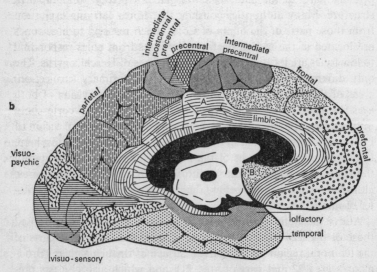

Figure 12 Chart of the hierarchical structure of cortical areas (after Campbell, 1905) (a) lateral surface, (b) medial surface

dominantly of a powerfully developed layer II and the layer III of cells. Just as was found in the systems of the visual cortex, they also convert the somatotopic projection of the auditory impulses into their functional organization. A detailed analysis of the function of these zones and the symptoms of disturbance of auditory perception arising in patients with lesions of these areas will be given below.

Finally, the same functional organization is also preserved, in principle, in the *general sensory (parietal) cortex*. Just as in the visual and auditory cortex, it is based on *primary* or *projection* zones (Brodmann's area 3), the substance of which also consists mainly of neurons of layer IV, possessing high modal specificity, while their topography is distinguished by the same precise somatotopic projection of individual segments of the body which I mentioned and, on account of which, stimulation of the upper part of this zone causes the appearance of sensations in the lower limbs, stimulation of the middle portions gives rise to sensations in the upper limbs on the contralateral side, and stimulation of points in the lower part of this zone produces corresponding sensations in the contralateral areas of the face, lips and tongue.

Above these primary zones of the general sensory (parietal) cortex are superposed its *secondary* (Brodmann's areas 1, 3 and 5 and part of area 40); like the secondary zones of the visual and auditory cortex these zones consist mainly of associative neurons of layers II and III, and their stimulation leads to the appearance of more complex forms of cutaneous and kinaesthetic sensation. The patterns accompanying local lesions of these zones will be discussed in detail later.

The principal modally-specific zones of the second brain system, which we are at present discussing, are thus built in accordance with a single *principle of hierarchical organization*, originally formulated as long ago as 1905 by Campbell (Figure 12), and which applies equally to all these zones, each of which must be regarded as the *central, cortical apparatus of a modally-specific analyser*. Views regarding the cytoarchitectonic structure of the human brain were later substantially clarified and sharpened, and in Figure 13 I give an up-to-date version of Brodmann's map of the cortical areas which, with some variations, have been accepted through the work of the Moscow Brain Institute.

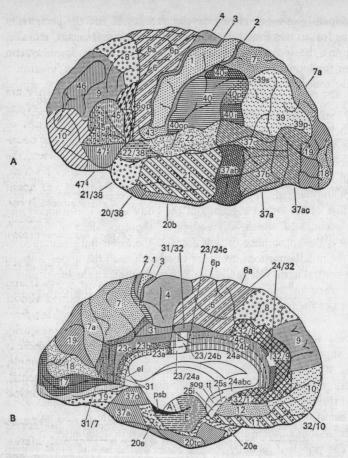

Figure 13 Map of the cytoarchitectonic areas (after Brodmann and the Moscow Brain Institute) (A) lateral surface, (B) medial surface

All the zone described above are in fact adapted so as to serve as an *apparatus for the reception, analysis and* (as we shall see) *the storage of information arriving from the outside world* or, in other words, *the cerebral mechanisms of modally-specific forms of gnostic processes.*

As we have discussed, human gnostic activity never takes place with respect to one single isolated modality (vision, hearing, touch); the perception – and still more, the representation – of any object is a *complex* procedure, the result of polymodal activity, originally expanded in character, later concentrated and condensed. Naturally, therefore, it must rely on the combined working of a complete system of cortical zones.

It is the *tertiary* zones of this second brain system or, as they are generally called, the *zones of overlapping* of the cortical ends of the various analysers, which are responsible for enabling groups of several analysers to work concertedly. These zones lie on the boundary between the occipital, temporal, and post-central cortex; the greater part of them is formed by the inferior parietal region which, in man, has developed to a considerable size, occupying just about one-quarter of the total mass of the system we are describing. It can therefore be considered that the tertiary zones or, as Flechsig described them, the 'posterior associative centre', are *specifically human structures.*

As we now know, the tertiary zones of the posterior regions of the brain consist almost entirely of cells of the associative layers II and III of the cortex and, consequently, that they are concerned almost entirely with the function of *integration of excitation arriving from different analysers.* There is reason to suppose that the great majority of neurons in these zones are multimodal in character, and there is evidence to show that they respond to general features (for example, to the character of spatial arrangement, the number of components), to which neurons of the primary, and even the secondary, cortical zones are unable to respond.

These tertiary structures of the posterior zones of the cortex include Brodmann's areas 5, 7, 39 and 40 (the superior and inferior zones of the parietal region), area 21 of the temporal region, and areas 37 and 39 of the temporo-occipital region.

The function of these tertiary structures will be discussed in more detail, when, on the basis of analysis of psychological experiments and clinical material, I shall show that the principal role of these zones is connected with the *spatial organization* of discrete impulses of excitation entering the various regions and with the conversion of *successive stimuli into simultaneously processed groups,* the only possible mechanism for that synthetic character of perception which Sechenov originally discussed many years ago (Luria, 1963; 1966b; 1970c).

This work of the tertiary zones of the posterior cortical regions is thus essential, not only for the successful integration of information reaching man through his visual system, but also for the _transition from direct, visually represented syntheses to the level of symbolic processes_ – or operations with word meanings, with complex grammatical and logical structures, with systems of numbers and abstract relationships. It is because of this that the _tertiary zones of the posterior cortical region play an essential role in the conversion of concrete perception into abstract thinking_, which always proceeds in the form of _internal_ schemes, and for the _memorizing of organized experience_ or, in other words, not only for the reception and coding of information, but also for its storage.

We have therefore every reason for regarding the whole of this functional system of the brain as a system for the reception, coding and storage of information.

From what has just been said it is possible to distinguish _three basic laws_ governing the work structure of the individual cortical regions composing the second brain system and which also apply to the next functional unit.

The first is the _law of the hierarchical structure of the cortical zones._ The relationships between the primary, secondary and tertiary cortical zones, responsible for increasingly complex synthesis of incoming information, are a clear enough illustration of this law.

The relationships between these primary, secondary and tertiary cortical zones composing this system do not, of course, remain the same, but _change in the course of ontogenetic development_.

In the young child, as has been shown, the formation of properly working secondary zones could not take place without the integrity of the primary zones which constitute their basis, and the proper working of the tertiary zones would be impossible without adequate development of the secondary (gnostic) cortical zones which supply the necessary material for the creation of major cognitive syntheses. A disturbance of the lower zones of the corresponding types of cortex in infancy must therefore lead inevitably to incomplete development of the higher cortical zones and, consequently, as Vygotsky (1934; 1960) expressed it, the main line of interaction between these cortical zones runs 'from below upward'.

Conversely, in the *adult* person, with his fully formed higher psychological functions, the *higher cortical zones have assumed the dominant role*. Even when he perceives the world around him, the adult person organizes (codes) his impressions into logical systems, fits them into certain schemes; *the highest, tertiary zones of the cortex thus begin to control the work of the secondary zones* which are subordinated to them, and if the secondary zones are affected by a pathological lesion, the tertiary zones have a compensatory influence on their work. This relationship between the principal, hierarchically organized cortical zones in the adult led Vygotsky to the conclusion that in the late stage of ontogeny the main line of their interaction runs 'from above downward', and that the work of the adult human cerebral cortex reveals not so much the dependence of the higher zones on the lower as the opposite – dependence of the lower (modally specific) zones on the higher.

This suggests that the *hierarchical principle of the working of individual zones of the second brain unit* is the first fundamental law which provides a clue to its functional organization.

The second law governing the work of this functional unit, and one which follows logically from the facts just described, can be expressed as the *law of diminishing specificity of the hierarchically arranged cortical zones composing it*.

The primary zones of each part of the cortex in this system, as was mentioned earlier, possess *maximal modal specificity*. This property is a feature both of the primary (projection) areas of the visual (occipital) cortex and of the primary (projection) areas of the auditory (temporal) or general sensory (postcentral) cortex. The fact that they contain a very large number of neurons with highly differentiated, modally-specific functions confirms this view.

The *secondary* cortical areas, in which the upper layers with their associative neurons are predominant, possess this modal specificity *to a much lesser degree*. While preserving their direct relationship to the cortical ends of the corresponding analysers, these areas, which Polyakov (1966) preferred to call projection-association areas, retain their modally specific *gnostic* function, integrating in some cases visual (secondary occipital areas), in other cases auditory (secondary temporal areas), and in yet other cases tactile (secondary parietal areas) information. However, the fact that these zones, with their predominance of multi-modal neurons and neurons with short axons, play the principal role in the *conversion of the somatotopical projection into the functional organization* of incoming information, indicates that the high level of specialization of the cells of these zones is considerably less, and that the transition to them marks a significant step forward along the path of 'diminishing modal specificity'.

This modal specificity is represented to an even lesser degree in the *tertiary* zones of this second brain unit.

The fact that these cortical areas can be described as 'zones of overlapping' of the cortical ends of the various analysers is itself sufficient to show that the modal specificity of its components is less highly represented, and that although one can point to the simultaneous (spatial) syntheses performed by these zones of the cortex it is virtually almost impossible to suggest that they are modally-specific (visual or tactile) in character. This applies to an incomparably lesser degree to the higher, symbolic levels of work of these zones, with the transition to which the function of the tertiary zones becomes to some extent '*supramodal*' in character.

The *law of diminishing specificity* is thus another aspect of the already familiar law of hierarchical structure of individual cortical areas forming this second brain system and responsible for the transition from discrete reflection of particular modally-specific cues to the integrated reflection of more general and abstract schemes of the perceived world.

At this point it is imperative to mention that the principles I have expressed above are in contradiction, to some extent, with Pavlov's statement that the cortical projection zones are the 'most highly differentiated' in their structure, whereas the zones surrounding them are the 'diffuse periphery', performing the same functions but with less precision.

The fact that the primary cortical zones are characterized by the highest 'modal specificity' is not in question. However, it cannot be accepted that the surrounding secondary and tertiary zones can be dismissed merely as a 'diffuse periphery, preserving the same functions but in a less perfect form'.

My argument starts from the concept that the secondary and tertiary cortical zones, with their predominance of multimodal and associative neurons and with the absence of any direct connection with the periphery, possess, not less perfect and lower functional properties but, on the contrary, more perfect and higher functional properties than the primary cortical zones; that, despite the diminishing specificity (or perhaps, by virtue of this diminishing specificity) they become capable of playing an *organizing, integrative role in the work of the more specific areas,* thus acquiring a key position in the organization of the functional systems essential for complex gnostic processes. Unless this principle is taken into account, it would be impossible to understand all the clinical facts concerning disturbances of function arising in local brain lesions which will be described.

It remains to consider the *third fundamental law* governing the work of the second brain system and, indeed, the work of the cortex as a whole. This can be expressed as the law of the *progressive lateralization of functions,* implying their progressive transfer from the primary cortical areas to the secondary and, ultimately, to the tertiary areas.

The *primary* cortical *areas* of both cerebral hemispheres, whose structure is based on the principle of somatotopical projection, are known to have *identical roles.* Each of them is the projection of contralateral receptor surfaces, and there is no question of any dominance of the primary areas of either hemisphere. The situation is different with regard to the *secondary* and, still more, with the *tertiary areas.* With the appearance of *right-handedness* (which is associated with *work,* and which evidently relates to a very early stage in man's history), and later with the appearance of another related process, namely *speech,* some degree of *lateralization of functions* begins to take place, which has not been found in animals but which in man has become an important principle of the functional organization of the brain.

The left hemisphere (in right-handed persons) has become *dominant;* it is this hemisphere which begins to be responsible for speech functions, whereas the right hemisphere, unconnected with the activity of the right hands or with speech, has remained *subdominant.* This *principle of lateralization of functions* has naturally become a new and decisive principle of the *functional organization of the cerebral cortex.*

The left (dominant) hemisphere (in right handers) begins to play an essential role not only in the cerebral organization of speech, but also in the *cerebral organization of all higher forms of cognitive activity connected with speech* – perception organized into logical schemes, active verbal memory, logical thought – whereas the right (non-dominant) hemisphere either begins to play a subordinate role in the cerebral organization of these processes or plays no part whatsoever in their course.

This principle of lateralization of higher functions in the cerebral cortex begins to operate only with the *transition to the secondary* and, in particular, to the *tertiary zones* which are principally concerned with the *coding* (or functional organization) of information reaching the cortex, and performed in man with the aid of speech.

It is for that reason that the *functions of the secondary and tertiary zones of the left (dominant) hemisphere start to differ radically from functions of the secondary and tertiary zones of the right* (non-dominant) hemisphere. It is for that reason that the great majority of symptoms of disturbance of higher psychological processes described in patients with local brain lesions refer to symptoms arising as the result of lesions in the secondary and tertiary zones of the dominant (left) hemisphere, whereas the symptomatology of lesions of these same zones in the non-dominant (right) hemisphere has received far less study and analysis. This leading role of the left (dominant) hemisphere, like the principle of progressive lateralization of functions, sharply distinguishes the organization of the human brain from that of animals, whose behaviour is not organized with the close participation of speech activity. This is one of the most important features distinguishing the human brain as the organ of his mental activity, and this unique organization of the human brain has very recently been the subject of close scrutiny by a number of investigators (see the survey by Drew *et al.*, 1970).

However, it must be remembered that the absolute dominance of one (the left) hemisphere is not by any means always found, and the law of lateralization is only relative in character. According to recent investigations (Zangwill, 1960; Subirana, 1969), only one-quarter of all persons are completely right-handed, and slightly more than one-third show marked dominance of the left hemisphere, whereas the rest are distinguished by relatively slight dominance of the left hemisphere, and in one-tenth of all cases the dominance of the left hemisphere is totally absent. When the main clinical picture of changes in higher mental processes in lesions of individual cortical zones is discussed, we shall have occasion once again to convince ourselves of the truth of this situation.

Let us briefly summarize what has been said. The second functional system of the cerebral cortex is a system for the *reception, coding and storage of information*. It is located in the posterior divisions of the cerebral hemispheres and it incorporates visual (occipital), auditory (temporal) and general sensory (parietal) regions of the cortex.

The organization of the structures forming this system is *hierarchical*, for they are subdivided into *primary* (projection) areas, receiving the corresponding information and analysing it into its elementary components, *secondary* (projection-association) areas, responsible for the coding (synthesis) of these elements and converting somatotopical projections into functional organization, and the *tertiary* zones (or zones of overlapping), responsible for the concerted working of the various analysers and the production of supramodal (symbolic) schemes, the basis for complex forms of gnostic activity.

These hierarchically organized zones of the cortex constituting second brain systems work according to the principle of *diminishing modal specificity and increasing functional lateralization*. These two principles are the means whereby the brain can carry out its most complex forms of work, lying at the basis of the whole type of human cognitive activity, linked by its origin with work and structurally with the participation of speech in the organization of mental processes.

This concludes our examination of the most general principles governing the structure and work of the second functional unit of the brain.

The unit for programming, regulation and verification of activity

The reception, coding and storage of information constitute only one aspect of human cognitive processes. Another of its aspects is the organization of conscious activity. This task is linked with the third of the fundamental functional systems of the brain, responsible for programming, regulation and verification.

Man not only reacts passively to incoming information, but creates *intentions*, forms *plans* and *programmes* of his actions, inspects their performance, and *regulates* his behaviour so that it conforms to these plans and programmes; finally, he *verifies* his conscious activity, comparing the effects of his actions with the original intentions and correcting any mistakes he has made.

All these processes of conscious activity require quite different brain systems from those which we have already described. Whereas even in simple reflex tasks there are both afferent and effector sides as well as a feedback system, acting as a controlling servo-mechanism, special neuronal structures of this type are even more essential to the work of the brain when regulating complex conscious activity. These tasks are met by the structures of the third brain unit, whose functions we have just described.

The structures of the third functional unit, the system for programming, regulation and verification, are located in the *anterior regions* of the hemispheres, anteriorly to the precentral gyrus (Figure 14).

The outlet channel for this unit is the *motor cortex* (Brodmann's area 4), layer V of which contains the giant pyramidal cells of Betz, fibres from which run to the spinal motor nuclei and from thence to the muscles, forming the parts of the *great pyramidal tract*. This cortical area is projectional in character and, as is well known, its topographical structure is such that its superior parts are the origin of fibres leading to the lower limbs, its medial parts of fibres leading to the upper limbs of the contralateral side, while its lower parts give rise to fibres running to the muscles of the face, lips and tongue. The principle of widest representation of organs of greatest value and requiring the most accurate regulation in this zone has already been mentioned.

The motor projection cortex cannot work in isolation; all a person's movements require to some extent or other a *tonic background*, provided by the basal motor ganglia and the fibres of the *extra-pyramidal* system. The importance of this system, which ensures a plastic background for all voluntary movements, has been the subject of many excellent investigations, and there is no need to discuss it in particular here.

The primary (projection) motor cortex, as I have said, is only the outlet channel for motor impulses or, as that great authority on the

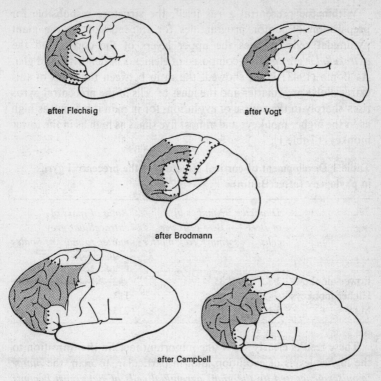

after Flechsig

after Vogt

after Brodmann

after Campbell

Figure 14 Diagram showing arrangement of the frontal (prefrontal) zones of the brain

investigation of movement, Bernstein, has said – 'the anterior horns of the brain'. The motor composition of the impulses which it sends to the periphery must naturally be well prepared and incorporated into certain programmes, and only after preparation in this manner can impulses sent out through the precentral gyrus give rise to the necessary purposive movements.

This preparation of the motor impulses cannot be undertaken by the pyramidal cells themselves; it must be carried out both in the structures of the precentral gyrus itself, and also in the structures of the superposed *secondary* areas of the motor cortex, which prepare the motor programmes and only then transmit them to the giant pyramidal cells.

Within the precentral gyrus itself, the structure responsible for preparation of motor programmes for transmission to the giant pyramidal cells includes the upper layers of the cortex and the *extracellular grey matter*, composed of elements of dendrites and glia. As Bonin (1943; 1948) showed, the ratio between the mass of this extracellular grey matter and the mass of cells of the precentral gyrus rises sharply in the course of evolution, for in man it is twice as high as in the higher monkeys and almost five times as high as in the lower monkeys (Table 1).

Table 1 **Development of cortical structure of the precentral gyrus in phylogeny** (after Bonin)

	Diameter of Betz cells	Number of Betz cells per mm^3 grey matter	Ratio of mass of extracellular grey matter to mass of bodies of Betz cells
Lower monkeys	3·7	31	52
Higher monkeys			113
Man	6·1	12	233

These results clearly show one important fact: in the transition to the higher levels of evolution and, in particular, to man, the *motor impulses generated by the giant pyramidal cells of Betz must become increasingly controlled*, and it is this control which is effected by the powerfully developed systems of extracellular grey matter, consisting of dendrites and glia.

The precentral gyrus is, however, only a projection area, an effector apparatus of the cortex. A decisive role in the preparation of the motor impulses is played by the superposed secondary and tertiary zones, governed by the same principles of hierarchical organization and diminishing specificity which I mentioned when discussing the principles governing the functional organization of the system for reception, coding and storage of information. The main difference now is that whereas in the second, afferent system of the brain the processes go from the primary to the secondary and tertiary zones; in the third, efferent system the processes run in a descending direction, starting at the highest levels of the tertiary and secondary zones, where the motor plans and programmes are formed, and then passing through the structures of the primary motor area, which sends the prepared motor impulses to the periphery.

The second feature distinguishing the work of the third, efferent unit of the cortex from that of its second, afferent unit is that the unit itself does not contain a number of different modally-specific zones representing individual analysers, but consists entirely of systems of efferent, motor type, and is itself under the constant influence of structures of the afferent unit. The role played by these afferent systems in the structure of movements will be examined when we discuss the interaction between the principal functional units of the brain.

As I have mentioned, the role of the principal *secondary* zone of the third unit is played by the *premotor* areas of the frontal region. Morphologically they adhere to the same 'vertical' type of striation (Polyakov, 1965; 1966) characteristic of the motor cortex, but differ in the incomparably greater development of the upper layers of small pyramidal cells; stimulation of these parts of the cortex gives rise not to somatotopically defined twitches of individual muscles, but to groups of systemically organized movements (turning the eyes, head, or whole body and grasping movements of the hands), evidence of the integrative role of these cortical zones in movement organization.

Another important point is that although stimulation of the precentral gyrus evokes localized excitation, spreading only to nearby points, excitation of the premotor areas of the cortex, as the neuronographic experiments of McCulloch (1943) showed, spreads to the more distant parts, including the postcentral areas and, conversely, these parts of the premotor areas are themselves excited by stimulation of distant parts of the afferent cortex.

On the basis of all these facts, the premotor areas can be classified among the secondary divisions of the cortex, and they can be considered to play the same organizing role with respect to movements as is played by the secondary zones of the posterior divisions of the cortex, which convert somatotopical projection into functional organization. We shall return to the consideration of clinical pictures affecting the movements of patients with lesions of the premotor cortex (part 2, ch. 6).

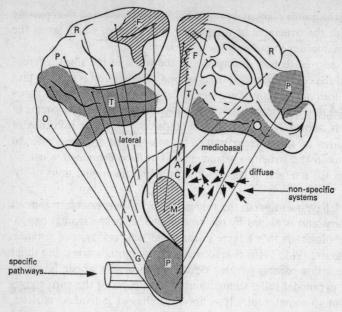

Figure 15 Diagram of the prefrontal regions of the brain with subjacent structures (after Pribram)

The most important part of this third functional unit of the brain, however, is the *frontal lobes* or, to be more precise, the *prefrontal divisions of the brain* which, because they do not contain pyramidal cells, are sometimes known as the *granular frontal cortex*. It is these portions of the brain, belonging to the tertiary zones of the cortex, which play a decisive role in the formation of intentions and programmes, and in the regulation and verification of the most complex forms of human behaviour.

A distinguishing feature of the prefrontal region of the brain is that it has a very rich system of connections both with lower levels of the brain (the medial and ventral nuclei and pulvinar of the thalamus and with other structures) (Figure 15) and with virtually all other parts of the cortex (Figure 16). These connections are two-way in character and the prefrontal divisions of the cortex structures they make are in a particularly favourable position both for the reception and synthesis of the complex system of afferent impulses arriving from

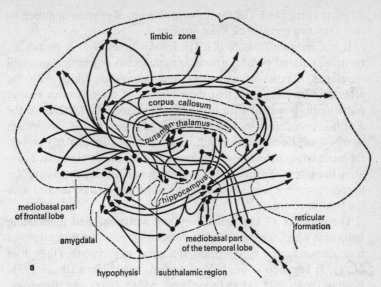

Figure 16a Connections of the frontal lobes with other brain structures (after Polyakov)

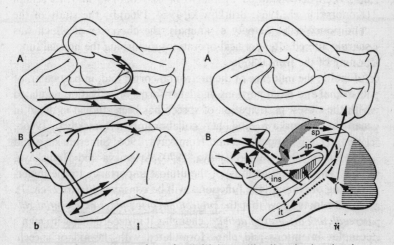

Figure 16b Connections of the frontal lobes with other brain structures (b) after Nauta. (i) efferent connections; (ii) afferent connections, (A) medial surface (B) lateral surface

all parts of the brain and for the organization of efferent impulses, so that they can regulate all these structures.

It is important to note that the frontal lobes and, in particular, their medial and basal portions are connected by particularly well developed bundles of ascending and descending fibres with the reticular formation, and that these regions of the neocortex receive particularly powerful streams of impulses from the systems of the first functional unit, by which they are 'charged' to the appropriate energy tone; on the other hand, they can have a particularly powerful modulating influence on the reticular formation, giving its activating impulses their differential character, and making them conform to the dynamic schemes of behaviour which are directly formed with the frontal cortex.

The presence of both inhibitory and activating and modulating influences which the frontal lobes exert on the reticular formation has been demonstrated by electrophysiological experiments (French *et al.*, 1955; Segundo *et al.*, 1955; Pribram, 1960; Narikashvili, 1963; Nauta, 1964; 1971; Hernández-Peón, 1966; Bureš and Burešova, 1968; Durinyan *et al.*, 1968). The presence of inhibitory influences of the frontal (especially the orbital) cortex on lower structures has also been demonstrated by the work of Konorski and his school (Konorski *et al.*, 1964; Brutkowski, 1964; 1966) by the study of the conditioned-reflex activity of animals, the character of which was sharply altered after surgical operations disturbing the normal functioning of the frontal lobes.

Finally, the influence of the prefrontal cortex and, in particular, of its medial and basal portions on higher forms of activation regulated with the closest participation of speech has been studied in detail in man by Homskaya and her collaborators (Homskaya, 1966b, 1969; 1972; Baranovskaya and Homskaya, 1966; Simernitskaya and Homskaya, 1966; Simernitskaya, 1970; Artemeva and Homskaya, 1966). These investigations, of the utmost importance to the understanding of frontal lobe functions, will be considered (part 2, ch. 7).

These facts show that the *prefrontal cortex plays an essential role in regulating the state of activity,* changing it in accordance with man's complex intentions and plans formulated with the aid of speech. This role of the frontal lobes in the regulation of states of activity which are the background for behaviour is one of the most important ways in which the prefrontal regions of the brain participate in the organization of human behaviour.

Finally, it must also be noted that the prefrontal regions of the cortex do not mature until very late in ontogeny, and not until the child has reached the age of four to seven years do they become finally prepared for action.

This fact is clear from the successive increase in area occupied by the prefrontal divisions of the cortex in ontogeny and also from the rate of development in size of the constituent nerve cells.

Recent observations relating to the dynamics of development of the prefrontal cortex are illustrated in Figure 17. As the figure shows, the rate of increase in area of the frontal regions of the brain rises sharply by the age of three and a half to four years, and this is

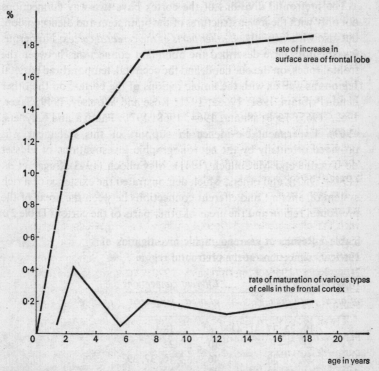

Figure 17 Rate of increase in area of the frontal lobes and rate of increase in size of nerve cells in ontogeny (after Moscow Brain Institute)

followed by a second jump towards the age of seven to eight years. The first of these periods is marked by a significant increase in the rate of growth of the cell bodies contained in the prefrontal regions of the cortex. When discussing the role of the prefrontal cortex in the formation of complex programmes, to which the child's behaviour begins to become subordinated at these ages (Luria, 1961; 1969b), we shall appreciate once again the whole importance of this fact.

As I have previously stated, the prefrontal divisions of the brain, which undergo powerful development in the later stages of evolution and which, in man, occupy up to one-quarter of the total mass of the brain, also have other functions more directly connected with the organization of human activity.

The prefrontal divisions of the cortex have two-way connections not only with the lower structures of the brain stem and diencephalon, but also with virtually *all other parts of the cerebral cortex*. Numerous investigators have described the abundant connections between the frontal lobes, on the one hand, and the occipital, temporal and parietal regions as well as with the limbic regions of the cortex, on the other hand (Pribram, 1961; 1966a; 1971; Rose and Woolsey, 1949; Sager, 1962; 1965; 1968; Nauta, 1964; 1968; 1971; Pandya and Kuypers, 1969). Experimental evidence in support of this statement was provided originally by the neuronographic investigations of Dusser de Barenne and McCulloch (1941), McCulloch (1943), Sugar *et al.* (1948; 1950;), and others, which demonstrated the existence of a rich system of afferent and efferent connections between the areas of the prefrontal region and the areas of other parts of the cortex (Table 2).

Table 2 **Results of neuronographic investigation of cortical connections at the prefrontal region**

Afferent connections		*Efferent connections*	
of area	*with area*	*of area*	*with area*
8	19, 22, 37, 41, 42	8	18
9	23	10	22
10	22, 37, 38	46	6, 37, 39
44	41, 42, 22, 37	47	38
47	36, 38	24	31, 32

There is thus conclusive evidence that the prefrontal regions of the cortex are tertiary cortical structures, in intimate communication with nearly every other principal zone of the cortex, and if it were necessary to mention any particular feature distinguishing the prefrontal regions of the brain from the tertiary zones of the posterior regions, it would be that the *tertiary portions of the frontal lobes are in fact a superstructure above all other parts of the cerebral cortex, so that they perform a far more universal function of general regulation of behaviour* than that performed by the posterior associative centre, or, in other words, the tertiary areas of the second functional unit.

The morphological details concerning the structure and connections of the frontal lobes which are described above explain the contribution made by these structures of the third brain unit to the general organization of behaviour. Early observations on animals from which the frontal lobes have been removed, undertaken by such classical authorities on physiology and neurology as Bianchi (1895; 1921), Franz (1907), Bekhterev (1905–7), Pavlov (1949a, 1949b), and which were later developed and supplemented by the work of Jacobsen (1935), Malmo (1942), Anokhin (1949), Pribram (1954; 1959b; 1960), Rosvold and Delgado (1956), Rosvold (1959), Mishkin *et al.* (1955; 1956; 1958), and Konorski and his collaborators (1952; 1964), showed the depth to which the animal's behaviour is altered after extirpation of the frontal lobes.

As Pavlov pointed out originally, no disturbances in the work of the individual sense organs can be detected in such an animal: its visual and kinaesthetic analysis remains intact; however, its rational, goal-directed behaviour is profoundly upset. The normal animal always aims at a certain goal, inhibiting its response to irrelevant, unimportant stimuli; the dog with destroyed frontal lobes, on the other hand, responds to all irrelevant stimuli; when it sees leaves which have fallen on the garden path, it seizes them, chews them, and spits them out; it does not recognize its master, and is distracted by all irrelevant stimuli; it responds to any element of the environment by uninhibitable orienting reflexes, and its distractions by these unimportant elements of the environment disturb the plans and programmes of its behaviour, making it fragmentary and uncontrolled. Sometimes the animal's planned, goal-directed behaviour is interrupted by the senseless repetition of established inert sterotypes. Dogs without their frontal lobes which Anokhin and Shumilina observed, having once taken food from two feeding bowls located on their right and left sides, began to perform prolonged and stereotyped 'pendulum' movements, shifting from one feeding bowl to the other time and time again, not regulating their behaviour by the obtaining of food as reinforcement (Shumilina; see Anokhin, 1949).

On the basis of facts such as these, Pavlov stated that the frontal lobes play an essential role in the 'synthesis of goal-directed movements' (1949a, p. 295), and Bekhterev postulated that the frontal lobes play an important role in 'the correct assessment of external impressions and the goal-directed choice of movements in accordance with such an assessment', thereby performing 'psychoregulatory activity' (Bekhterev, 1905-7, pp. 1464-8). Finally, Anokhin concluded from these observations that the frontal lobes play an essential role in the 'synthesis of environmental information', thereby providing the 'preliminary triggering afferentation of behaviour' (Anokhin, 1949).

Subsequent investigations have led to further clarification of the details and to progress in the analysis of these functions of the frontal lobes.

The early observations of Jacobsen (1935) showed that a monkey after extirpation of the frontal lobes can perform simple behavioural acts successfully under the control of direct impressions, but cannot synthesize information arriving from the different parts of a situation not received in one visual field and, therefore, it cannot carry out complex behavioural programmes requiring support on the mnestic plane. Further experiments by a number of workers have shown that extirpation of the frontal lobes leads to the breakdown of delayed responses and to inability to subordinate the animal's behaviour to an internal programme (for example, a programme based on a successive change or alteration of signals). The most recent analysis has provided a closer insight into the mechanisms of these disturbances and has shown that destruction of the frontal lobes leads, not so much to a disturbance of memory as to a disturbance of the ability to inhibit orienting reflexes to distracting stimuli: as the experiments of Malmo (1942), Pribram (1959a; 1960), Weiskrantz (1964) and others have shown, such an animal cannot perform tasks involving delayed responses under ordinary conditions, but can do so provided that irrelevant, distracting stimuli are removed (if the animal is kept in total darkness, if tranquillizers are administered, and so on).

As a result of these observations it has thus been established that *destruction of the prefrontal cortex leads to a profound disturbance of complex behavioural programmes* and to marked *disinhibition of immediate responses to irrelevant stimuli,* thus making the performance of complex behavioural programmes impossible (Konorski and Lawicka, 1964; Brutkowski *et al.,* 1957; Brutkowski, 1966).

The role of the prefrontal cortex in the synthesis of systems of stimuli and the creation of a *plan of action* is manifested not only in relation to currently acting stimuli, but also in the formation of active behaviour directed towards the future.

The observations of Pribram have shown that an animal with intact frontal lobes can tolerate long pauses while awaiting appropriate reinforcement, and that its active responses are strengthened only with the approach of the time when the expected stimulus should appear; by contrast, an animal deprived of its frontal lobes cannot maintain such a state of 'active anticipation' and, during a long pause it immediately responds with a mass of movements which it cannot relate to the end of the pause or to the time of the anticipated stimulus (Figure 18). It can thus be concluded that the frontal lobes of the brain are among the vital structures responsible for the orientation of an animal's behaviour *not only to the present, but also to the future,* and that they thus are responsible for the most complex forms of active behaviour.

Finally, attention must be drawn to yet another important function of the frontal lobes in the regulation and verification of behaviour. As a result of recent work, it can no longer be held that the scheme of the reflex arc can adequately reflect all that is essential in the structure of behaviour, but that it must be replaced by the scheme of *a reflex ring or reflex circle* in which, besides reception and analysis of stimuli from the external environment and a response to them, it is also necessary to take into account the *reverse influence which the effect of the action has on the animal's brain.* This feedback mechanism or 'reverse afferentation', as an essential component of any organized action, has been closely studied by several investi-

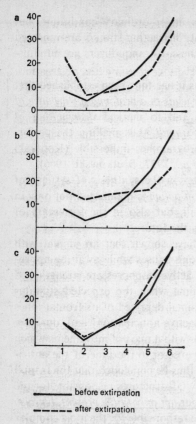

Figure 18 Disturbance of the expectancy response in monkeys after extirpation of the frontal lobes (after Pribram) (a) extirpation of the occipital lobes; (b) extirpation of the frontal lobes; (c) control. The numbers 1–6 denote 20-second intervals until expected reinforcement, given after the 3rd minute

— before extirpation
---- after extirpation

gators (Anokhin, 1935; 1955–71; Bernstein, 1935; 1957; 1966; Miller, Galanter and Pribram, 1960), and it has been described by Anokhin as the 'action acceptor' apparatus, without which any form of organized action is impossible.

Numerous observations show that the most complex forms of 'action acceptor' are associated with the frontal lobes, and that the *frontal lobes not only perform the function of synthesis of external*

92 Functional Organization and Mental Activity

stimuli, preparation for action, and formation of programmes, but also the function of allowing for the effect of the action carried out and verification that it has taken the proper course.

This fact was established by observations showing that destruction of the frontal lobes makes the animal unable to assess and correct errors it has made, and that for this reason the behaviour of an animal without its frontal lobes loses its organized and purposive character (Pribram, 1959b; 1960; 1961). Recent work has added yet another important fact to our understanding of the functional organization of the frontal lobes.

Investigations (Gross and Weiskrantz, 1964; Brutkowski, 1964) have shown that the frontal lobes of an animal are *not a homogeneous structure* and that whereas some parts of the frontal lobes (the sulcus principalis, areas homologous to those parts of the human frontal lobe on the lateral, convex surface of the brain) are directly concerned with the regulation of *motor* processes, other areas (homologous to the medial and basal portions of the human frontal lobes) evidently subserve a different function, for their destruction does not lead to disturbance of motor processes.

We shall see again how important this is for the understanding of the methods of work of the human frontal lobes.

The *human frontal lobes* are much more highly developed than the frontal lobes even of the higher monkeys; that is why in man, through the progressive corticalization of functions, processes of programming, regulation and verification of conscious activity are dependent to a far greater extent on the prefrontal parts of the brain than the processes of regulation of behaviour are in animals.

For reasons which will be obvious, the opportunities for experimenting on man do not compare with those on animals; however, extensive material has now been collected, as a result of which much more complete information than hitherto is now available on the role of the prefrontal cortex in the regulation of human mental processes.

The chief distinguishing feature of the regulation of human conscious activity is that this regulation takes place with the close participation of *speech*. Whereas the relatively elementary forms of regulation of organic processes and even of the simplest forms of behaviour can take place without the aid of speech, *higher mental processes are formed and take place on the basis of speech activity*, which is expanded in the early stages of development, but later becomes increasingly contracted (Vygotsky, 1956; 1960; Leontiev, 1959; Zaporozhets, 1960; Galperin, 1959). It is therefore natural to seek the programming, regulating and verifying action of the human brain primarily in those forms of conscious activity whose regulation takes place through the intimate participation of speech.

In the last decade, some incontrovertible facts have been obtained to show that these forms of regulation are effected in man with the close participation of the frontal lobes. Some years ago, Grey Walter (Walter *et al.*, 1964; Walter, 1966) showed that every act of *expectancy* evokes characteristic slow potentials in the human cerebral cortex, which increase in amplitude with an increase in the likelihood of materialization of the expected stimulus, decrease with a decrease in the likelihood, and disappear as soon as the task of awaiting the stimulus is discontinued (Figure 19). Characteristically these waves, which he called 'expectancy waves' appear primarily in the *frontal lobes of the brain*, from which they spread throughout the rest of the cortex.

Almost simultaneously with this discovery, the Soviet physiologist Livanov, with his collaborators (Livanov *et al.*, 1964; 1967), confirmed this intimate participation of the prefrontal regions of the brain in the most complex forms of activation evoked by intellectual activity by a different method.

By recording the action potentials reflecting excitation of fifty, or sometimes as many as 120 or 150 simultaneously working points of the brain by means of a special multichannel apparatus, they showed that these complex mental tasks lead to the appearance of a large number of synchronously working points in the *frontal lobes* (Figure 20a,b), that the same picture is found in a patient with the paranoid form of schizophrenia, permanently in a state of compulsive excitation (Figure 20c), and that these synchronously working points in the frontal lobes disappear after administration of chlorpromazine, which abolishes this state of compulsive excitation (Figure 20d).

These two independent series of investigations show conclusively that the *frontal cortex participates in the generation of activation processes* which arise as the result of the most complex forms of conscious activity and are effected with the immediate participation of speech.

These facts become clear if it is remembered that it is these parts of the cerebral cortex (as was indicated above) which are particularly rich in connections with the descending activating reticular formation, and they demonstrate that the *frontal lobes in man participate directly in the state of increased activation which accompanies all forms of conscious activity*. They also suggest that it is the prefrontal zones of the cortex which evoke this activation and enable the complex programming, control, and verification of human conscious activity, which require the optimal tone of cortical processes, to take place.

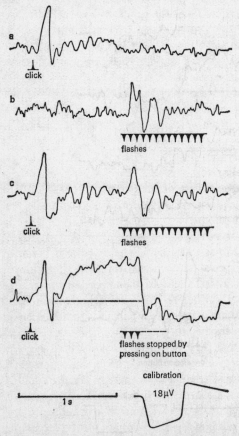

Figure 19 Dynamics of the 'expectancy waves' (after Grey Walter)

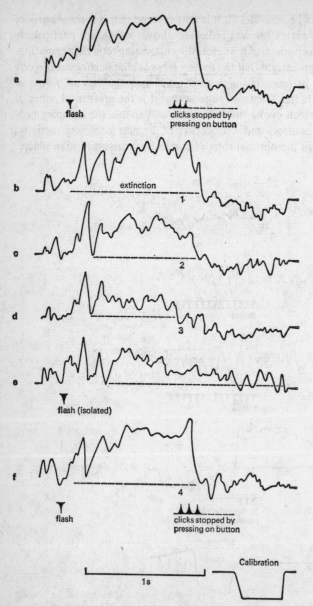

a

flash   clicks stopped by
         pressing on button

b

extinction
1

c

2

d

3

e

flash (isolated)

f

4

flash   clicks stopped by
         pressing on button

1s   Calibration

Figure 19 – continued

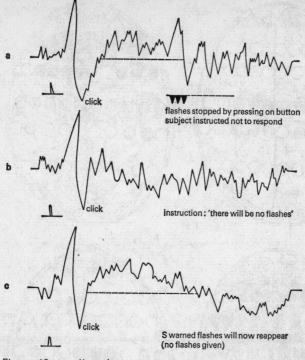

a

click

flashes stopped by pressing on button
subject instructed not to respond

b

click

instruction: 'there will be no flashes'

c

click

S warned flashes will now reappear
(no flashes given)

Figure 19 – continued

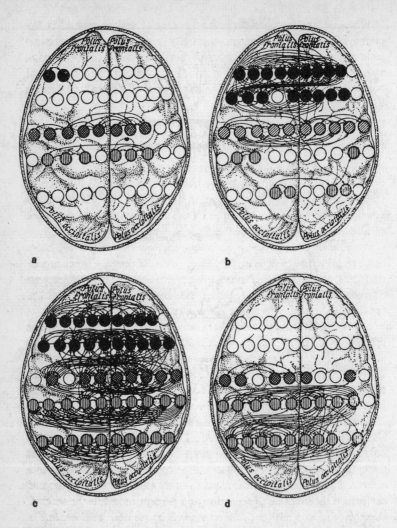

Figure 20 Changes in correlation between synchronously working points of the frontal region during intellectual activity (after Livanov, Gavrilova and Aslanov): (a) resting state; (b) solution of a difficult problem; (c) patient with paranoid schizophrenia in a state of excitation; (d) after administration of chlorpromazine

When we analyse changes in the process of activation and in the course of goal-directed conscious activity in patients with local brain lesions, we shall be able to cite much factual evidence of the decisive role of this functional brain unit, and, in particular, of its prefrontal zones, in the programming, regulation and verification of human mental processes.

Interaction between the three principal functional units of the brain

We have examined modern ideas regarding the three principal functional units of the brain and have tried to show the role of each of them in the organization of complex mental activity. We must now consider a fact which is essential to the understanding of the work of all the functional units of the brain we have examined.

It would be a mistake to imagine that each of these units can carry out a certain form of activity completely independently – for example, that the second functional unit is entirely responsible for the function of perception and thought, whiie the third is responsible for the function of movement and for the construction of action.

It will be clear from what has been said already regarding the *systemic structure of complex psychological processes* that this is not so. Each form of conscious activity is always a *complex functional system* and takes place through the *combined working of all three brain units*, each of which makes its own contribution. The well established facts of modern psychology provide a solid basis for this view.

Many years have passed since psychologists regarded mental functions as isolated *faculties*, each of which could be localized in a certain part of the brain. However, the time has also passed when it was thought that mental processes could be represented by models of a *reflex arc*, the first part of which was purely afferent in character and performed the function of sensation and perception, while the second, effector part, was entirely concerned with movement and action.

Modern views regarding the structure of mental processes are completely different in character and are based more on the model of a *reflex ring* or *self-regulating system*, each component of which embodies both afferent and effector elements, so that on the whole, *mental activity assumes a complex and active character* (Leontev, 1959).

As an example let us examine the structure, first, of perception and, second, of movement or action. We shall do so only at the most general level, for we shall make a more detailed analysis of the structure and cerebral organization of these processes in the last part of this book.

It would be a mistake to imagine that sensation and perception are purely passive processes. Sensation has been shown to include motor components, and in modern psychology sensation and, more especially, perception are regarded as active processes incorporating both afferent and efferent components (Leontev, 1959). Adequate proof that sensation is complex and active in character is given by the fact that even in animals it incorporates a process of selection of biologically significant features, while in man it also includes the active coding influence of speech (Bruner, 1957; Lyublinskaya, 1959).

The active character of the processes in the perception of complex objects is more obvious still. It is well known that perception of objects not only is polyreceptor in character and dependent on the combined working of a group of analysers, but also that it always incorporates active motor components. The vital role of eye movements in visual perception was described originally by Sechenov (1874–8), but it is only recently that psychophysiological investigations have shown that the stationary eye is virtually incapable of the stable perception of complex objects and that such perception is always based on the use of active, searching movements of the eyes, picking out the essential clues (Yarbus, 1965; 1967), and that these movements only gradually become contracted in character in the course of development (Zaporozhets, 1967; Zinchenko *et al.*, 1962).

These facts clearly show that *perception takes place through the combined action of all three functional units of the brain*; the first provides the necessary cortical tone, the second carries out the analysis and synthesis of incoming information, and the third provides for the necessary controlled searching movements which give perceptual activity its active character.

We shall see how this complex structure of perception explains why it can be disturbed by lesions of different and widely separated brain systems. The situation is similar with regard to the structure of *voluntary movement and action*.

The role of the efferent mechanisms in the structure of movement is obvious; however, Bernstein (1947) showed that movement cannot be controlled by efferent impulses alone, and that organized movement requires a constant flow of afferent impulses, providing information on the state of the joints and muscles, the position of the segments of the moving system, and the spatial coordinates within which the movement takes place.

Clearly, therefore, *voluntary movement and, more especially, manipulations of objects are based on the combined working of different parts of the brain.* The systems of the first brain unit supply the necessary muscle tone, without which coordinated movement would be impossible, the systems of the second unit provide the afferent syntheses within the framework of which the movement takes place, and the systems of the third unit subordinate the movement and action to the corresponding plans, produce the programmes for the performance of motor actions, and provide the necessary regulation and checking of the course of the movements without which their organized and purposive character would be lost.

We shall see the contribution made by each area of the brain to the construction of movement and we shall obtain some idea of the complexity of the system of their cerebral organization.

It is clear that *all three principal functional brain units work concertedly*, and that it is only by studying their interactions, when each unit makes its own specific contribution, that an insight can be obtained into the nature of the cerebral mechanisms of mental activity.

We have described the principal functional units located in the brain and have shown how they work together. The next step is to make a detailed analysis of the contribution made by each area of the brain to the construction of mental processes and of the cerebral organization of complex forms of human conscious activity. These matters will be dealt with in the next two parts of this book.

Part Two
Local Brain Systems and their Functional Analysis

I have shown above that human mental processes are complex functional systems entailing the combined working of individual areas of the brain. At the same time I showed that in order to analyse their cerebral organization it is essential to determine the contribution made by each area of the brain to this complex functional system and to establish which factors of mental activity are the responsibility of which brain systems. Finally, I discussed the chief sources of our knowledge of the cerebral basis of mental activity and I showed that of these three sources – the comparative anatomy of the brain, methods of stimulation and methods of destruction of its individual areas – with respect to the analysis of the functional organization of the human brain it is the last which is evidently the most important.

These considerations lead us to the *clinical study of local brain lesions* and to the analysis of *changes arising in human mental processes where there are local lesions of individual areas of the brain* as the principal ways of obtaining the answers to our questions and also of discovering the contribution made by a particular brain area to the organization of human mental activity. However, despite the importance of this method, it must not be imagined that it provides a direct and simple road to the solution of our problems. As we have seen above, a local brain lesion does not lead to the direct 'loss' of a particular mental condition; this was the view held by the supporters of 'narrow localizationism'. A pathological focus arising as the result of a wound, of haemorrhage, or of a tumour disturbs the normal working of a given brain area, abolishes the conditions necessary for the normal working of the particular functional system, and thus leads to *reorganization* of the working of the intact parts of the brain, so that the disturbed function can be performed in new ways.

These basic facts, well known to every clinician, make it extremely difficult to draw conclusions on the role of the affected area in the normal organization of the disturbed form of activity from the symptoms arising in local brain lesions.

There is another factor which increases the difficulty of using local brain lesions in order to analyse the contribution made by each brain area to the organization of mental processes.

In practice, no local brain lesion is so precisely demarcated that it destroys only one narrowly localized group of nerve cells. On the other hand, a pathological focus in the brain only very rarely *destroys all the nerve elements* within that zone. As a rule some elements are completely destroyed whereas others continue to function, although they function under pathologically changed conditions, sometimes depressed or inhibited by the pathological process and sometimes stimulated or excited by it. These facts naturally cause substantial variation in the symptoms arising as the result of local brain lesions, so that topographically the same focus may lead to symptoms of a completely different character.

Again, it must be remembered that a local brain lesion is *never narrowly localized* in character. As a rule, every pathological focus is surrounded by a pathologically changed 'perifocal zone', in which the nerve tissue has to function under conditions altered by changes in the haemodynamics and in the flow of cerebrospinal fluid (leading to ischaemia in some cases and to oedema in others). These changes vary from case to case and from phase to phase, so that the study of the *dynamics* of the disease begins to assume special importance (Smirnov, 1946; 1948).

Finally, any pathological focus as a rule gives rise to far-reaching *reflex effects*, which were described in the early part of this century by Monakow (1910; 1914) as manifestations of 'diaschisis' and which have subsequently been investigated by physiologists. These investigations have revealed interesting phenomena such as the appearance of 'mirror foci of excitation' (Morrell, 1967), and they have demonstrated the wide extent of spread of the influence of an apparently narrowly localized focus.

All these features add considerably to the difficulty of drawing conclusions on the role of the affected area in the structure of a given psychological process from the study of local brain lesions. However, despite all these limitations, investigation of the effect of local brain lesions on the dynamics of psychological processes remains not only a possible method, but in fact the principal method of studying the cerebral organization of mental activity.

If we describe, in a sufficiently large number of cases, the changes in human mental processes which arise through local brain lesions, carefully qualify the facts discovered, and pick out the basic factors leading to their appearance, and if we then compare all the changes arising in these cases with the processes that remain intact (or in other words, if we analyse not only symptoms, but entire syndromes of the lesion), we can make substantial progress towards identifying these aspects of a specific mental activity which are directly connected with a specific area of the brain and towards establishing the contribution made by that area of the brain to the construction of human mental processes.

This method, the basic method of the new scientific discipline of *neuropsychology*, is the one which I shall use throughout the second part of this book. I shall give preference to analysis of the functions of the dominant (left) hemisphere, which are better known, although definite predominance of the left hemisphere over the right is not found in every case but, according to Subirana (1969), in only 63·1 per cent of cases.

We shall study consecutively the changes in mental processes arising in lesions of the occipital (visual), temporal (auditory), parieto-temporo-occipital, premotor and frontal divisions of the brain, describe them as thoroughly as possible, and complete our description with an analysis of the changes produced by lesions of the limbic region (medial parts of the cortex), and the deep brain structures (structures of the brain stem); finally, we shall consider a number of unsolved problems including the still inadequately studied question of the functions of the non-dominant (right) cerebral hemisphere. This is the basic plan of this second part of the book.

Chapter 3
The Occipital Regions and the Organization of Visual Perception

As I have already mentioned, the occipital zones of the brain constitute the cortical centre of the visual system; naturally, therefore, a lesion of these zones must give rise primarily to a disturbance of the processing of visual information and this must be reflected in those mental processes in which visual analysis and synthesis play a direct part.

Let us examine very briefly the disturbances of these functions which arise in lesions of the occipital region of the brain and attempt to describe the characteristic features of lesions affecting individual parts of this region.

Primary areas of the occipital cortex and the elementary functions of vision

The primary areas of the occipital cortex are those where fibres from the retina terminate; these fibres run initially in the optic nerve and then cross over in the chiasma (the decussation of the two visual centres), and continue their course in the optic tract; the optic tract of the right hemisphere includes fibres carrying excitation received by the left halves of the visual field of both eyes, while the optic tract of the left hemisphere includes fibres carrying excitation received from the right halves of the visual field of both eyes; the fibres of the optic tract relay in the lateral geniculate body, and then are arranged fanwise within the temporal region, where they are aptly described by the term 'optic radiation', to terminate in the primary (projection) area of the occipital cortex (Figure 21).

It is clear that because of this arrangement of the optic pathway's fibres a lesion of the optic nerve (b) leads to blindness in one eye, a lesion of the optic chiasma in its medial portions (c) leads to loss of

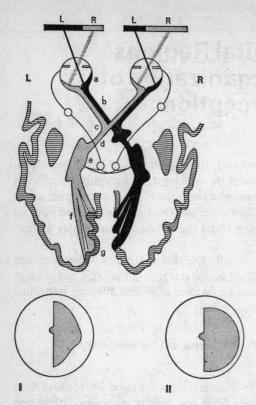

Figure 21 Diagram of the visual pathways of the brain: (a) retina;
(b) optic nerve; (c) chiasma; (d) optic tract; (e) lateral geniculate body;
(f) optic radiation; (g) primary visual area of the cortex (i) and (ii)
corresponding halves of the visual fields.

both outer (temporal) fields of vision, while lesions of the optic tract
(d), the optic radiation (f) or the visual cortex of one hemisphere (g)
lead to loss of the opposite fields of vision or, to use the term employed in neurology, to contralateral homonymous hemianopia.

At the same time, it must be remembered that fibres of the optic
nerve, the optic tract and the optic radiation (Figure 22) all carry
excitation in a strict somatotopical order (Figure 23), and that lesions
of some of these fibres or of part of the projection zone of the visual
cortex lead to the loss of strictly defined parts of the visual field or to

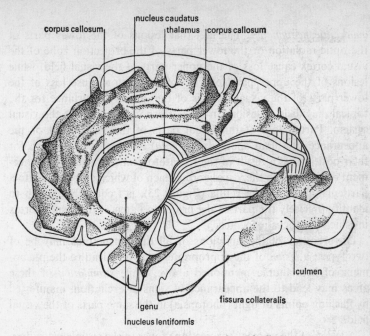

Figure 22 Diagram of the optic radiation (after Pfeiffer)

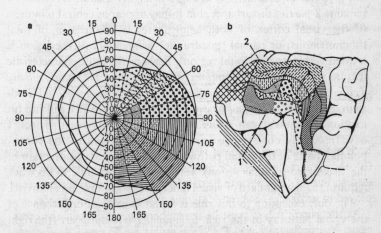

Figure 23 Scheme of retinal projections on the visual cortex and somatotopical character of primary areas of the visual cortex (Brodmann's area 17) (after Holmes): (a) visual field; (b) visual cortex; (1) lower lip of calcarine fissure, (2) upper lip of calcarine fissure

quadrantic hemianopia. The fact that lesions of the lower parts of the optic radiation or the lower parts of the projection zone of the visual cortex cause loss of the upper parts of the visual field, while lesions of the upper parts of the optic radiation cause loss of the lower parts of the visual field, is of the utmost importance for the topical diagnosis of lesions in the corresponding areas of the visual system. Partial loss of individual parts of the visual field or the appearance of 'blind spots' (*scotomata*) is equally important, for their position, as a result of the somatotopical character of arrangement of elements in the visual cortex, each of which corresponds to a particular point of the retina (Figure 23), is frequently enough to identify precisely the part of the projection area of the visual cortex in which the focus is located.

Disturbances of the functions of all these structures may be of two types; a *lesion* of the appropriate areas may lead to the phenomena of hemianopia mentioned above, while *stimulation* of these areas may lead to the appearance of signs of excitation, manifested by flashing points of light (photopsia) in the same parts of the visual field.

A lesion of the primary (projection) zones of the visual cortex does not give rise to such serious changes in higher mental processes; it remains a *partial* disturbance, but it may appear as central blindness (if the visual cortex of both hemispheres is affected) or of total (homonymous) or partial (quadrantic) hemianopia (if the lesion is located within one occipital region). Perhaps the most characteristic feature is that the manifestations of partial loss of the visual field are well compensated both by functional adaptations of the retina (Goldstein and Gelb, 1920) and by movements of the eyes: by shifting his fixation the patient can easily compensate for his visual defect. I have frequently observed patients in whom a lesion of the corresponding parts of the visual pathway has caused gross contraction of the visual field (tubular vision), yet who have been able to do work requiring a high standard of visual function (for example, an archivist).

The only exception to this rule is found in cases of disturbance of the visual pathway in the *right (non-dominant) hemisphere* (the right visual cortex or the deep parts of the right occipital or temporal region, including the structures of the lateral geniculate body). In these cases, as was pointed out many years ago (Holmes, 1919;

Brain, 1941; Luria and Skorodumova, 1950) a distinctive phenomenon of *right-sided fixed hemianopia* arises. An analysis of this
phenomenon will be given later when we examine the disturbances
arising in lesions of the right (non-dominant) hemisphere: the patient
does not notice the defects of the visual field, does not compensate
for them by eye movements, and while he can see only the right side
of a picture or text shown to him, he attributes the defects of his
vision to defects in the material presented. For example, he reads
only the right half of a text, fails to understand what it is about, and
assumes that it is meaningless; such patients characteristically begin
to read or write or draw on the right half of the paper only, and
symptoms of this type immediately suggest that the lesion is located
in the right occipital region.

This phenomenon, sometimes described as *unilateral spatial*
agnosia (Brain, 1941; Ajuriaguerra and Hécaen, 1960; Korchazhinskaya, 1971), can also develop in patients with lesions in the deep
parts of more complex regions of the right hemisphere, and we shall
examine it again later.

Secondary zones of the occipital cortex and optico-gnostic functions

The secondary zones of the occipital cortex differ considerably from
the primary (projection) zones over which they are placed both in
their structure and in their functions. The distinguishing feature of
the secondary zones of the occipital cortex is that the fourth (afferent)
layer of cells, receiving stimuli from the retina, is much smaller here
than in the primary zones (Brodmann's area 17); conversely, the
upper associative layers (II and III), consisting mainly of cells with
short axons, now constitute the greater part of the thickness of these
secondary or 'projection-association' zones (areas 18 and 19), which
have recently been named the *intrinsic cortical areas* (Rose and
Pribram).

A section through the layers of the zone between the primary (17)
and secondary (18) areas of the occipital cortex, taken from Brodmann's classical work (1909), is illustrated in Figure 24. It clearly
demonstrates the radical changes which take place in the cytoarchitectonic structure of the cortex from the primary to the secondary
zones. If it is remembered that the elements of the upper layers of

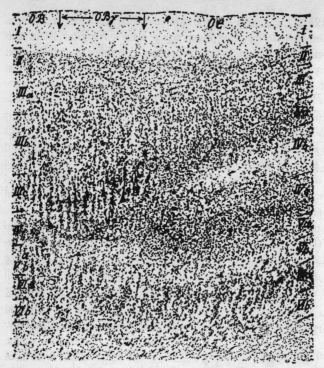

Figure 24 Cytoarchitectonic structure of the primary and secondary visual cortex (section through the boundary between Brodmann's areas 17 and 18) (after Brodmann)

the cortex, which are so powerfully represented in the secondary zones of the visual (occipital) region, not directly connected with fibres from the retina and subserving a predominantly integrative (coding) role, the importance of these zones in the organization of visual perception will be clearly apparent.

The secondary zones of the occipital cortex have also undergone substantial changes by comparison with the primary zones in the course of evolution. Whereas in lower monkeys (with their powerfully developed visual cortex) its primary (projection) area (Brodmann's area 17) is much more extensive than the secondary zone, in man this ratio is reversed, and the secondary visual zone (Brodmann's area 18) is now distinctly larger than the primary visual cortex. The actual figures, given in Table 3, clearly show that the role of systems responsible not for the reception, but for the coding (analysis and synthesis) of incoming visual information, is considerably increased in man by comparison with his antecedents on the scale of evolution.

Table 3 **Relative areas of primary and secondary visual cortex in a series of primates** (percentages to the total area of the occipital cortex; after Filimonov, 1949)

	Area 17	*Area 18*
Galago	66	25·4
Guenon	41·1	32·2
Orang-Utan	39·6	30·5
Man	25·4	37·7

This hypothesis is confirmed by analysis of the morphological and physiological data and also by clinical observations.

The morphological studies of the Moscow Brain Institute showed that the distribution of nerve cells in the cortex of the primary and secondary occipital zones (areas 17 and 18) differs very considerably. Whereas cells of afferent layer IV are distinctly predominant in the primary visual cortex (area 17), these cells are much less numerous in the secondary visual cortex (area 18) where most cells are located in the upper 'associative' layers (II and III). This feature is evident from the figures given in Table 4.

Table 4 **Number of cells in some layers of the primary and secondary occipital** (visual) **cortical zones** (areas 17 and 18) **in man and their percentages of the total number of cells in these areas** (after Moscow Brain Institute,).

Area	*Layers*			*Total*
	II–III	*IV*	*V*	*number*
17	143·4	166·4	49·3	538·2
	(25·9%)	(33·1%)	(8·9%)	
18	392·1	152·9	75·9	756·8
	(51·9%)	(20·2%)	(10·2%)	

This conclusion is also confirmed by physiological investigations conducted at the neuronal level. The complex function of the secondary zones of the visual (occipital) cortex is also revealed by later neurophysiological investigations.

The neuronographic studies of McCulloch and his collaborators (1943), show that stimulation of the secondary zones of the visual cortex spreads over much wider areas than stimulation of its primary zones, sometimes even crossing over to the corresponding areas of the opposite hemisphere (Figure 25).

The morphological and physiological features distinguishing the structure of the secondary zones of the visual cortex also determine

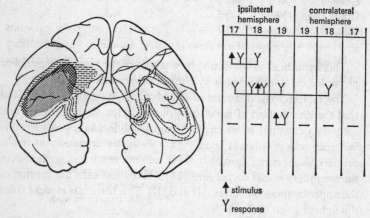

Figure 25 Results of neuronographic experiments with stimulation of the primary and secondary zones of the visual cortex (after McCulloch)

the role which it plays in organizing complex visual perception. This was clearly shown in experiments carried out in the past by leading neurologists and neurosurgeons (Pötzl, Foerster, Penfield) during operations on these cortical zones. Their observations (which have already been mentioned) show that stimulation of the *primary* zones of the occipital cortex by a weak electric current evoked the appearance of elementary visual hallucinations in the patient (who perceived flashes of light, tongues of flame and coloured spots). These phenomena, moreover, appeared in strictly defined parts of the visual field (stimulation of the right occipital region led to the appearance of these 'photopsias' in the left part, while stimulation of the left occipital cortex led to their appearance in the right part of the visual field, and so on).

The results of stimulation of the *secondary* zones of the visual cortex were completely different. In these cases electrical stimulation of a certain point of the cortex gave rise, not to elementary visual sensations, but to complex recognizable visual hallucinations (images of flowers, animals, familiar persons and so on). Sometimes such stimulation caused the appearance of a complex sequence: the patient saw his friend approaching and beckoning him with his hand and so on. These hallucinations, it must be noted, were not restricted to a certain part of the visual field, and they were meaningful rather than topical in character.

These hallucinations naturally reflected the subject's previous visual experience, and consequently, stimulation of the secondary visual cortical zones activated traces of those integral visual images which were stored in this part of the human cortex (Figure 26).

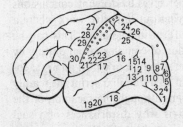

1– 6 elementary visual hallucination
7–11 complex visual hallucination
12–15 complex spatial displacement
16–17 acoustico-verbal hallucination
18–20 lingual hallucination
21–23 hallucination to the tongue
24–26 vestibular phenomena
27–30 production of sounds and words
o sensory hallucination

Figure 26 Character of visual hallucinations, etc. arising in response to stimulation of the primary and secondary zones of the visual cortex (after Pötzl, Foerster, Penfield, and others)

It follows that the secondary zones of the visual cortex, with their complex structure and their facility for the extensive spread of excitation, play the role of *synthesizing visual stimuli, coding them, and forming them into complex systems.* It can therefore be concluded that the function of the secondary zones of the occipital cortex is to *convert the somatotopical projection of incoming visual excitation into its functional organization.* Consequently, these zones play a decisive role in the provision of a higher level of processing and storing of visual information.

Further evidence of the way in which the secondary occipital zones synthesize visual excitation and thus create the physiological basis for complex visual perception is given by observations on changes in visual processes arising in patients with local lesions of the secondary zones of the visual cortex.

These observations show that local lesions of these parts of the occipital cortex neither lead to hemianopia or to loss of part of the visual field, nor diminish visual acuity. The essential symptom associated with a lesion of these zones is *disturbance of the integral perception of complete visual complexes,* the *inability to combine individual impressions into complete patterns*, and the consequent development of the phenomenon of *inability to recognize complete objects or their pictorial representations.*

A patient with a lesion of the secondary visual zones is not blind; he can still see the individual features and, sometimes, the individual parts of objects. His defect is that he *cannot combine these individual features into complete forms*, and he is therefore compelled to *deduce* the meaning of the image which he perceives by drawing conclusions from individual details and by carrying out intensive work where a normal subject perceives the whole form immediately. This can be expressed by saying that the perception of complex visual objects by such a patient begins to resemble the situation in which an archaeologist is attempting to decode a text in an unfamiliar script; he readily understands the meaning of each sign although the meaning of the whole text remains unknown. That is why disturbances of visual perception arising in lesions of the secondary visual cortex are not associated clinically with disturbances of the visual field or visual acuity, but are described by the term *visual agnosia.*

This is a description of a typical case of a patient with such a lesion. This patient carefully examines the picture of a pair of spectacles shown to him. He is confused and does not know what the picture represents. He starts to guess. 'There is a circle . . . and another circle . . . and a stick . . . a cross-bar . . . why, it must be a bicycle?' He looks at the picture of a cock with feathers of different colours in its tail, but not immediately recognizing the object as a whole he declares: 'this is a fire, here are the flames'. In cases of massive lesions of the secondary occipital zones the phenomena of visual agnosia may become more severe in character. In cases of more localized lesions of this zone they are less overt in form and are manifested only during the examination of more complex pictures or in tests of visual perception under more difficult conditions.

Such patients may take a telephone with a dial as a clock, and a couch upholstered in brown material as a trunk. They can no longer recognize outline drawings or silhouettes and are completely baffled if they are shown the outlines of figures overruled by a series of lines (Figure 27) or figures composed of separate elements and presented

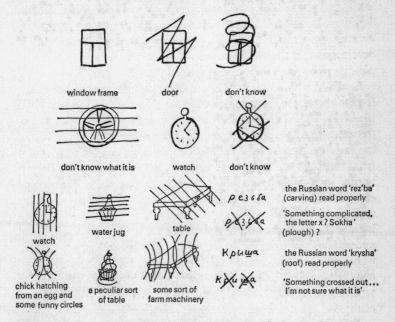

Figure 27 Perception of crossed-out figures by patients with optic agnosia

against an optically complex background (Figure 28). These defects of visual perception become particularly pronounced when the picture is presented only for a very short time or, in the case of a special test, by means of a tachistoscope, enabling the picture to be exposed for times of between 0·25 and 0·5 seconds.

The patient with visual agnosia is naturally unable not only to *perceive* whole visual forms but also to *draw* them. If he is instructed

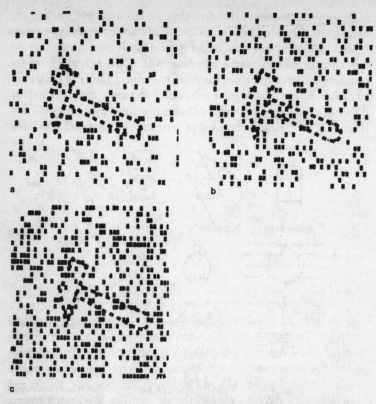

Figure 28 Obscured figures for the investigation of optic agnosia (a) (b) (c) increasing degree of 'obscuring' of the picture (after Tonkonogui)

to draw an object, he will be unable to depict it as a whole and he can only draw (or, more exactly, he can only depict) its individual parts, thus essentially giving a *visual list* of all the details where a normal subject would draw the complete picture. A series of typical illustrations showing the way in which such a patient constructs a drawing is given in Figure 29. The severest forms of visual agnosia are seen in patients with lesions of the secondary zones of *both* occipital lobes, but the features of such a breakdown of visual synthesis can also be observed clearly enough in patients with unilateral lesions.

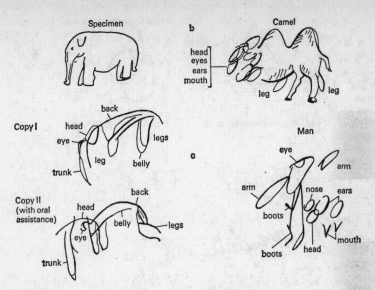

Figure 29 Drawings by patients with optic agnosia

It is essential to note that the disturbance of visual synthesis arising in lesions of the secondary zones of the occipital cortex remains a *partial* defect and does not affect other modalities in these patients or their intellectual processes. Although unable to perceive whole objects visually, they can still recognize them by touch, and they have little difficulty in performing complex intellectual operations, they understand the meaning of stories, they can use logico-grammatical relationships, perform calculations, and so on. The physiological mechanisms lying at the basis of these disturbances of visual perception are still not adequately understood; however, one group of facts allows for substantial progress in this field.

As long ago as 1909 the Hungarian neurologist Bálint (1909) made an observation which shed considerable light on the mechanisms at the base of these disturbances of visual gnosis. While observing a patient with a bilateral lesion of the anterior zones of the occipital cortex (at its boundary with the inferior parietal region) he found that this patient had a definite and distinctive *decrease in his range of visual perception*. This disturbance differed from cases of constriction of the visual field arising in lesions of the optic tract or the primary

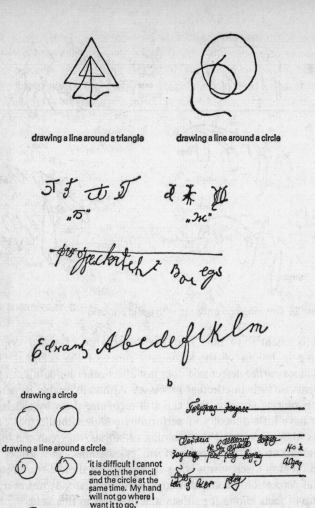

Figure 30 Disturbance of optico-motor coordinates in cases of simultaneous agnosia (a) encircling and drawing; (b) writing

zones of the visual cortex by the fact that it was measured in *units of meaning rather than in units of space*; this patient could see *only one object at a time* regardless of its size (no matter whether it was a needle or a horse), and he was completely unable to perceive two or more objects simultaneously. Similar observations were later made by Holmes (1919) and by Hécaen, Ajuriaguerra and Massonet (1951), and they have been studied in detail in special experimental investigations (Luria, 1959a; Luria, Pravdina-Vinarskaya and Yarbus, 1961).

These observations have shown that patients of this type are in fact unable to perceive two objects simultaneously, especially if they are presented only for a very short time (using a tachistoscope) and if there is no opportunity for a change of fixation. They cannot place a dot in the centre of a circle or cross, because they can perceive only the circle (or the cross), or the pencil point at any one time; they cannot trace the outline of an object or join the strokes together during writing; if they see the pencil point they lose the line, or if they see the line they can no longer see the pencil point (Figure 30). Because of this functional narrowing of the visual field and its limitation to one object, this phenomenon has been called *simultaneous agnosia*. The accompanying disturbance of opticomotor coordination (or *fixation ataxia*) was explained on the assumption that instead of the *two* excited points present in each normal visual field (one at the centre of the field, reflecting information reaching the subject and the other at the periphery of the visual field, giving information on its relationship to peripheral visual objects and evoking an orienting reflex, which leads to an organized shift of fixation), only *one* excited point remains in their field of vision, and the second (the peripheral), directing the potential movement of fixation, has disappeared. This state of affairs has been verified in experiments to record the eye movements of such a patient when examining a particular geometric shape (Luria, Pravdina-Vinarskaya and Yarbus, 1961), where these eye movements, unlike in a normal subject, were severely disorganized and ataxic (Figure 31b).

This syndrome has been subjected to extensive experimental analysis. Pribram (1959a) has shown that monkeys who have had bilateral removal of the inferior temporal gyri, respond to fewer of an array of objects that are simultaneously presented. Butters (1970)

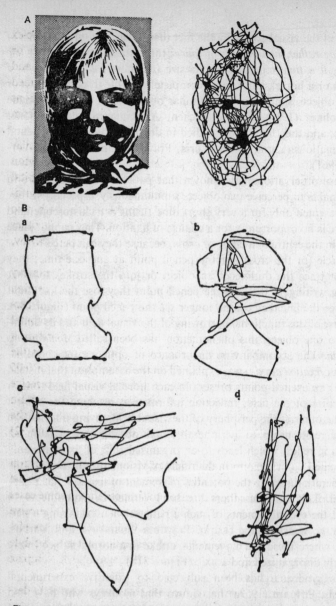

Figure 31 Eye movements during the examination of (A) complex images and (B) geometrical shapes: (a) normal subject (b) (examining a sphere and bust); patient with simultaneous agnosia; (c) (d) (examining the same figures)

has shown that this defect extends to attending features of complex figures: normal monkeys are less likely to be impaired when one or another feature is removed. Pribram and his co-workers (Spinelli and Pribram 1967; Gerbrandt, Spinelli and Pribram 1970) have performed physiological experiments to show that this effect is due to alterations in attention which are mediated by a corticofugal mechanism from the inferior temporal cortex that influences the visual process.

In his 'Wednesday Clinics', Pavlov discussed facts of a similar nature described originally by Pierre Janet. He gave this phenomenon a physiological interpretation, suggesting that the cells of the occipital (visual) cortex of this patient were so weakened by the pathological process that 'they are unable to deal simultaneously with two stimuli, that one excited point exerts an inhibitory effect on the other excited point, thus making it apparently non-existent' (Pavlov, 1949b).

On the basis of this hypothesis I have suggested that if excitatory processes can be fixed in the affected occipital cortex by an injection of caffeine, a substantial improvement in the process of visual perception should be obtained (provided that the lesion of the occipital cortex is partial in character). Tests of this nature carried out on a patient with a bilateral bullet wound of the anterior zones of the occipital region gave precisely this effect. After an injection of 0·05 ml of 1 per cent caffeine solution, the patient was able to perceive *two* (and in some cases *three*) objects simultaneously for a certain period of time (thirty to forty minutes, the duration of action of the caffeine), and the features of visual ataxia disappeared (Figure 32) (Luria, 1959a).

The facts so far described still do not directly answer the question of the physiological mechanisms of every disturbance of visual perception. Nevertheless there is reason to suppose that in some cases of classical visual agnosia, in which the patient can still perceive simple shapes, such as a ball, but is unable to identify complex pictures, there is also a narrowing of visual perception down to a single criterion, and it is this which makes the recognition of complex visual structures impossible.

Admittedly, there is reason to suppose that the mechanisms described above relate to those forms of visual agnosia which were

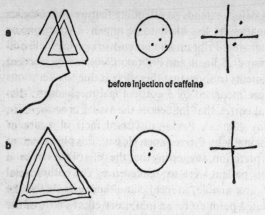

before injection of caffeine

30 minutes after injection of caffeine

Experiment requiring drawing a line around a shape and
placing a dot in the centre of a shape

Figure 32 Disappearance of the signs of optic ataxia in a patient with a
bilateral wound of the anterior zones of the occipital region after injection
of caffeine (tests involving placing a dot in the centre of a circle and a
cross, and tracing outlines): (a) before injection of caffeine; (b) 30 min.
after injection of caffeine

originally described by Lissauer (1898) as 'apperceptive mental
blindness', and that there are other cases, which the same neurologist described by the term 'associative mental blindness', in which
the patient continues to perceive the whole visual picture but is
simply unable to *recognize* it and to determine its meaning; but the
mechanisms of this condition are still unknown. When I discuss the
disturbance of visual representations in lesions of the temporo-
occipital regions of the brain, I shall take the opportunity to put
forward a number of suggestions for the psychological qualification
of this fact.

The disturbance of complex perception resulting from the neurodynamic characteristics of pathological lesions of the secondary
cortical zones, leading to a disturbance of afferent syntheses and to
the narrowing of the range of perception, is not limited to the
phenomena of visual agnosia arising in lesions of the secondary
occipital zones. Similar phenomena may occur in the *tactile perception* of patients with lesions of the *secondary zones of the parietal*

cortex. These phenomena have often been described by neurologists as *tactile asymbolia* (Wernicke, 1894), as *parietal tactile agnosia* (Nielsen, 1946), or as a disturbance of the synthesis of tactile sensations leading to defects of tactile perception of shape or, in other words, to *amorphosynthesis* (Denny-Brown *et al.*, 1952).

In all these cases, exhibiting a disturbance of the ability to distinguish shape by touch, known in clinical medicine as *astereognosis*, the basic defect is evidently not a special form of disturbance of symbolic processes, but inability to carry out the 'summation of spatial impressions' (Denny-Brown and Chambers, 1958); or a defect of the synthesis of individual tactile sensations, a special form of *narrowing of the range of tactile perception* developing as the result of increased mutual inhibition of separate excited points of the general sensory cortex associated with a pathological state of the secondary parietal zones. This hypothesis still requires special experimental verification, but there can be no dispute that the *pathological narrowing of the range of perception* arising in lesions of the secondary cortical zones is one of the general rules which can explain the important changes in perception which develop in these cases.

The phenomena of visual agnosia associated with lesions of the secondary occipital zones do not always follow exactly the same course, and clinical descriptions of other types of disturbances of perception depending on the localization of the lesion have been recorded.

I stated above that the transition from the primary to the secondary zones of the cortex obeys the laws of diminishing modal specificity and increasing lateralization of the forms of organization of mental activity connected with these zones. Whereas the first of these laws implies that the functions of the secondary cortical zones lose the character of somatotopical projection of the corresponding sensory structures, the second law has the result that the *secondary zones of the left* (*dominant*) *hemisphere differ substantially in the character of their activity from the secondary zones of the right* (*non-dominant*) *hemisphere*. As proof of these differences, the *secondary cortical zones of the left hemisphere retain their intimate connection with speech*, whereas the secondary cortical zones of the right hemisphere do not possess this connection.

This state of affairs is clearly reflected in the character of the *visual agnosia* which arises in lesions of the secondary zones of the left and right occipital regions. A lesion of the secondary zones of the temporal region of the *left* (dominant) hemisphere very often causes a disturbance of the *recognition of letters* and a corresponding *disturbance of reading* (optic alexia): the patient either can no longer recognize letters in general or he confuses letters of similar outline (for example, N and M or H and K), he cannot recognize more complicated letters (such as G or Q), and he is therefore unable to read. Difficulty in the recognition of complex visual objects may also be apparent, but sometimes this is relatively less pronounced.

Lesions of the corresponding zones of the *right* (*non-dominant*) *hemisphere* give rise to a different picture. In these cases the disturbance of recognition of letters is much less marked and sometimes is absent altogether. Instead, *direct visual perception* is much more severely disturbed, and in particular, signs of *agnosia for objects* may be present. In lesions of the right occipital zones a particularly conspicuous feature is the symptom of *agnosia for faces* or *prosopagnosia* (Pötzl, 1937; Faust, 1947; Bodamer, 1947; Hécaen and Angelergues, 1963; Chlenov and Bein, 1958; Bornstein, 1962; Kok, 1967). Patients with this symptom cannot even recognize very familiar faces, they cannot identify a portrait shown to them, and frequently they recognize a friend only by his voice and not by direct visual impression. We still do not know the physiological mechanisms of this defect, but it must also be a disturbance of synthesis of the features distinguishing one person from another, in this case without any participation of the logical codes of languages.

Some forms of disturbance of visual perception arising in lesions of the right hemisphere are quite distinctive in character and they can serve as reliable evidence for the topical diagnosis of the lesion. In these cases the patient shows none of the signs of narrowing of visual perception or inability to synthesize individual features into a complete visual image; he draws objects or pictures shown to him without difficulty; the basic defect lies in their *incorrect identification* or in the attribution of the wrong *ownership*. One such patient, for example, even recognized a shawl and could distinguish the flowers woven on it, but she did not recognize it as *her own* and helplessly asked: 'Whose shawl is this?' Another patient, with an extensive atrophic lesion in the right occipital region, when shown a picture of some soldiers on a tank exclaimed: 'Why, of course, it is all my family, my husband, sons and sisters'.

The internal mechanisms of these disturbances of memory remain unexplained; all that is clear is that the patient is unaware of his defect (it exists against the background of *anosognosia*) and makes no effort either to identify a picture shown to him or to correct his mistakes. We shall deal with these defects again below when we discuss the mental disorders arising in lesions of the right hemisphere.

Chapter 4
The Temporal Regions and Organization of Auditory Perception

We have examined the functional organization of the occipital regions of the brain and their role in the formation of visual perception. We shall now examine the functional organization of the temporal regions and their role in auditory analysis and synthesis in the same way.

As I have mentioned already, the functional organization of each modally-specific zone of the brain (visual, auditory, tactile) preserves certain common features and, despite differences associated with their particular modality, it is constructed in accordance with the same principle. Let us now consider the functional organization of the temporal (auditory) cortex in more detail.

Primary zones of the temporal cortex and the elementary functions of hearing

The auditory cortex occupies the lateral (convex) portions of the temporal region of the brain and, just as in the case of the visual (occipital) region, it is divided into primary (projection) and secondary auditory zones. The auditory pathway carrying acoustic impulses arises in the organ of Corti in the cochlea of the inner ear. Individual parts of this organ evidently resonate to sound waves of different pitch, and the nerve fibres transmitting these impulses retain their organized, somatotopical character. They run in the auditory pathway, decussate partially in the medial lemniscus, relay in the medial geniculate body and terminate in the primary (projection) zones of the auditory cortex, in the transverse gyrus of Heschl.

A feature common to the organization of these projection zones of the auditory system and those of the visual cortex is that this cortical zone also has a somatotopical structure, in which fibres carrying excitation produced by high tones are in the medial portions and fibres carrying excitation from low tones are in the lateral portions.

The organization of the projection zones of the auditory cortex differs from that of the occipital (visual) cortex in that there is no complete representation of each ear (or of some of the auditory fibres) in one (the opposite) hemisphere. The fibres of each organ of Corti are represented in both projection zones of the auditory cortex, and they are merely represented predominantly in the opposite hemisphere. For this reason cases of complete central deafness, which can arise only in the case of lesions of both gyri of Heschl, are very rare.

Unilateral lesions of Heschl's gyrus are compensated to such an extent by the second, intact gyrus that it was a long time before the precise symptoms for the diagnosis of these unilateral lesions of the primary auditory cortex could be described clinically. It is only very recently, as a result of the work of the eminent Soviet physiologist Gershuni (1968) and of Karasseva and Baru (Karasseva, 1967; Baru and Karasseva, 1970), that substantial information has been obtained about the mode of working of these parts of the temporal region and that reliable symptoms have been identified for the diagnosis of its lesions.

In these experiments the subject was presented with tones of 1000 Hz and of different durations (1, 2, 4, 45, 120 and 1200 ms) and the thresholds of discrimination were measured. To do this, the sounds were presented initially at intensities of 1, 5, 10, 15, ..., 45 and 50 dB until the threshold was approached, when the intensities were varied by 1 dB at a time. The thresholds of tonal discrimination were recorded monaurally (for each ear separately). These investigations showed that the temporal projection cortex not only *transmits* acoustic excitation to the cortex, but also *prolongs and stabilizes its action*, making it more constant in character and amenable to control. That is why, although unilateral lesions of the primary auditory zones of the cortex and adjacent zones did not produce total loss of hearing and did not reduce the acuity of auditory perception of ordinary sounds, signs of a disturbance of the sensitivity of auditory perception or, in other words, an *increase in the threshold of auditory sensation*, were observed if the subject was presented with ultrashort sounds with a duration of only 1–5 ms. When tested under

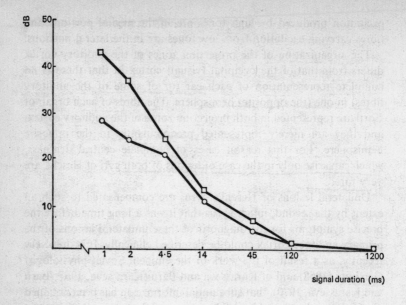

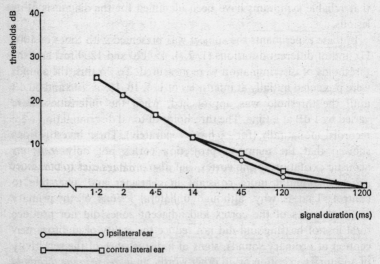

Figure 33 Changes in threshold of auditory perception of tones differing in duration: (a) by a normal subject; (b) by a patient with a unilateral lesion of the superior temporal zones (after Karasseva)

these conditions, patients with a unilateral lesion of the superior temporal zones showed definite *elevation of the threshold of auditory sensation in the opposite ear,* and this was sometimes virtually the only symptom on which a topical diagnosis of the lesion could be based (Figure 33).

This is a fact of the utmost importance, and it remains to all intents and purposes the only available fact characterizing the function of the primary zones of the auditory cortex.

The secondary zones of the temporal cortex and acoustico-gnostic functions

As I said above, the secondary zones of the auditory cortex (occupying the lateral, convex portions of the temporal lobe in man, corresponding to Brodmann's area 22 and part of area 21) have the same structure as the secondary zones of other sensory areas. They consist predominantly of cortical layers II and III, the greater part of which is composed of cells with short axons; they retain their modally-specific (auditory) character but are not somatotopical in structure; excitation evoked in them spreads over much wider areas than excitation of individual points of the primary cortex; finally, electrical stimulation of these zones in the patient on the operating table (Penfield and Jasper, 1959) evokes much more localized auditory sensations (musical sounds, voices, and so on). We are thus in a position to understand the facts obtained from observing the changes arising in auditory processes in patients with *local lesions* of the secondary auditory zones.

Pavlov's experiments originally showed that a lesion of the temporal cortex in an animal does not cause loss of hearing but disturbs the animal's ability to form differential reflexes to combined acoustic stimuli (Elyasson, 1908; Kryzhanovsky, 1909; Babkin, 1910; Kudrin, 1910). Similar results have been obtained more recently by American workers (Butler, Diamond and Neff, 1957; Goldberg, Diamond and Neff, 1957) who showed that after extirpation of the temporal cortex the animal can still distinguish simple sounds but can no longer differentiate between combinations of sounds.

In man, with the characteristically well-developed secondary zones of his auditory cortex, these phenomena naturally were manifested much more clearly, and investigations (Traugott, 1947; Kaidanova, 1954; 1967; Babenkova, 1954; Kabelyanskaya, 1957) showed that in patients with very small lesions of the secondary zones in the left temporal region ability to distinguish simple sounds was intact, differentiation of simple sounds was only slightly impaired, but differentiation of combinations of sounds was virtually impossible (Figure 34).

Similar results were obtained in a special study of differentiation between groups of two or three high-frequency tones and differentiation between complex acoustic rhythms in patients with a lesion of the temporal cortex. If rhythmic series of taps were presented to these patients rapidly, they were unable to distinguish or reproduce them (Semernitskaya, 1945).

These facts show conclusively that the *secondary zones of the auditory cortex play a vital role in the differentiation of groups of simultaneously presented acoustic stimuli and also of consecutive series of sounds of different pitch or rhythmic acoustic structures.*

They also reflect an essential, but by no means the most important, aspect of the work of the secondary zones of the human temporal cortex. Their importance lies in the fact that they are the fundamental apparatus for the analysis and synthesis of the *sounds of speech*, the quality which distinguishes human hearing from the hearing of animals.

Human speech, which is organized into a *phonemic system of language*, uses sounds of a special type and sharpness of hearing alone is not enough to distinguish between them. The sounds of speech constitute a system in which only certain characteristics are essential to the differentiation of the meaning of words, while others do not possess this role. For a person speaking Russian, it does not matter whether the word 'more' is pronounced with a short or a long 'o': the meaning of the word is not affected in any way; on the other hand, if anyone speaking German were to pronounce 'Satt' as 'Saat', 'Stadt' as 'Staat' or 'Hütte' as 'Hüte' he would give a completely different meaning to the word. The same is true of certain consonants which differ in their fricative characteristics; these distinctions are of no importance in Russian or German, but in English the words 'vine' and 'wine' have completely different meanings.

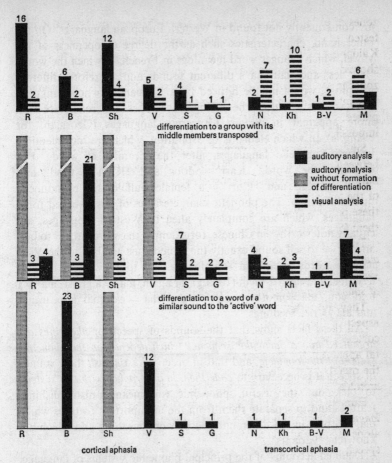

Figure 34 Disturbance of auditory differentiation in patients with lesions of the left temporal region (after Kabelyanskaya)

The phonemic systems of different languages differ very considerably, and features found in some languages do not exist in others. Perhaps the best examples are those of hardness and softness (designated by ') or of stress and absence of stress in the Russian language, when the words *pyl'* and *pyl* and *byl* and *byl'*, and also the words *byl* and *bil'* or *zámok* and *zamók* have quite different meanings, whereas such differences between sounds are meaningless and are consequently not found in Western European languages. On the other hand, characteristics such as the degree of openness of the vowel, which changes word meanings in French, in which the words 'le', 'les' and 'lait' have different sounds and, therefore, different meanings, would not be noticed by a Russian, in whose language these sounds would not be distinguished. These differences are even more apparent in certain Caucasian languages (Georgian, for example), in which elements of aspiration, which are imperceptible in Indo-European languages, alter the meaning of words. For example, the words 'Kari' = door and 'K'ari' = wind, and 'Puri' = bread and 'P'uri' = a female buffalo are pronounced quite differently. The phonetic characteristics of the so-called tonal languages, which are completely alien to Western languages, are equally noteworthy: in Chinese, for example the words m_a = to buy and m^a = to sell sound exactly the same to us, as also do the Vietnamese words ta = I, tá = a dozen, tà = to be wicked, tǎ = to describe, and tạ = 1 picul (100 kg), or again, ma = a ghost, mà = I told you, má = mother, mǎ = grave, mạ = external appearance and mã = rice seedlings.

All these facts show that the sounds of speech or *phonemes are organized into a particular sequence which depends on the phonemic system of the language*, and that in order to *distinguish* these sounds of speech it is necessary to *code them in accordance with this system*, to pick out the useful, phonemic (or meaning-distinguishing) features and to separate them from the unimportant features which play no part in the differentiation of word meaning and which are known as 'variants'.

Detailed accounts of the principal phonemic systems of language, using systems of *oppositions* (such as 'b' and 'p', 'd' and 't'), have been given by eminent linguists such as Troubezkoi (1939) and Jakobson (Jakobson and Halle, 1956) and these descriptions now constitute the essential basis for the understanding of the laws governing the perception of the sounds of human speech.

It is an essential fact that the secondary zones of the temporal cortex – and, because of the law of progressive lateralization, the temporal cortex of the dominant (left) hemisphere – are *specially adapted for the analysis and synthesis of the sounds of speech* or, in other words, for *qualified speech hearing*.

The work of neuroanatomists (Blinkov, 1955) has shown that the secondary zones of the temporal cortex are joined by numerous U-shaped connections with the lower region of the postcentral and premotor areas or, in other words, with all brain systems concerned with the production of articulated speech (Figure 35). It can thus participate in the *system for the cerebral organization of speech* and,

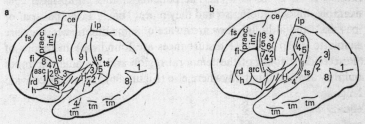

Figure 35 Connections of secondary zones of the temporal region with postcentral and premotor zones (after Blinkov). Synaptic map of connections of individual bundles of fibres entering the superior longitudinal (arcuate) fasciculus. Identical numbers on surface of corresponding brain areas denote connections of each bundle of fibres with the cortex: (a) connections between temporal and inferior frontal gyrus; (b) connections between temporal lobe and precentral gyrus

in particular, it can distinguish those phonemic signs on which the sounds of speech are built.

It is not, therefore, surprising to learn that *in local lesions of the secondary zones of the left temporal lobe in man the ability to distinguish clearly between the sounds of speech is lost*, and the patient develops a phenomenon described by the term *acoustic agnosia* or, on the basis of the speech disturbances, by the more widely known term *sensory aphasia.*

Patients with these disturbances still retain their sharpness of hearing, and as special investigations (Frankfurter and Thiele, 1912; Bonvicini, 1929; Katz, 1930) have shown, they do not exhibit any partial loss of tones in any part of the scale. Perception of sounds associated with objects (the clinking of dishes, the ringing of a glass) also remains intact. Important disturbances arise only when they have to *distinguish between the sounds of speech*. In more massive lesions of the left central lobe all the sounds of speech are perceived as unarticulated noise (the babbling of a brook, the rustling of leaves);

in more localized lesions this defect assumes less marked forms, and the patients are unable only to distinguish between closely similar 'oppositional' and 'correlating' phonemes differing *only in one feature* (for example, resonance), but can still clearly detect the quality of timbre and intonation of speech. This defect can easily be seen by asking the patient to repeat pairs of oppositional phonemes, such as d—t, b—p, or s—z. The patients of this group have considerable difficulty doing so and they repeat 'ba—pa' as 'pa—pa' or 'ba—ba', and although they are aware of some differences, they are unable to grasp it. These disturbances are found *only* in lesions of the secondary zones of the temporal region and the adjacent zones and they are not found anywhere else (Figure 36); they thus provide

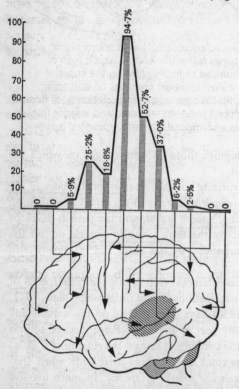

Figure 36 Disturbance of phonemic hearing in lesions of the left temporal region (scheme based on investigation of 800 cases) (after Luria)

a reliable basis for the topical diagnosis of local lesions in the corresponding zones.

It is interesting that disturbances of phonemic hearing which are the direct result of a lesion of the secondary zones of the temporal cortex, by virtue of the law of increasing lateralization arise only in *lesions of the left temporal region*, and are never found in lesions of the right temporal lobe. For this reason lesions of the right temporal lobe, which is unconnected with the speech system, may either remain asymptomatic or produce only disturbances of perception of complex rhythmic combinations or combinations of sound of different frequencies, and are manifested sometimes as a *disturbance of the hearing of music*, which has been called *sensory amusia*. These differences between the functions of the left (dominant) and right (non-dominant) temporal regions are among the most fundamental differences observed in the functional organization of cortical systems and they have important consequences for the smooth course of mental processes.

A disturbance of phonemic hearing and the phenomena of *acoustic agnosia* are only part (admittedly, the main part) of the syndrome produced by lesions of the secondary zones of the left temporal lobe. If the lesion disturbs the normal working of those parts of the secondary auditory cortex of the left hemisphere which are further from the primary auditory zones and occupy the region of the middle temporal gyrus (or are located in the depth of the left temporal lobe), phonemic hearing may remain intact or be disturbed only relatively slightly, and the defect assumes the form of a *disturbance of audio-verbal memory* or of *distinctive acoustico-mnestic disorders*. The principal feature is that the patient cannot retain even a short series of sounds, syllables or words in his memory, but begins to confuse their order, or states that some of the elements of the series presented to him simply disappear from his memory. If such a patient is presented with a series of three or four syllables (bu—ra—mi or ko—na—fu—po) or a series of the same number of words (house—wood—chair or night—cat—oak—bridge) he will be unable to repeat more than one or two of them, and sometimes only the first or the last; he says that he could not keep the rest in his memory or that he had 'forgotten'. This disturbance still remains *modally specific* in character, and if the same patient is presented with a group of drawn figures or even of written words he will be able to remember them quite well enough (Luria and Rapoport, 1962; Klimkovsky, 1966).

A closer analysis of this phenomenon shows that this disturbance of audio-verbal memory is based on *increased mutual inhibition of* auditory traces, a characteristic defect of a pathological state of the temporal cortex (Luria, Sokolov and Klimkovsky, 1967b) and similar in type to the phenomenon which we have previously observed in cases of simultaneous optic aphasia, leading to the distinctive *narrowing of the range of successive acoustic perception*. This hypothesis can be confirmed if the series of acoustic elements is presented *at longer intervals*, thereby reducing the mutually inhibitory effect of neighbouring elements. In such cases, as Tsvetkova (unpublished investigation) has shown, the traces of each acoustic stimulus have sufficient time for consolidation, so that the corresponding acoustic series can be adequately retained.

Systemic effect of disturbances of the hearing of speech in lesions of the secondary zones of the left temporal region

Disturbances of phonemic hearing and of audio-verbal memory produced by a lesion of the secondary zones of the left temporal lobe are partial and modality-specific in character, and by virtue of the law of 'double dissociation', they leave intact the other functions disturbed by lesions in other situations. These include the functions of visual perception, grasping of logico-grammatical relationships, mathematical operations, and so on. However, several complex psychological processes are severely disturbed under these conditions, and these disturbances, closely connected with the disorder of speech hearing, are *secondary* or *systemic* in character. These disturbances include disorders of the *understanding* of speech, the *naming* of objects and the *recalling* of words, and distinctive disturbances of *writing* to which special attention must be paid.

Loss of the ability to distinguish between closely sounding phonemes inevitably leads to difficulty in the understanding of spoken speech or, as we now customarily call this defect, to the *alienation of the meaning of words*. Words in the native tongue whose phonemic composition can no longer be perceived with adequate differentiation cannot now be understood clearly. For example, if the word 'golos' (voice) sounds to this patient sometimes like 'kolos' (an ear of corn), sometimes like 'kholost' (unmarried) or 'kholst' (cloth), naturally he will no longer be able to grasp its meaning and his attitude towards words of his native tongue will begin to resemble that to words in a foreign language. This is the basic symptom of what is now widely known clinically as *sensory or acoustico-gnostic aphasia*.

The second result of a disturbance of phonemic hearing is that, having lost the necessary support of a differentiated phonemic system of language, the patient finds it difficult to *name objects* and to *recall the necessary words*, making mistakes in both cases, mixing closely related phonemes. Instead of the word 'kolos' he will say something like: 'let me see ... khorst ... gorst ... khōros ... kóros ...' and so on. Characteristically, prompting the first syllable in these cases does not help the patient, and without a precise system of phonemes he cannot take advantage of it. For example, in an attempt to find the word 'rascheska' (comb) one such patient did not respond to prompting with 'ras ...', 'rasche ...', 'rasches ...'. This inability to profit by prompting of the beginning of the word, which is explained by the imprecision of the patient's phonemic system, is an important accessory feature for the topical diagnosis of lesions of the left temporal lobe.

The third result of the fundamental defect is a *disorder of the patient's speech*. Being unable to find support in the phonemic system of the language, and exhibiting a defect in the stability of acoustic traces, such a patient naturally cannot grasp coherent speech, and his spontaneous expressions assume the character of an incoherent assortment of words, some of which are severely defective in their phonemic structure, while the others are replaced by similar but inadequate words. Characteristically, the patient is not clearly aware of the defects in his own coherent speech, and cannot of course correct them, so that his speech becomes converted into what has been called a 'word salad', in which the nominative components (the substantives) are almost completely absent, and all that are left are either interjections or habitual expressions such as: 'let me see ... how does it ... confound it all ... I know but I can't ...' and so on.

Finally, although the phonemic and lexical aspects of the coherent speech of these patients are grossly disturbed, characteristically the *intonational and melodic aspect of their speech as a rule remains intact*, and by its aid the listener can understand the meaning of the patient's apparently incoherent speech. Who, listening to a flow of words such as 'well now... I mean ... so ...we ... now ... went...went ... suddenly ... now this ... like this ... bang! ... and then – nothing... nothing... and since... little by little ... better still ... quite ... and now ... do you see?' – completely devoid of substantives, could guess that a person wounded in the temporal region was describing how they were going, how the exploding shell stunned him, how he lost consciousness, and how his consciousness gradually returned, although his speech still remained difficult?

The last direct result of disturbance of phonemic hearing is *loss of the ability to write*, characteristic of patients with lesions of the left temporal lobe. Such patients cannot distinguish the necessary acoustic content of a word, they begin to confuse similarly sounding phonemes and they can no longer analyse complex combinations of sounds (the running together of consonants, for example). Their writing is thus converted into a series of frustrated attempts to find the required sounds and letters composing the word, with many corrections, but with complete inability to write words properly. An example of the difficulties in active writing or writing from dictation is shown in Figure 37, and it is in sharp contrast with the patient's ability to copy words presented by sight.

A characteristic exception from this defect is the patient's ability to write familiar words (for example, his signature), which do not require analysis of their acoustic content and have become a stable motor stereotype. This conversion of the writing of words from a process requiring precise acoustic analysis into a motor automatism, with a completely different psychophysiological structure and depending on a completely different series of cortical zones, is a clear example of the *change in structure and cerebral organization of a process in the course of its functional development* (Luria, Simernitskaya and Tubylevich, 1970).

Learning processes are only partly disturbed in the patients of this group. The recognition of such firmly impressed visual stereotypes as 'USSR', 'Moscow', '*Pravda*' and so on, which have in fact become

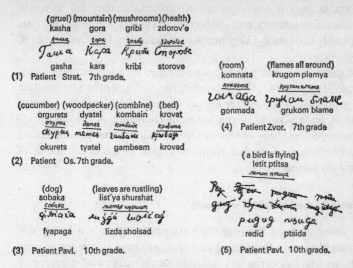

(gruel) (mountain) (mushrooms) (health)
kasha   gora   gribi   zdorov'e

gasha   kara   kribi   storove
(1) Patient Strat. 7th grade.

(cucumber) (woodpecker) (combine) (bed)
orgurets   dyatel   kombain   krovat

okurets   tyatel   gambeam   krovad
(2) Patient Os. 7th grade.

(dog)   (leaves are rustling)
sobaka   list'ya shurshat

fyapaga   lizda sholsad
(3) Patient Pavl. 10th grade.

(room)   (flames all around)
komnata   krugom plamya

gonmada   grukom blame
(4) Patient Zvor. 7th grade

(a bird is flying)
letit ptitsa

redid   ptsida
(5) Patient Pavl. 10th grade.

Figure 37 Handwriting of patients with lesions of the left temporal lobe

converted into *optical ideograms*, remains unaffected in these patients. On the other hand, reading words which have not become fixed in this way or words of complex meaning whose perception requires acoustic analysis is severely disturbed. I shall never forget a case in which a man wounded in the temporal region could easily read his surname 'Levsky' written on an envelope addressed to him, but was completely unable to read the much simpler word 'lev' (lion), which was not fixed to the same degree in his memory.

I have already mentioned that the understanding of logical relationships and of operations such as written calculations can still remain relatively unimpaired in patients with lesions of the left temporal region. However, this does not mean that the operations of *reasoning* remain completely intact in such patients. If these operations require the performance of a number of intermediate links, which must be retained in the 'operative memory', patients with a lesion of the left temporal lobe will be unable to perform them, and although these patients retain their aim, their reasoning will be discontinuous and fragmentary in character. That is why, although they can still grasp single logical relationships sufficiently well, these patients easily lose the sequence of operations, they fail to retain individual components, and the process of orderly reasoning becomes profoundly disturbed. (This problem is discussed in detail in Luria, 1973).

All these facts, which have been described by many writers (Luria, 1947; 1971; Bein, 1947; 1964; Ombrédane, 1951, and others), constitute the syndrome of *temporal (or sensory) aphasia*, which arises in lesions of the secondary zones of the *left temporal region*. A careful neuropsychological analysis of this syndrome will help us to understand the contribution of the left temporal region to the construction of mental processes.

Variants of the 'temporal syndrome'

Like other parts of the brain, the temporal region is a highly differentiated system. Depending on the localization of the lesion (and on its severity) disturbances differing in character and degree may therefore arise.

A lesion of the *superior zones* of the left temporal region can give rise to the picture of sensory aphasia which I have just described. It is based on a disturbance of phonemic hearing, and its secondary (or systemic) results are difficulty in the understanding of the meaning of words, a disturbance of the naming of objects, defects of coherent speech, disturbances of writing, and difficulties of a special kind in performing consecutive intellectual operations, whose apparent severity is determined by the extent to which these operations rely on stable and differentiated traces of the operative audio-verbal memory. It is a characteristic fact that lesions of the left temporal lobe, producing substantial disturbances of *speech hearing*, do not give rise to similar disturbances of *musical hearing*. This is reflected both in the integrity of the intonational-melodic components of the speech of patients with sensory aphasia and in the integrity of their singing, which is in sharp contrast with their disturbed phonemic hearing. In individual cases, a severe disturbance of speech hearing arising from a lesion of the systems of the left temporal region in a composer of music left the musical hearing intact to such a degree that, although suffering from severe sensory aphasia, the patient could still write intricate musical compositions (Luria, Tsvetkova and Futer, 1965).

Disturbances arising in lesions of the *middle zones* of the left temporal region or in lesions lying in the *depths of the left temporal lobe* and causing destruction of the auditory cortex only secondarily are distinguished by essentially different features.

Prolonged observations (Luria, 1947; 1962; 1966a; 1971; Klim kovsky, 1966) have shown that such lesions lead not so much to a disturbance of phonemic hearing and auditory analysis as to a marked disturbance of audio-verbal *memory*, and they assume the form of *acoustico-mnestic aphasia*. These disturbances are not significantly reflected in analysis of the acoustic content of words, they do not produce any marked degree of 'alienation of word meaning', and in some cases no appreciable disorders of writing, but they do give rise to definite disturbances of the *retention of word series*, sometimes discernible in tests in which the subject has to remember a series of two or three elements (Klimkovsky, 1966; Luria, 1971; Luria, Sokolov and Klimkovsky, 1967b).

In such cases the patient as a rule will easily retain *one* word (or even *one* short phrase) and is able to reproduce it after an interval of one to two minutes. However, retention even of a short *series* of words, presented aloud, causes considerable difficulty and the patient can reproduce only the first word, stating that the others are very quickly forgotten, or the last word, when the first elements of the presented series are apparently forgotten. Special observations (Luria, Sokolov and Klimkovsky, 1967a) have shown that sometimes the subject reproduces the *last* word of the series initially, and only later reproduces the preceding word. This phenomenon can perhaps be explained by a tendency for the most recent traces to be reproduced first (the *recency* factor described by a number of workers) and, as a rule, this tendency is not exhibited when the patient is asked to reproduce a series presented in writing, or even if he is asked to transcribe an auditory into a visual series by writing down a series presented to him aloud. Characteristically defects such as these are also observed in tests involving the reproduction of long phrases and anecdotes in which the last part is omitted although the general meaning is usually preserved.

Special investigations (Luria, 1971; 1973), have shown that in all these cases the defect is *not so much the instability of audio-verbal traces themselves* as a *pathologically increased inhibitability of the audio-verbal traces*. This arises both during the mutual action of the components of an audio-verbal series and also under the influence of irrelevant and interfering factors, but does not affect the integrity of mnestic traces of other modalities (Luria and Rapoport, 1962; Klimkovsky, 1966; Luria, Sokolov and Klimkovsky, 1967a) (Figure

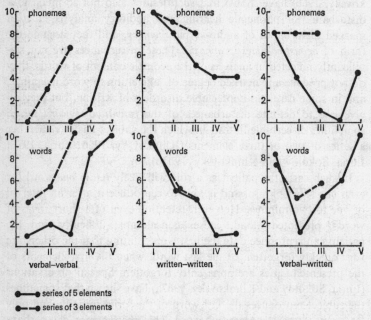

● series of 5 elements
●--● series of 3 elements

Figure 38 Differences in recall of series of words and numbers presented audibly and visually in patients with acoustico-mnestic aphasia (after Luria, Sokolov and Klimkovsky)

38). It remains a characteristic feature, as was described above, that, on the presentation of an audio-verbal series with longer intervals between its elements, this mutual inhibition between the elements can be reduced and the integrity of an audio-verbal series, imprinted in the memory 'little by little' (or under conditions favouring increased consolidation of individual traces), is increased (Tsvetkova, unpublished investigations).

144 Local Brain Systems and their Functional Analysis

The syndrome of acoustico-mnestic aphasia naturally leads to marked disturbances of discursive intellectual operations, based on the defect of operative memory already described. No special discussion will be devoted here to the analysis of these forms of disturbance of memory and intellectual operations in patients with lesions of the middle zones of the temporal region and with acoustico-mnestic aphasia.

The disturbances arising in lesions of the *posterior zones of the left temporal region*, on its boundary with the occipital region, are of particular interest. The cardinal symptom of these lesions is a disturbance both of the *nominative function of speech* (the naming of objects) and of the ability to evoke *visual images* in response to a given word. This is manifested not only by great difficulty in finding the meaning of a given word (which this time is based not so much on a disturbance of phonemic hearing as on a disturbance of the link

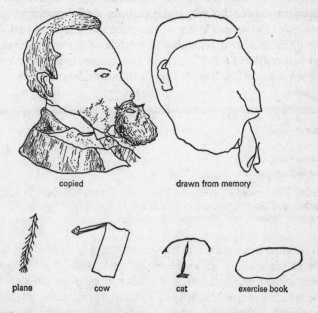

copied   drawn from memory

plane   cow   cat   exercise book

(after being shown a corresponding drawing)   drawn to order (without examples)

Figure 39 Disturbance of the ability to draw a named object and of the ability to copy a named object (after Luria, Blinkov, and Bein)

between the cortical zones of the auditory and visual analysers), but also as gross *inability to draw a picture of an object named* although the patient is still perfectly capable of copying it (Figure 39). There is reason to suppose that these phenomena (to which the name optic aphasia has been given), arise through a disturbance of the concerted working of the visual and auditory analysers.

At this stage no special analysis will be given of the syndrome of the disturbances arising in lesions of the fronto-temporal zones of the left hemisphere, for this will be done in a later chapter.

All that has been described so far is concerned with disturbances arising in lesions of the *left* (dominant) temporal region. Unfortunately we still know very little about the symptoms arising in lesions of the *right* (non-dominant) temporal region. It is known that in such cases speech hearing remains intact, whereas *musical hearing* may suffer substantially, and this may be reflected, for example, in difficulty in reproducing rhythmic structures. However, this fact has not been proved conclusively and it requires special investigation.

Lesions of the *medial* zones of the temporal region, a part of a totally different system belonging to the first of the brain units described earlier (Part One, Chapter 2) and whose functions already have been discussed, will receive no further consideration here.

Chapter 5
The Parietal Regions and the Organization of Simultaneous Syntheses

We have discussed the functional organization and modes of work of the secondary zones of the cortex and, using the visual (occipital) and auditory (temporal) regions as examples, I have attempted to show the contribution made by each of them to the structure of mental processes. We have seen that although they are responsible for complex forms of human gnostic activity, these zones of the brain retain their modal specificity, and they can rightly be regarded as systems responsible for the highest levels of special mental forms of modality-specific activity.

However, there are other gnostic processes, playing a leading role in human conscious activity, which depend on the combined working of several analysers and thus permit the most complex forms of information analysis; they form the basis of the highest forms of human gnostic activity, and we must now examine them in detail. I refer to the zones of the cortex which lie between the occipital, temporal and central regions and which play a basic role in the organization of *complex simultaneous (spatial) syntheses*.

I shall not dwell at this stage on the character of the work of the secondary zones of the postcentral (parietal) region, which will be discussed in the next chapter, but I shall turn at once to an examination of the functions of the tertiary zones just mentioned.

The tertiary cortical zones and the organization of concrete spatial syntheses

The zones of the posterior regions of the brain that lie at the boundary between the occipital, temporal and postcentral regions of the hemisphere, where the cortical areas for visual, auditory, vestibular, cutaneous and proprioceptive sensation overlap are tertiary in function. Their centre is formed by Brodmann's areas 39 and 40 or the inferior parietal region, although there are no strong grounds for excluding the adjacent temporo-occipital formations of area 37 and 21 from it.

These zones, which preserve the transverse striation and the well-marked six-layer structure characteristic of all receptor zones, consist entirely of cells of the upper cortical layers, with short axons and predominantly associative functions; fibres run to them from the secondary thalamic nuclei, and the impulses which they carry have already been integrated at the lower levels.

These zones are formed only in man and they constitute the specifically human portions of the brain. They mature later than all other zones of the posterior regions of the cortex, and do not become fully operative until the seventh year of life. This suggests that the tertiary structures of the parieto-temporo-occipital region now to be described play a special role in *inter-analyser syntheses*, and that they are concerned with the integration of individual impulses within the same (visual, tactile) analyser as well as with the transfer of structures of excitation of one analyser to another. It is this 'supramodal' function which has been ascribed by many investigators to the inferior parietal cortex (Semmes, 1965; Semmes *et al.*, 1955; Geschwind, 1965; Butters *et al.*, 1970). All these hypotheses regarding the integrative function of the tertiary zones of the parieto-temporo-occipital cortex are confirmed by the results of physiological experiments and neuropsychological observations.

Electrical stimulation of these zones gives rise to no modally-specific effects, which forces the conclusion that most of the information about the role which they play in the organization of mental activity is to be obtained from a careful study of the changes arising in mental processes when they are disturbed by pathological lesions.

Lesions of the inferior parietal and parieto-occipital zones of the cortex do not give rise to modally-specific disturbances; vision, hearing and tactile and kinaesthetic sensation remain completely intact in these cases. However, analysis shows that patients with lesions of these zones develop very marked disorders of the reception and analysis of information.

The picture of these disturbances is largely similar to simultaneous agnosia. Patients with such lesions experience difficulty in grasping the information which they receive as a whole; they cannot fit together the individual elements of incoming impressions into a single structure; they cannot convert the consecutive presentation of the elements of a situation into the new quality of simultaneous perceptibility; they can no longer find their bearings in space and their attempt to do so is converted into a series of disconnected and fragmentary attempts at orientation. However, we must add one characteristic feature to the description of these defects, which is already familiar from our examination of simultaneous agnosia. Patients with lesions of the parieto-occipital region can no longer *find their bearings within a system of spatial coordinates* and, in particular, they can no longer distinguish correctly between *right* and *left*. The evident explanation of this disturbance is that excitation from the visual, vestibular and kinaesthetic spheres and, in particular, from the dominant (right) and non-dominant (left) hand meets in the tertiary cortical zones, and the lesion therefore presents as a complex group of clearly demonstrable disorders.

Patients with a lesion in this part of the cortex easily lose their direction in space. If they go out into the corridor, they cannot find their way back into the ward, but turn right instead of left; they cannot find their own bed; when they try to make their bed they find it an impossible task: instead of laying the blanket lengthwise, they place it crosswise; when they try to put on a dressing gown which the physician holds up for them they cannot find the proper sleeve and usually put their arm in the wrong one. They are quite incapable of telling the time by *the position of the hands of a clock* on which the hours are not numbered, and they have difficulty in distinguishing between symmetrical positions such as 'three o'clock' and 'nine o'clock'; they are quite unable to identify more complex positions of the hands or to illustrate some specified time on a blank dial.

All these patients – even those who in the past were sufficiently experienced – are unable to *find their bearings on a map*, but confuse the directions of east and west, and when asked to outline the position of well-known places on a map they make appalling mistakes (Figure 40). They make equally bad mistakes when they attempt to find coordinates in three dimensions: they confuse the horizontal, frontal and sagittal planes; when tested by the physician they are unable to reproduce the position of his hand correctly or to construct

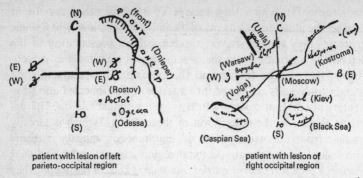

patient with lesion of left
parieto-occipital region

patient with lesion of
right occipital region

Figure 40 Disturbance of orientation on maps in patients with lesions of the parieto-occipital regions (spatial relations are confused)

a figure from its component elements which have to be fitted together in a precise position in space. Because of these difficulties, these patients exhibit the symptom known as constructional apraxia. Finally, a particularly pronounced manifestation of this disorder is that they have great *difficulty in drawing letters*. Unlike patients with lesions of the left temporal zones, the difficulty which these patients experience in writing is due, not to inability to distinguish clearly the sound or phoneme to be written, but inability to *retain the required spatial position of the lines forming the letter*, and as a result, their drawings (or copies) of letters become disorganized in character; sometimes, in less severe cases, the letter is replaced by its mirror image (Figure 41).

In the severest cases all these defects are manifested during the *direct reproduction* of three-dimensional structures. In less severe cases they are manifested only when the patient tries to reproduce a required spatial position *from memory*, or when he is given the task of consciously transferring certain spatial relationships (for example, when he is asked to raise the same hand, or to reproduce the position of the hand, of a person sitting face to face with him, or to *mentally reverse* the perceived spatial relationship of a geometrical figure on the table in front of the investigator so that it bears the same relationship to himself). Disturbances of spatial orientation of this type may arise in lesions both of the left (dominant) hemisphere, in which case they are particularly marked, and of the right (non-dominant) hemisphere.

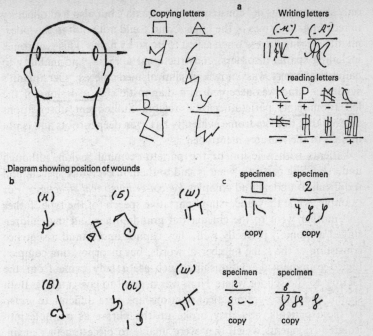

Figure 41 Optico-spatial disturbances of writing in patients with lesions of the parieto-occipital region: (a) a patient with a bilateral wound of the occipital region; (b) and (c) a patient with a wound of the left parieto-occipital region

Appreciable differences begin to appear only when from studying disturbances in *concrete* space we move on to more complex forms of disturbance of orientation in logical, 'quasi-spatial' relationships. This brings us to the neuropsychological analysis of the most complex and specifically human forms of gnostic activity.

The tertiary cortical zones and organization of symbolic (quasi-spatial) syntheses

Neurologists observed many years ago that patients with a lesion of the parieto-occipital zones of the left (dominant) hemisphere have difficulty in the analysis not only of concrete, but also of symbolic relationships. Patients with the simplest forms of this disturbance not only showed signs of 'constructional apraxia', but also had difficulty in recalling the names of the fingers, and could not point to the index, middle, or ring fingers when asked to do so by name. This syndrome, including spatial disorders, constructional apraxia, and inability to name the fingers was known in clinical medicine as 'Gerstmann's syndrome' and was accepted as a diagnostic sign of lesions of the left (dominant) parieto-occipital region. Subsequent observations showed that this syndrome evidently has even deeper roots and is not limited to the features mentioned.

Patients with a lesion of the parieto-occipital region, although understanding perfectly what is said to them in everyday speech, find it difficult to understand complex *logical-grammatical structures*. For example, while they understand narrative speech (of the type 'father and mother went to the cinema but grandmother and the children stayed at home') perfectly well, they cannot understand a sentence consisting of the same number of words, but incorporating complex logico-grammatical relationships (such as 'a lady came from the factory to the school where Nina was a pupil to give a talk'). Both spatial and logico-grammatical relationships were difficult to grasp by these patients, and they broke up the phrase as a whole into isolated fragments which they were unable to piece together again. Even such an apparently simple sentence, taken from a child's elementary reading book, as 'there is a bird's nest on the branch of a tree' confused them utterly, and they were completely unable to understand the relationship between the four words branch, tree, nest and bird, all included in the same sentence.

Further investigations (Luria, 1946: 1947: 1970e) led to considerable progress and to the discovery of the basic models of the syntactic structures (syntagmas) which are incomprehensible to patients with lesions of the parieto-occipital zones of the left hemisphere. These were the basic syntagmas expressing logical relationships or, to use the term suggested originally by the young Swedish linguist, Svedelius (1897), 'communications of relationships', which he distinguished from simple narrative speech or 'communications of events'. These 'communications of relationships' were grammatical structures which arose last of all in the history of the language and are expressed in languages such as Russian either with the aid of inflexions (formulating case relationships), prepositions (expressing relationships of space, sequence, or more complex logical concepts) and, finally, by means of word order. A common feature of all these constructions was that none of them was represented in the concrete form and that consequently all, in various ways, coded *logical* and not concrete relationships.

A typical example of these models is the structure of the attributive genitive case [for example 'brat (brother) otts*a*' (*of* the father), i.e. the father'*s* brother; 'khozyain (master) sobak*i*' (*of* the dog), i.e. the dog'*s* master], which, by contrast with simpler constructions such as the partitive genitive 'kusok (piece) khleb*a*' (*of* bread)), cannot be visualized in concrete terms but expresses certain *abstract* relationships. Another example is given by constructions with prepositions expressing either relationships of space – 'krest *pod* kvadratom' (cross *below* square), 'kvadrat *pod* krestom' (square *below* cross) – or relationships of time – 'vesna *pered* letom' (spring *before* summer) or 'leto *pered* vesnoi' (summer *before* spring). Finally, other examples are constructions in which the rearrangement of identical words formulates different relationships – such as 'plat'e zadelo veslo' (the dress caught on the oar) or 'veslo zadelo plat'e' (the oar caught on the dress).

In all these constructions, identical words included in different relationships receive different values, and the *grammatical codes* denoting the different grammatical relationships begin to assume a decisive role.

A characteristic feature of patients with <u>lesions of the left inferior parietal</u> (or parieto-temporo-occipital) system is that although they <u>*have a good understanding of the meaning of individual words, they cannot grasp the meaning of the construction as a whole*</u>; they painstakingly attempt to fit the individual elements of the construction together and often declare that constructions incorporating identical words (for example, 'brat ottsa' – the father's brother – and 'otets brata' – the brother's father) have the same meaning, for they *cannot appreciate the meaning of the logical-grammatical relationships expressed by these constructions*. It is easy to see that the meaning of constructions such as 'Solntse (the sun) osveshchaetsya (is lit) zemleyu (by the earth) or 'Zemlya (the earth) osveschaetsya (is lit) solntsem (by the sun), or of constructions in which the word order differs from the order of meaning (for example 'I had breakfast after I had read the newspaper') is completely beyond the grasp of these patients, and that they are completely unable to understand the meaning of more complex constructions such as 'Olga is paler than Sonia but darker than Kate'.

Clinicians (van Woerkom, 1925; Head, 1926; Conrad, 1932; Zucker, 1934) described these difficulties many years ago and called this symptom 'semantic aphasia'. However, only now is it becoming clear that this disturbance is the same defect of perception of simultaneous spatial structures, but transferred to a higher (symbolic) level.

It is a very interesting fact that patients with lesions of this region of the cortex exhibit disturbances of the naming of objects and in recalling desired words. Some of the essential mechanisms of these defects, which have been described collectively as 'semantic aphasia', will be discussed (see part 3, ch. 12, p. 13).

The far-reaching prospects of discovery of the physiological nature of cerebral organization of complex gnostic activity afforded by the analysis of these disturbances will be readily apparent.

The disturbances of internal 'quasi-spatial' syntheses we have just mentioned are even more obvious in the disturbance of _mathematical operations_ observed in patients of this group. Arithmetical operations, which in the early stages of learning are discursive in character, and are then converted into actions based on internal spatial schemes known as tables, are always dependent on the integrity of simultaneous syntheses with a similar structure to external spatial operations. This is reflected both in the columnar structure of multiple-digit numbers, in which the value of each number is determined by its place in the group as a whole, and also in the internal operations of arrangement of the columns necessary to understand the meaning of the number; finally, it is reflected in operations of addition and subtraction (not to mention more complex mathematical operations), which can only be carried out if the numerical schemes are retained in the operative memory and the operations are checked as they are performed (Luria, 1946, 1947, 1970e; Tsvetkova, 1972). To subtract 7 from 31, as a rule we begin by rounding the first number and obtain the result $30 - 7 = 23$. We then add the remaining unit, placing it in the right-hand column, and obtain the result $23 + 1 = 24$. The operation is much more complex when we subtract a number of two digits (for example, 51−17), when, besides observing the conditions just mentioned, we have to carry over from the tens column and to retain the double system of elements in the operative memory.

It is these operations which are completely impossible for patients with lesions of the left parieto-occipital zones. When they attempt to perform the first part of the operation described above (30 − 7 = 23) they do not know whether to put the residual '1' on the left or the right, or in other words whether to add it or to take it away. In relatively localized cases, these disturbances are manifested only in more complex operations (subtraction of two-digit from two-digit or subtraction of one-digit from two-digit numbers, requiring carrying over from the tens column, with intermediate splitting of the diminuend into its component parts); in cases of more massive lesions, these disturbances assume a gross character and the patients are unable to perform even elementary mathematical operations. Characteristically in all these cases the purposive character of the activity remains intact; both the basic problem and the general plan of its solution are undisturbed, and only the *executive* part of the calculation, requiring integrity of the differentiated 'quasi-spatial' organization of the action, is lost.

This symptom of *acalculia* has been known for a long time in the patients with local brain lesions; however, it is only with the introduction of neuropsychological methods of analysis of primary disorders and of symptom qualification into clinical neurology that the true nature of these disturbances has begun to be clarified.

Disturbances of simultaneous ('quasi-spatial') syntheses at the mnestic and speech or symbolic level invariably lead to marked disturbances of gnostic operations and intellectual processes, and it will be clear that these patients will have considerable difficulty not only in formulating thoughts but also in carrying out complex intellectual operations. However, it remains a characteristic feature of all these cases that intellectual activity remains largely intact: the patients retain their motives; the basic problem is well retained, the aim of their attempts is still present, and sometimes they may possess a general scheme for the required solution. They experience difficulty only when performing the corresponding *operations*. Although they grasp the general meaning of a school exercise, they are hopelessly perplexed by the grammatical wording of the conditions which it incorporates. They cannot understand the meaning of the expressions 'so much larger' and 'so many times more', or of formulae such as 'there were so many metres of cloth, of which so many were used', and as a result, they are completely unable to solve the problem although its general meaning is perfectly clear to them (Luria and Tsvetkova, 1967).

This dissociation between the integrity of intellectual *activity* and disturbance of intellectual *operations*, between the integrity of the general *purpose* and the disturbance of concrete *meanings*, together with the complete awareness of their own defects, are the features which distinguish this syndrome found in patients with lesions of the parieto-occipital zones of the left hemisphere, leading to the disintegration of simultaneous 'quasi-spatial' syntheses.

The tertiary cortical zones and processes of speech memory

We must now examine the last problem, that of the role of the tertiary (parieto-occipital) zones of the cortex in speech memory.

One of the earliest symptoms to be described in lesions of the parieto-occipital zones of the left (dominant) hemisphere was a disturbance of the *naming of objects*. These defects were studied by many investigators (Lotmar, 1919; 1935; Isserlin, 1929–32; Goldstein, 1927; 1948) and the condition was described as *amnestic aphasia*.

The features of amnestic aphasia outwardly have much in common with the disturbances of speech memory which I described when dealing with the disturbances arising in lesions of the middle zones of the temporal region. The patient also has difficulty when asked to name an object; he tries just as painstakingly to find the name required and is equally unable to do so. However, close analysis shows that the features of amnestic aphasia arising in lesions of the left parieto-occipital region differ significantly from the disturbances of audio-verbal memory found in lesions of the left temporal lobe. The weakness of the acoustico-verbal traces and the instability of the differential acoustic basis of speech are completely absent in these cases, as one very simple test convincingly demonstrates: if a patient with a lesion of the left parieto-occipital region is prompted with the first sound or first syllable of the forgotten word, he will immediately recall the word and pronounce it without any acoustico-verbal difficulties. It thus follows that the amnestic aphasia arising in these patients has no basis in a disturbance of audio-verbal memory, and we must look for other mechanisms which may be responsible for it.

The first clue to the causes of this disturbance of the nominative function is given by psychological analysis of the normal process of name recall. When we name a certain object, when we attach a verbal label to it, we in fact *include it in a definite system of values* – we give it a *classification*. Every word in essence is a *code*, which distinguishes its significant features ('teapot', 'steam-ship', 'baker', 'ruler') and places the specified object in a certain *category* (Morton, 1970; Kintch, 1970a; 1970b). However, this process requires the integrity of certain *semantic schemes*, and it is these simultaneously existing schemes which are disturbed in lesions of the tertiary zones of the left parieto-occipital (or parieto-temporo-occipital) regions. That is why such an apparently simple thing as the naming of an object is so severely disturbed, and presents the same difficulty as any normal person would have if asked to recall the name of a person not yet properly fixed in the memory and incorporated in a rigid semantic system.

However, the difficulty of recalling objects observed in these patients has additional pathophysiological mechanisms. When affected by a pathological lesion, the cerebral cortex is usually in an abnormal inhibitory or 'phasic' state in which, as had already been mentioned, the 'law of strength' is upset and weak stimuli begin to evoke the same reactions as strong. Naturally under these conditions a well stabilized and dominant value will no longer be distinguished from irrelevant and weaker connections, and these irrelevant connections will start to appear just as easily as the required name. If such a patient attempts to find, for example, the word 'bol'nitsa' (hospital), he may come up with 'militsiya' (Police), because of their common suffix, or with the word 'shkola' (school), as another public institution, or again with the words 'Red Army' (through the chain: Hospital – Red Cross – Red Army). The appearance of a *flood of equally probable possibilities* prevents the discovery of the required dominant word (Luria, 1972). This appearance of an irrelevant word, resembling the required word either in its morphology, in its meaning or in its phonetic composition, is known as *paraphasia* (in the first two cases, 'verbal', and in the last case 'literal'). It indicates considerable neurodynamic disturbances in the functioning of the pathologically changed parieto-occipital (or parieto-occipito-temporal) cortex, and it suggests that it is along these lines that an explanation will be found of this hitherto unexplained phenomenon.

Recently a further attempt has been made to explain the disturbance of speech memory in lesions of the left parieto-occipital region. This explanation was suggested by Tsvetkova (1972), and is as follows. The difficulty in finding names is concentrated mainly on the naming of *objects*, and it is much less frequently observed in the naming of *qualities* or *actions*. This is clear from the time spent in finding words in each of these groups and from the number of names of objects, qualities and actions which the subject can recall in a certain period of time. Tsvetkova found that patients with lesions of the tertiary (parieto-occipital) cortex spend on average 2·5 seconds (with a scatter from 1·4 to 7 seconds) in recalling words denoting qualities (adjectives); 9·3 seconds (with a scatter from 2·6 to 20 seconds) on words denoting actions (verbs), 15 seconds (with a scatter from 4 to 35 seconds) on names of objects (nouns). This emphasis on difficulties in the naming of objects raises the question whether in such cases there may be certain special difficulties associated with the naming of *concrete objects* and not arising during the naming of qualities and actions. The fact that most words substituted for the desired word belong to the same *general category* also shows that the difficulties are connected with the actual naming of concrete objects. Therefore, it is not the abstract category but the naming of the concrete object which is disturbed.

Tsvetkova's later experiments revealed the essential mechanisms of these difficulties. She found that patients with amnestic aphasia of the type I have described exhibit marked defects in their *visual representations* of the corresponding objects and that they could not distinguish the systems of characteristic features embodied in an object. When, therefore, they were asked to identify the picture of an object drawn in a stylized manner, to draw an object, or to complete the drawing of an object started by someone else, or even to give a description of its details, they revealed unexpected defects (Figure 42).

These experiments suggest that yet another mechanism may be

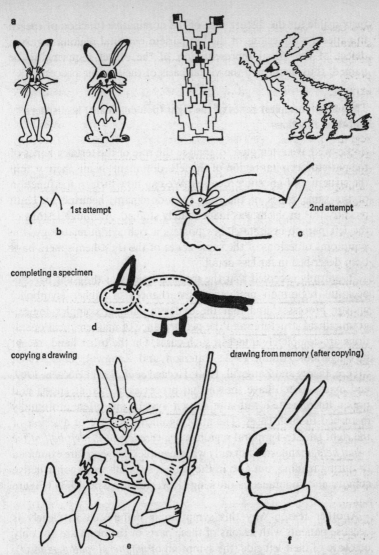

Figure 42 Examples of the drawing of objects and completion of unfinished drawings of objects by patients with amnestic aphasia: (a) drawings shown to the patient for identification, (b-f) completion of the task under various conditions (with or without the possibility of copying, etc.) (after Tsvetkova)

responsible for the disturbance of the nominative function of speech in patients with lesions of the left parieto-occipital region, namely a defect of the visual representation of the object requiring to be named, thus disturbing the visual basis of the naming process.

The parieto-occipital zones of the right (non-dominant) hemisphere and their functions

So far we have attempted to analyse the role of the tertiary zones of the parieto-occipital region of the left (dominant) hemisphere within the structure of gnostic processes. We can now turn to the function of the same zones of the right (non-dominant) hemisphere. Until recently this problem was inadequately studied. Although lesions of the left parieto-occipital lobes possess a rich symptomatology, the symptoms of lesions of the same zones of the right hemisphere have been described in far less detail.

It is firmly accepted that the massive lesions of the right parieto-occipital region do not cause disturbances of higher (symbolic) gnostic processes, and that the understanding of complex logical-grammatical structures and the performance of mathematical operations are completely intact in such cases. On the other hand, recent investigations (Brain, 1941; Paterson and Zangwill, 1944; 1945; McFie, Piercy and Zangwill, 1950; Hécaen *et al.*, 1951; Hécaen, 1969, and many others) have shown that processes of spatial gnosis and praxis unconnected with the speech system are often profoundly disturbed in such cases. The most significant feature of a lesion of the right parieto-temporal region is *unawareness of the left half of the visual field*, manifested not only when complex drawings are examined or during reading, but also in the patient's spontaneous constructive activity and spontaneous drawing (Korchazhinskaya, 1971) (Figure 43).

Another reason why this symptom is manifested so clearly is because patients with lesions of these parts of the brain are not only unaware of their left side (the symptom of *unilateral spatial agnosia*), but they do not notice their mistakes and exhibit in a special form the symptom of failure to perceive their own defects (*anosognosia*) which is characteristic of many patients with lesions of the right hemisphere, a matter to which we shall refer again.

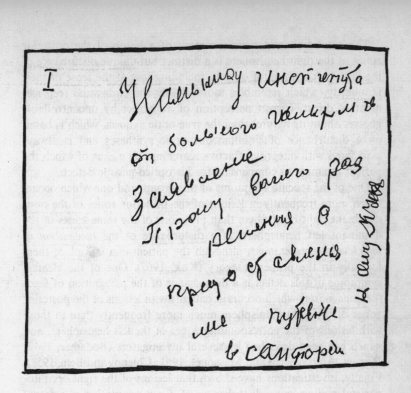

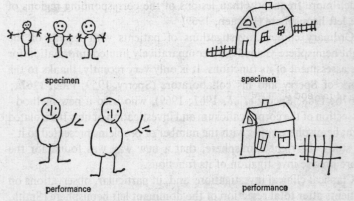

specimen   specimen

performance   performance

Figure 43 Loss of the left half of the field of vision in the functions of patients with left-sided spatial agnosia: (a) writing; (b) drawing

The second characteristic symptom of a lesion of the posterior zones of the right hemisphere is a distinct but unique disturbance of the visual recognition of objects, including loss of the sense of their familiarity, which resembles more closely the *paragnosia* (replacement of direct, correct perception of an object by uncontrollable guesses about its nature) than the true optic agnosia, which is based on a disturbance of simultaneous optic syntheses and is always associated with integrity of active searching, by means of which the patient attempts to compensate for his optico-gnostic defects.

One of the specific symptoms of this group, and one which occurs much more frequently in lesions of the posterior zones of the non-dominant right hemisphere than in lesions of the same zones of the dominant left hemisphere, is a disturbance of the *recognition of individual representations*, although the patient can still place them logically in the proper category (Kok, 1967). One of the clearest symptoms of this defect is a disturbance of the recognition of faces (*prosopagnosia*), which occurs in patients with lesions of the posterior zones of the right hemisphere much more frequently than in those with lesions of the corresponding zones of the left hemisphere, and which has been described by several investigators (Bodamer, 1947; Hécaen, Ajuriaguerra and Massonet, 1951; Chlenov and Bein, 1958). Finally, investigations have shown that lesions of the right occipito-parietal regions cause disturbances of direct orientation in external space, phenomena of constructional apraxia and similar defects much more frequently than lesions of the corresponding regions of the left hemisphere (Hécaen, 1969).

Ordinary clinical investigations of patients with lesions of the right hemisphere yielded only comparatively limited information for the assessment of its functions. It is only very recently, thanks to the work of Sperry and his collaborators (Sperry, 1959; 1966; 1967a; 1967b; 1968; Sperry *et al.*, 1967; 1969), who used a new method – dissection of the corpus callosum and investigation of how the isolated right hemisphere copes with the number of problems presented to it – to study the right hemisphere, that a new way was found for the more precise investigation of its functions.

Classical clinical investigations and, in particular, observations on patients after total resection of the dominant left hemisphere (Smith, 1966; 1969; Smith and Burkland, 1966), as well as the observations of Sperry, have confirmed the view that any complex mental function is effected by the combined activity of both hemispheres, but that each hemisphere makes its own particular contribution to the construction of mental processes (Ananev, 1952).

Despite the extreme shortage of reliable evidence regarding the function of the non-dominant hemisphere, a number of general principles governing its role can now be stated. Two facts must be regarded as firmly established. One of them was discovered long ago and there is no question whatever about its validity, while the other was discovered only very recently and requires further verification.

The first fact is that the non-dominant (right) hemisphere, despite its complete symmetry with the left, *plays no part in the organization of speech activity* and that its lesions, even if extensive, *do not affect speech processes*. The non-dominant hemisphere naturally can neither perform complex speech and intellectual functions, nor even participate in the construction of complex motor acts (Sperry *et al.*, 1967; 1969). Characteristically, however, as Sperry's observations show, the isolated right hemisphere, which is inadequate for action such as the naming of objects, remains capable not only of perceiving objects directly, but also of a diffuse type of differentiation between the meanings of words; similar conclusions can be drawn from observation on patients after total resection of the dominant left hemisphere (Smith, 1966).

Important and interesting data, which provide indirect information on the function of the right hemisphere in the organization of human mental processes, are given by observations on patients with massive lesions of the right hemisphere. For instance, right-handed persons with a lesion of the non-dominant right hemisphere exhibit no disturbances of speech, writing, reading and arithmetic, and even if the lesion is situated in those zones (temporal, parieto-occipital and inferior zones of the premotor region) whose lesions, if located in the left hemisphere, would give rise to gross manifestations of aphasia, it leaves the speech functions of the patient with a lesion in the right hemisphere completely unaffected. These differences are not confined to speech itself; patients with a lesion of the corresponding zones of the non-dominant hemisphere likewise exhibit no defects of processes formed on the basis of speech: it is often impossible to detect any disturbance of logical reasoning in them, and their understanding of logical-grammatical structures, as well as their formal logical operations, remain unimpaired.

These findings suggest that the right hemisphere plays a different role in the organization of mental processes and that the disturbances of mental activity associated with its lesions must be sought in a sphere far removed from the verbal or logical-grammatical organization of consciousness.

The second fact was discovered comparatively recently as a result of some elegant statistical investigations conducted by Teuber and his collaborators (Teuber *et al.*, 1960).

They showed that the *functional organization of the non-dominant right hemisphere is much less differentiated in character than that of the dominant left hemisphere*. For instance, whereas disturbances of cutaneous and deep sensation of the *right* upper limb occur *only* in lesions of the postcentral zones of the left hemisphere, the same disturbance of cutaneous and kinaesthetic sensation in the left upper limb may arise in the presence of much more widespread lesions of the non-dominant, right hemisphere. This lower functional differentiation of the cortical structures of the right hemisphere, without any participation in fine speech processes, is evidently one of its leading (although still inadequately investigated) characteristics, analysis of which could yield much new and valuable information.

Certain difficulties arise in the investigation of the role of the non-dominant hemisphere in the organization of mental processes.

Recent work (Zangwill, 1960; Hécaen and Ajuriaguerra, 1963; Subirana, 1952; 1964; 1969) has shown that dominance of the left hemisphere in right-handed individuals is by no means as absolute as might be supposed, and that many transitional stages exist from absolute dominance of the left hemisphere, through ambidexterity, to absolute dominance of the right hemisphere (which itself is quite uncommon); the decision that an individual is right-handed or left-handed is thus to a large extent relative.

This diagnostic problem has been made easier by the results of experiments (Wada, 1949; Wada and Rasmussen, 1960) in which sodium amytal was injected into the left and right carotid arteries.

What facts are now known regarding the role of the non-dominant, right hemisphere in the organization of mental activity, and what changes are found in the course of mental processes when that hemisphere is affected by a pathological lesion?

Nearly a century ago, Hughlings Jackson postulated that the right hemisphere, although unconnected with any speech functions or with logical forms of organization of consciousness dependent on speech, participates directly in perceptual processes and is responsible for more direct, visual forms of relationships with the outside world (Jackson, 1874).

This hypothesis failed to attract due attention for many decades, and it is only recently that it has begun to be appreciated. First of all it was noticed that the right hemisphere is directly concerned with the analysis of direct information received by the subject *from his own body* and which, it can easily be understood, is much more closely connected with direct sensation than with verbally logical codes.

This provides an explanation for the fact that lesions of the right hemisphere lead much more frequently (according to Hécaen, 1969, seven times more frequently) than lesions of the left hemisphere to disturbances of the normal sensation of the subject's own body or, to use the term generally employed in neurology, to a disturbance of the body schema.

Very similar to these symptoms is the distinctive ignorance of the opposite (left) side of the body and the ignorance of the left side of space, connected with it, observed in patients with lesions of the right hemisphere and which form the syndrome known in clinical neurology as unilateral spatial agnosia.

This phenomenon, described in turn by Brain (1941), McFie, Piercy and Zangwill (1950), Critchley (1953), Piercy, Hécaen and Ajuriaguerra (1960), Benton (1961; 1965; 1967) and Korchazhinskaya (1971), which has subsequently been further investigated by the schools of Zangwill and of Hécaen (1969), can manifest itself in various spheres.

As was mentioned above, in lesions of the posterior zones of the right hemisphere (especially of the deep structures) this syndrome is manifested as left-sided fixed hemianopia (Luria and Skorodumova, 1950), or inattention towards the left side (Holmes, 1919; Brain, 1941; McFie, Piercy and Zangwill, 1950; Critchley, 1953; Warrington, James and Kinsbourne, 1966), while in lesions of the middle zones of the right hemisphere it is manifested particularly as inattention to the left side of the body and is seen most clearly when the experimenter touches symmetrically opposite parts of the body at the same time; in such cases the patient has no diminution of cutaneous sensation, but is definitely unaware of or indifferent to anything touching the left half of the body, or even to the left of a pair of tactile stimuli on the same side of the body (Teuber, 1962; Weinstein *et al.*, 1964).

However, in these cases *unawareness* of the opposite side is not the only disturbance of sensation of the subject's own body. In many cases a lesion of the right hemisphere causes a true *disturbance of the body schema,* in which the patient's head and one upper or lower limb is perceived by him as disproportionately large or smaller than the other, or deformed. Such disturbances of the body schema and the 'apraxia of dress' associated with it have been studied by a number of workers, including Hécaen (1969). He found that they occur four or five times more frequently in lesions of the non-dominant right hemisphere than in lesions of the left.

The gnostic disturbances arising in lesions of the right hemisphere are not, however, confined to the patient's body schema but they sometimes extend also to his spatial orientation. The patient frequently cannot orient himself normally in space and familiar spatial relationships become strange; sometimes these defects prevent the patient from reproducing constructions when required to do so, when they manifest themselves as constructional agnosia and apraxia. As several investigators (Hécaen and Angelergues, 1963; Piercy, Hécaen and Ajuriaguerra, 1960; Benton, 1961; 1967; 1969) have shown, these defects are more common in patients with lesions of the right, than of the left, dominant hemisphere.

Finally, lesions of the right hemisphere (and, in particular, of its posterior zones) very often lead to a distinctive disturbance of the recognition of objects (Kimura, 1963; Hécaen and Angelergues, 1963; Kok, 1967) which externally may resemble the picture of optic agnosia but which, in fact, is characterized by loss of the sense of familiarity and a disturbance of the direct recognition of individual (not included in particular logical codes) objects, or even people. This phenomenon, described in clinical practice by Bodamer (1947), Pötzl (1937), Hoff and Pötzl (1937), Chlenov and Bein (1958) and others has been called prosopagnosia. The disturbances of visual perception arising in lesions of the right hemisphere may possibly be characterized also by lack of control over the patient's searches when assessing an object, as a result of which they exhibit the character of *paragnosias* (uncontrolled guesses), they are accompanied by marked changes in all the patient's activities, and in this way they differ in their psychological structure from the true optic agnosias which I have described above (part 2, ch. 3) and which I shall discuss again later (part 3, ch. 9). This feature is closely related to the basic phenomenon to which we shall return again shortly.

The gnostic disturbances arising in lesions of the right hemisphere are characterized by a much less marked modal specificity and they are much more frequently global and polysensory in character (de Renzi and Spinnler, 1966a; 1966b; Hécaen, 1969). This is explained by the more diffuse functional organization of the cortex of the right hemisphere which I have mentioned above.

However, it is not the gnostic disorders just described which are of the greatest importance so far as the functions of the right hemisphere are concerned, but the general *perception by the patient of his own body and his own personality*; accordingly, by far the most important symptom of a lesion of the right hemisphere is the remarkable *absence of perception by the patient of his own defects*, a condition known for many years in clinical practice and to which the name *anosognosia* has been given.

The essence of this phenomenon is that a patient with a lesion of the right hemisphere affected by paralysis 'does not notice' this paralysis; a patient unaware of the left side of space or with a disturbance of the recognition of objects 'does not notice' these defects and, accordingly, does not compensate for them but behaves just as if these defects were not there. The behaviour of a patient with a lesion of the right hemisphere thus resembles in certain special features the behaviour of a patient with the frontal syndrome (see part 2, ch. 7), from which, however, it differs, in particular in the much greater degree of integrity of the patient's intentions and his plans of behaviour.

The symptom of anosognosia may perhaps be explained on the assumption that the right hemisphere is not concerned with those forms of analysis of the patient's own behaviour which evidently take place with the aid of complex speech mechanisms. However, the nature and internal mechanisms of this important symptom have not been adequately studied and require careful analysis.

We now come to the last group of symptoms associated with lesions of the right hemisphere, which are seen most clearly in patients with deep lesions of the right hemisphere, and whose nature also remains insufficiently studied.

I refer to changes in personality and consciousness, which are particularly severely affected in patients with these lesions. Such patients have unimpaired speech, but they lack the precise analysis of the direct flow of information about their own body; their perception of the direct situation is often defective, but they cannot adequately assess their defects. For this reason, in patients with deep lesions of the right hemisphere it is particularly common to find evidence of disorientation in the surroundings, or evidence of confusion and disturbances of direct consciousness, which the patient tries to conceal by his intact speech, thereby making the confusion even more conspicuous.

I shall never forget a group of such patients with deep lesions (tumours and aneurysms) of the right hemisphere, who were under my care and who showed severe loss of direct orientation in space and time. They firmly believed that at one and the same time they were in Moscow and also in another town. They suggested that they had left Moscow and gone to the other town, but having done so, they were still in Moscow where an operation had been performed on their brain. Yet they found nothing contradictory about these conclusions. Integrity of the verbal-logical processes in these patients, despite the profound disturbance of their direct self-perception and self-evaluation, led to a characteristic over-development of speech, to verbosity, which bore the character of empty reasoning and which masked their true defects.

These still completely unstudied defects lead us to one of the fundamental problems – to the role of the right hemisphere in direct consciousness. However, because the study of this highly important problem has so far been neglected, we can do no more at this stage than to mention it. It will receive a detailed analysis in a special series of papers which are in preparation for publication.

Chapter 6
Sensorimotor and Premotor Zones and the Organization of Movement

So far we have examined the work of the zones of the cerebral cortex which form the second functional brain unit and participate in the reception, analysis and storage of information. We must now turn to those systems of the brain which prepare and carry out the functions of movement.

In the early stages of mammalian development, the cortical systems preparing for movement were not so clearly subdivided between two units, and a single *sensorimotor* region, consisting of afferent (kinaesthetic) cells and motor cells proper, could be distinguished in the cortex. In the late stages of development, in primates and, in particular, in man, differentiation took place and the two parts of the functionally single system, one for the preparation of movements and the other for carrying them out, became clearly separated. The posterior zones of the sensorimotor cortex, providing the kinaesthetic basis of movement, became separated into the *postcentral* region, maintaining its afferent functions and forming a part of the second brain unit, while the anterior zones, including the *motor and premotor* areas, took over special responsibility for the efferent organization of movement, and they both form a part of the third brain unit.

Since this group of zones as a whole continues as a structurally differentiated, but single system for the preparation and execution of movements, we shall examine its functional organization in a single chapter, dealing first with the afferent and later with the efferent part of the system.

Postcentral cortical zones and the afferent organization of movement

The postcentral (cutaneo-kinaesthetic) zones lie posteriorly to the central sulcus and have the typical parvocellular and granular structure of the second brain system. In the primary zones of this region (Brodmann's area 3), just as in all projection zones, afferent layer IV of the cortex is predominant, and exhibits a clearly somatotopical structure. It is well known that fibres carrying impulses from the contralateral lower limbs run to the upper parts of this zone, some of them reaching its medial surface, fibres carrying impulses from the upper limbs run to the middle part, and fibres carrying impulses from the face, lips, and tongue run to the lower part of this cortical zone. This projection is functional rather than geometrical in character, because the more important a particular region of peripheral receptors, the greater the need for control over its corresponding motor segments and the greater the area occupied by its projection in these cortical zones.

Clearly a local *lesion* of these regions of the brain must cause the *loss (or a decrease) of sensation* in the corresponding segments of the body. However, although this is the most direct and obvious result of such a lesion, it is by no means the only result. As I have already said (and as I shall discuss again in a special context), a *normal flow of cutaneo-kinaesthetic afferent impulses is the essential basis of movement*. It gives motor impulses their necessary destination, which is lost in lesions of the corresponding cortical zones. *A lesion of the posterior, postcentral cortical zones and their tracts thus gives rise to 'afferent paresis'* in which the potential strength of the muscles remains intact, but differential control over the limb is sharply reduced so that the patient cannot perform voluntary movements with his hand or foot which has lost its kinaesthetic sensation.

The mechanism of this *afferent paresis*, described originally by Foerster (1936), is that the motor impulses no longer have a precise, differentiated destination and they no longer reach the proper muscle groups. This can be seen by comparing the electromyogram of the flexor and extensor muscles of a normal person (Figure 44a) and of a person with a lesion (tumour) of the postcentral region (Figure 44b). The electromyograms illustrated clearly show that in the second case impulses reach the group of agonists and the group of antagonists simultaneously, so that the required movement cannot take place.

Just as with other modally specific zones of this brain unit, secondary zones are superposed above the primary (projection)

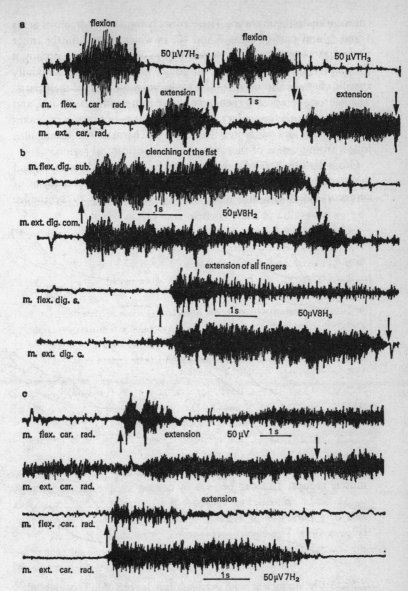

Figure 44 Electromyogram of flexion and extension movements:
(a) in a normal subject; (b) in a patient with a tumour of the postcentral
region of the cortex; (c) the same two months after operation (after
Zambran)

cutaneo-kinaesthetic cortex. These zones comprise Brodmann's areas 1 and 5, and part of areas 7 and 40, in which, just as in the other secondary zones, the upper layers of the cortex begin to occupy a substantial place and which, although preserving their modally specific character, lose the somatotopical organization of their parts. The neurons composing them respond to more complex stimuli, and stimulation of the secondary kinaesthetic zones of the cortex evokes more general and widespread sensations. Characteristic results also follow from a *lesion* of these zones of the postcentral region.

Gross disturbances of sensation may be absent in these cases, and the predominant feature may be a disturbance of complex forms of cutaneo-kinaesthetic sensation, leading to inability to synthesize

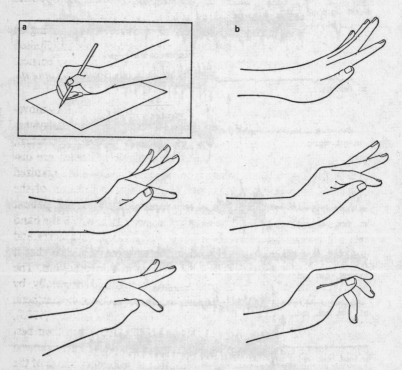

Figure 45 Disturbance of hand movements in lesions of the postcentral region (after Foerster) (a) disturbance of fine movements in writing; (b) the phenomenon of static ataxia.

individual stimuli into whole structures. As a result, in patients with a lesion of this cortical zone it is the most complex forms of active *tactile sensation* which are affected, giving rise to defects which have been analysed in detail during recent years by Soviet investigators (Ananev, 1959). The phenomenon which arises is analogous to the simultaneous optic agnosia and the object agnosia described in the section on the pathology of the secondary zones of the occipital cortex, and which has recently been given the descriptive name of *amorphosynthesis* (Denny-Brown, 1951; 1958). This is a disturbance of the ability to combine isolated tactile and kinaesthetic impressions into a single entity, and it evidently lies at the basis of the well-known clinical phenomenon of *astereognosis* (inability to recognize objects by touch), as a rule affecting the hand on the opposite side to the focus.

It would be a mistake to suppose that disturbances arising in lesions of the secondary zones of the postcentral cortex are limited to afferent or gnostic disorders. An essential feature of these cortical zones is that a *pathological lesion* in them is *invariably reflected in the course of movement.*

As I stated above, the organized performance of a voluntary movement (manipulation of an object) is largely dependent on the system of kinaesthetic afferent impulses on which it is based (Bernstein, 1947; 1967). Naturally, therefore, if kinaesthetic syntheses are disturbed, the direct afferent basis of the movement is lost and organized movement is therefore impossible. That is why in a lesion of the secondary zones of the postcentral kinaesthetic cortex, the patient develops a characteristic form of *afferent apraxia*, in which the hand does not receive the necessary afferent (kinaesthetic) syntheses and is unable to perform properly differentiated movements, so that it works in a coarse manner, lacking in fineness and precision. The manifestations of afferent apraxia were recognized originally by Liepmann (1905; 1920), who described them as 'acro-kinaesthetic apraxia', and subsequently by Kleist (1907; 1911), Pick (1905), Monakow (1910; 1914), Brun (1921) and Sittig (1931), but their best description of all was given by Foerster (1936), who clearly showed that the hand of a patient with a lesion of the secondary zones of the postcentral region is deprived of its complex synthetic afferentation and is unable to adapt itself adequately to the character of an object, so that the movements of such a patient lose their differentiated character. The specific character of the movements of what Foerster described as a 'spade-hand', which holds a needle and a large object in exactly the same way, will be clearly seen in Figure 45, illustrating changes in movement due to lesions of the postcentral region.

These disturbances could logically be called 'postural apraxia' or 'afferent kinaesthetic apraxia' (Luria, 1963; 1969a, 1969c) and regarded as reliable evidence of a lesion of the secondary zones of the postcentral kinaesthetic cortex. However, one essential factor requires special examination.

If a lesion of the secondary (kinaesthetic) zones of the postcentral region affects the *lower zones of this region of the left* (*dominant*) *hemisphere*, i.e. the region of secondary organization of kinaesthetic sensation in the face, lips and tongue, the kinaesthetic apraxia may manifest itself in a special manner in the organization of movements of the speech apparatus, leading to the distinctive disorder of speech which has been called *afferent motor aphasia* (Luria, 1962, 1964, 1969c, 1970a).

The basic feature of this syndrome is inability to determine immediately the positions of the lips and tongue necessary to articulate the required sounds of speech. Patients with massive lesions in this region do not know in what position to put the tongue and lips in order to pronounce the necessary sounds; patients with a less massive form of this disturbance begin to confuse only *similar* (differing in only one feature) *articulemes*; they may substitute palatoglossal articulations, so that they pronounce 'd' as 'l' or confuse similar labial articulations, pronouncing 'b' or 'p' as 'm'. The substitution of these sounds of different acoustic properties, yet similar in their articulation, provides firm evidence for the diagnosis of lesions of the inferior postcentral zones of the left hemisphere (Vinarskaya, 1971).

Characteristic secondary (systemic) results of this defect are special forms of *disturbance of writing*, involving the *substitution of similar articulemes*. The patient may write 'khadat' or 'khanat' instead of 'khalat', or 'snot' or 'slon' instead of 'stol' (Figure 46). This type of substitution of sounds with similar *articulation* distinguishes them from patients with lesions of the left temporal region, whose writing defect is predominantly one of confusion between similar *phonemes*.

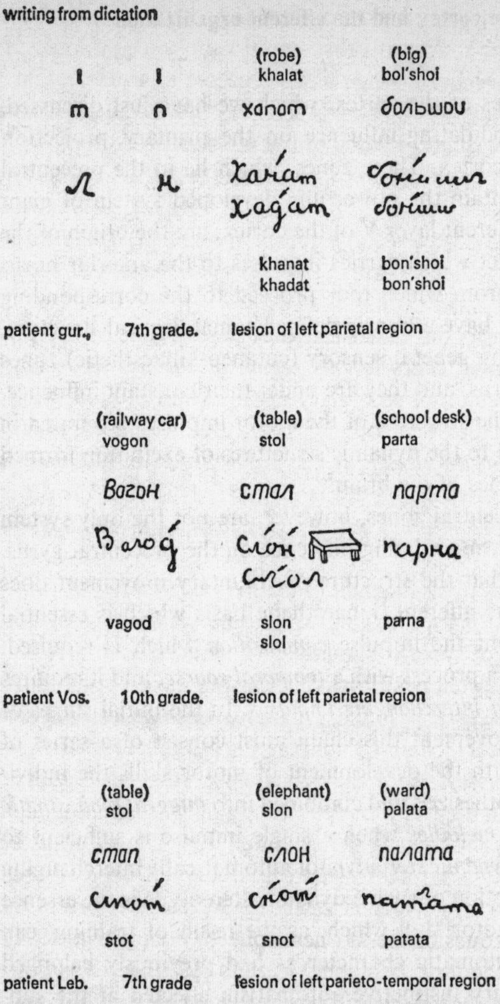

		(robe) khalat	(big) bol'shoi
I	I	халат	большои
m	n		

[handwritten] Xaváam / Xagam   / бои иш / бои иш

| | | khanat
khadat | bon'shoi
bon'shoi |

patient gur., 7th grade. lesion of left parietal region

	(railway car) vogon	(table) stol	(school desk) parta
	Вагон	стол	парта

[handwritten] Вагоɡ   Слон   парна / слол

| | vagod | slon
slol | parna |

patient Vos. 10th grade. lesion of left parietal region

	(table) stol	(elephant) slon	(ward) palata
	стол	слон	палата

[handwritten] слол   слон   палата

| | stot | snot | patata |

patient Leb. 7th grade lesion of left parieto-temporal region

Figure 46 Handwriting of patients with afferent motor aphasia

All the disorders described above are the result of a disturbance of the *afferent basis of movement*. They constitute one form of movement pathology in local brain lesions and they differ clearly from its other type, which is associated with the lesion of the premotor, and not the postcentral, zones of the brain.

Premotor zones of the cortex and the efferent organization of movement

The postcentral zones of the cortex, which we have just discussed, have a tuning or modulating influence on the primary, projection zones of the motor cortex. These zones, which lie in the precentral gyrus and which contain the powerfully developed system of giant pyramidal cells in afferent layer V of the cortex, are the origin of the pyramidal motor tract which carries impulses to the anterior horns of the spinal cord, from which they proceed to the corresponding muscle groups. They have a clearly defined somatotopical structure, like the corresponding general sensory (cutaneo-kinaesthetic) zones of the postcentral gyrus, and they are under their constant influence, with the result that the structure of the motor impulses generated in them is subordinated to the dynamic structures of excitation formed in the postcentral zones of the brain.

The afferent, postcentral zones, however, are not the only system exerting a regulatory, modulating influence on the precentral gyrus.

It is well known that the structure of voluntary movement does not rest solely on the afferent, kinaesthetic basis which is essential to give the movement the impulse *composition* which is required. Movement is always a process with a *temporal course*, and it requires a continuous *chain of interchanging impulses*. In the initial stages of formation of any movement this chain must consist of a series of isolated impulses; with the development of motor skills the individual impulses are synthesized and combined into *integral kinaesthetic structures* or *kinetic melodies* when a single impulse is sufficient to activate a complete *dynamic stereotype* of automatically interchanging elements. The production of such a dynamic stereotype is the essence of formation of a motor skill which, as the result of training, can acquire the same automatic character as had previously belonged only to the elementary instinctive automatism effected at the subcortical level or, as Bernstein (1947; 1967), the founder of the physiology of movement, calls it – the level of *motor synergisms*.

Above the system of subcortical synergisms, which is powerfully developed in lower vertebrates and incorporates the structures of the thalamus and the subcortical motor nuclei (the thalamo-strate system), are now superposed the systems of the cerebral cortex, the most important of which, so far as the present issue is concerned, are the *premotor zones* whose connections are shown diagrammatically in Figure 47.

The premotor region (Brodmann's areas 6 and 8) is the site of the mechanism which is superposed above the subcortical level of

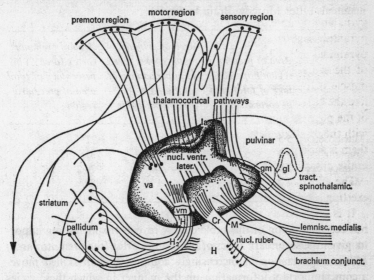

Figure 47 Diagram of connections of subcortical and cortical levels responsible for sensory and motor searches (after Papez and others)

the spinal system and also above the cortical systems of the precentral gyrus. In its structure it clearly retains the character of the *motor cortex* and its vertical striation, but it differs from the primary motor area in the powerful development of the small pyramidal cells of layers II and III, which gives it the typical structure of the *secondary* cortical zones.

An essential feature is that the premotor zone becomes powerfully developed only in the last stages of evolution of mammals. Whereas in lower monkeys the primary motor area (area 4) is sharply predominant and the premotor cortical zones (area 6) occupy only an insignificant place, in man these relationships are reversed, and the premotor cortex now occupies the greater part of the precentral region.

Thesec hanging relationships in phylogeny, with the increase in the relative size of the premotor zones, are clearly shown in Table 5.

Table 5 **Changes in relative area of precentral** (motor) **and premotor regions at subsequent stages of evolution of higher mammals** (after Moscow Brain Institute)

	Area of precentral region in percentage of total area of cortex	*Area of primary motor cortex (area 4) in percentage of total area of precentral region*	*Area of premotor cortex (area 6) in percentage of total area of precentral region*
Marmoset	5·5	79	21
Guenon	8·3	69	31
Chimpanzee	7·6	29·8	70·2
Man	8·4	12	88

An examination of this table clearly reveals the increasing importance of the secondary zones of the motor cortex (the premotor area) in the organization of increasingly complex human skilled movements. Important information on the manner in which these zones participate in motor functions is provided by anatomical, physiological and clinical analysis.

Morphological studies have shown that the distribution of cells varies from one layer of the motor cortex to another. According to the Moscow Brain Institute in the primary motor area (Brodmann's area 4) a much larger number of cells is concentrated in cortical layer V (the effector layer), whereas there are comparatively few cells in layers II and III (the associative layers). Meanwhile, in the secondary, premotor zones of the motor cortex (Brodmann's area 6) the number of cells in the upper layers of the cortex rises sharply, and the number of cells in the same layers in the still more complex tertiary cortical zones (Brodmann's area 10) is even greater. These results, which are summarized in Table 6, clearly demonstrate this situation and reflect the increasing role of the premotor, and then of the prefrontal zones in the organization of complex human motor behaviour.

Table 6 **Total number of cells in individual layers of the primary, secondary and tertiary zones of the human motor cortex** (in millions) (after Moscow Brain Institute)

	Total number	Layers II–III	Layer IV	Layer V
Area 4	520	30		10·6
Area 6	511	275		80·6
Area 10	917	386	94	177

These hypotheses are also confirmed by physiological findings. Stimulation of the premotor cortex spreads over relatively large areas of the cortex and evokes integrated movements successively incorporating rotation of the eyes and head, followed by rotation of the trunk to the opposite side and grasping movements of the hands. Adversive epileptic fits of this type are caused by factors producing permanent irritation (scars, for example) in the premotor region.[1]

Accordingly the premotor cortex is the site of the system adapted for *integration of efferent (motor) impulses in time*. Whereas the postcentral cortical zones are responsible for the *spatial distribution of motor impulses*, the premotor zones, based on motor synergisms at lower levels, are responsible for the *conversion of individual motor impulses into consecutive kinetic melodies*, and they thus introduce a second essential component into the organization of complex motor skills.

It is now possible to look for the symptoms which arise in patients with lesions of the premotor zones. The classical observations of Fulton (1935; 1943) and later of other neurologists (Foerster, 1936; Kleist, 1934), and a series of my own investigations conducted in 1943 (published in 1963, 1947, 1962, 1963, 1969c and 1970a) have shown that lesions of the premotor cortex give rise neither to paralysis nor to paresis of the contralateral limbs. Their basic symptom

1. Woolsey (1958) supposed that the premotor zone preserves the same principles of functional organization as the motor zone; the only difference is that in the premotor zone proximal parts of the extremities are represented while in the motor zone there is a representation of the distal parts. But this idea of the identity of the principles of the organization of both motor and premotor zones is not yet established for the human brain cortex.

is a definite *disturbance of skilled movements*, which are *no longer performed smoothly*, and each component of the skilled movement now requires its own isolated impulse. Clinically, the patient's handwriting is altered and every stroke of a letter requires a special effort; the typist loses the speed and smoothness of her work, the musician cannot play a tune smoothly, and the skilled worker is unable to carry out automatically the successive system of operations constituting a habitual motor act.

From the physiological standpoint, the smooth process of succession of innervations and denervations is lost in this defect, the electromyographic impulses leading to the initiation of the move-

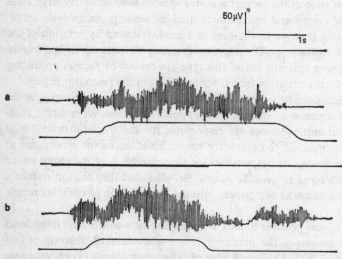

Figure 48 Pathological electromyogram and mechanogram in lesions of the premotor area: (a) disturbance of the initiation of movement (difficulty in activation); (b) disturbance of the end of movement (pathological inertia) (after Ioshpa and Homskaya)

ment become pathologically protracted, and they cannot be stopped at the correct time (Figure 48). The defect is manifested outwardly, in neuropsychological tests, as the patient's inability to perform a complex movement requiring a smooth succession of innervations, or to switch from one component of the movement to the next, so that the phenomena known to the clinican as '*inertia of motor stereotypes*'

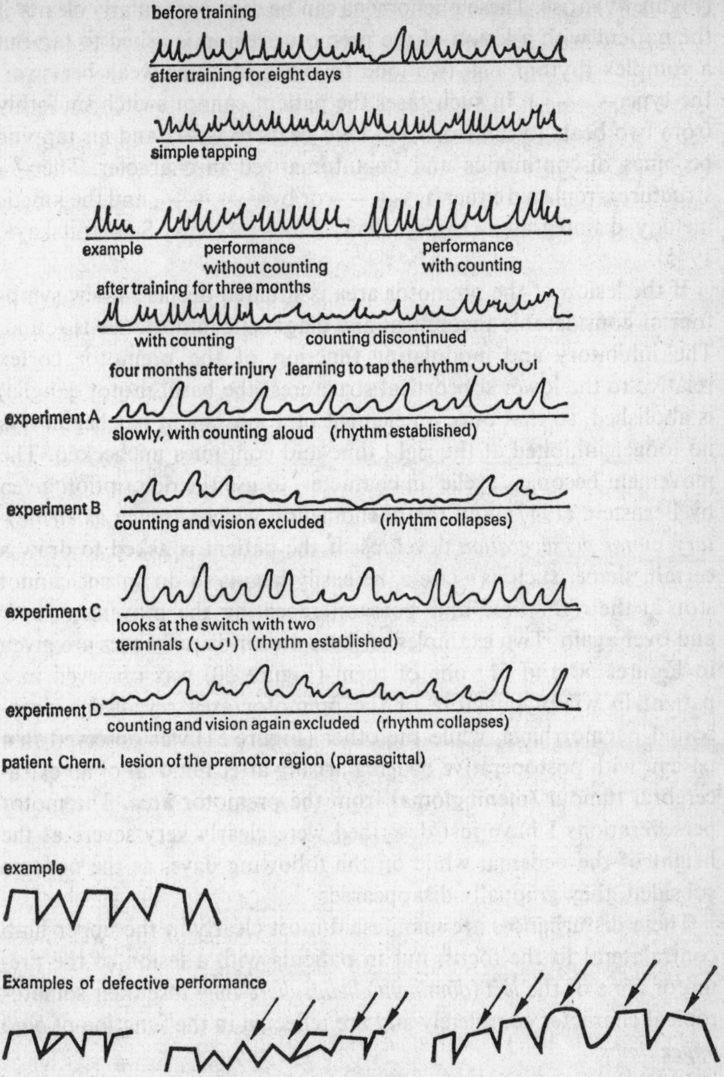

Figure 49 Inertia of elementary motor stereotypes during performance of graphic tests by patients with lesions of the premotor region

(Figure 49) arise. These phenomena can be seen particularly clearly if the patient with a lesion of the premotor region is asked to tap out a complex rhythm, e.g. two loud followed by three weak beats (of the type --... --...). In such cases the patient cannot switch smoothly from two beats to three or from loud beats to weak, and his tapping becomes discontinuous and de-automatized in character. The --... structure is replaced either by -- -- -- -- or by -- --- --- ---, and the kinetic melody disintegrates (Luria, 1963; 1966a; 1966b; Semernitskaya, 1945).

If the lesion of the premotor area is situated deeper, a new symptom of considerable theoretical and diagnostic importance is found. The inhibitory and modulating function of the premotor cortex relative to the lower subcortical structures (the basal motor ganglia) is abolished, so that once an element of a movement has begun it is no longer inhibited at the right time and continues unchecked. The movement becomes 'cyclic' in character, to use the description given by Bernstein (1947), and the phenomenon widely known as *elementary motor perseveration* develops. If the patient is asked to draw a certain shape, such as a circle, he easily begins to do so but cannot stop at the right time and goes on repeating the movement over and over again. Two examples of these motor disturbances are given in Figures 50 and 51: one of them (Figure 50) was observed in a patient in whom puncture of the premotor area revealed a deep-seated haemorrhage, while the other (Figure 51) was observed in a patient with postoperative oedema arising after removal of an extra-cerebral tumour (meningioma) from the premotor area. The motor perseverations I have just described were clearly very severe at the height of the oedema, while on the following days, as the oedema subsided, they gradually disappeared.

These disturbances are manifested most clearly in the upper limb contralateral to the focus, but in patients with a lesion of the premotor zone of the *left* (*dominant*) *hemisphere* they lose their somatotopical character completely and are reflected in the function of *both upper limbs*.

In all these cases, it is clear that the *intention* to perform the movement as well as the *general plan* of its execution remain intact, but the actual execution of the movement becomes freed from the restraining effect of the programme and all control over it is lost.

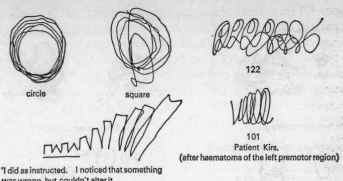

circle   square

122

101
Patient Kirs.
(after haematoma of the left premotor region)

'I did as instructed. I noticed that something
was wrong, but couldn't alter it.

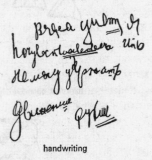

handwriting

Figure 50 Compulsive movements in drawing and writing in a patient
with a haematoma of the left premotor region: (a) drawings and
numbers; (b) writing

We must now examine a symptom of fundamental significance.
In cases in which the lesion affects the *inferior zones* of the premotor
area of the left (dominant) hemisphere the phenomena of disturbance
of the smooth switching from one motor element to another and the
appearance of pathological motor perseverations which I have just
described start to show more in the patient's speech than in the
movement of his hands, so giving rise to a distinctive phenomenon
which I prefer to call *efferent (or kinetic) motor aphasia* (Luria, 1947;
1962; 1966a; 1966b; 1966c; 1966d; 1970a). In contrast to the afferent
(kinaesthetic) asphasia already described, in this condition the discovery of the required articulations and the pronunciation of
individual, isolated sounds of speech present no appreciable difficulty to the patients.

a

second post-operative day

 circle

 triangle

third post-operative day

 circle

 triangle

fourth post-operative day

(near end of experiment, after 15 minutes)

circle

triangle

cross

circle

fifth post-operative day

 circle

 triangle

b

second post-operative day

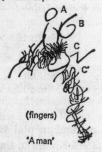

(fingers)

"A man"

A. draws head and trunk
B. draws a second man
C. draws sterotyped lines
C'. with the paper moving

third post-operative day

fingers

legs

fourth post-operative day

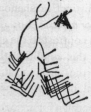

fifth post-operative day

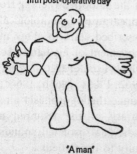

"A man"

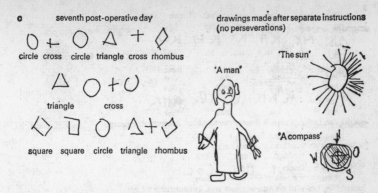

circle cross circle triangle cross rhombus

triangle   cross

square square circle triangle rhombus

drawings made after separate instructions
(no perseverations)

'A man'

'The sun'

'A compass'

Figure 51 Motor performance in the postoperative period (removal of a meningioma from the premotor area): (a) copying shapes (second-fifth days after operation); (b) drawing a man (the same days); (c) drawing shapes and a man on the seventh day after operation

The disturbance becomes apparent when such patients have to *switch from one articulation to another* (as when pronouncing a polysyllabic word or a combination of words). In this case the process of denervation of the preceding articuleme and the smooth switching to the next articuleme is profoundly disturbed, signs of *pathological inertia of an existing articulation* arise, and the smooth pronunciation of a polysyllabic word becomes impossible. In an attempt to pronounce the word 'mukha' the patient articulates the first (labial) syllable 'mu' properly, but cannot change to the next (retroglosso-laryngeal) syllable 'kha' and instead of the word required he can only say: 'mu. . . m . . . m . . . mu . . . ma'. This disturbance of the kinetic organization of articulations is the basis of the form of motor aphasia described originally by Broca (1861a; 1861b), which differs sharply in its physiological mechanisms from the 'aphraxic'afferent motor aphasia I have described.

Disturbances of this type are found not only in the spoken speech of patients with lesions of the lower zones of the left premotor region, but also in their *writing*, in which the order of the elements is lost and the smooth transition from one component of a word to another and the retention of the required sequence are impossible, and in which *the pathological perseveration of a word once written* is clearly apparent, so that these patients cannot write properly (Figure 52).

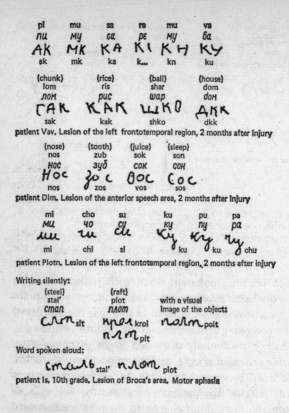

patient Vav. Lesion of the left frontotemporal region, 2 months after injury

patient Dim. Lesion of the anterior speech area, 2 months after injury

patient Plotn. Lesion of the left frontotemporal region, 2 months after injury

Writing silently:

Word spoken aloud:

patient Is. 10th grade. Lesion of Broca's area. Motor aphasia

Writing silently:

Writing a word spoken aloud:

okno (window)

patient Min. Engineer. Lesion of the right speech area (left-handed subject). Motor aphasia

Figure 52 Handwriting of patient with efferent (kinetic) motor aphasia

The study of the functions of the premotor cortical zones thus provides a clear insight into the mechanisms of one of the most complex of clinical phenomena: disturbance of the motor aspect of speech.

Chapter 7
The Frontal Lobes and the Regulation of Mental Activity

With the description of the functions of the motor cortex we have in fact begun the detailed analysis of the functional organization of the third principal brain unit; the one responsible for the programming, regulation and verification of human activity.

I have said that the frontal lobes of the brain and, in particular, their tertiary formations (including the prefrontal cortex) were the latest parts of the cerebral hemispheres to be formed, and that while they are hardly visible in lower animals, they become appreciably larger in primates, and in man they occupy up to one-quarter of the total mass of the cerebral hemispheres, but they do not attain maturity in the child until between four and seven years of age.

I also said that the prefrontal zones, or the frontal granular cortex, consist entirely of cells of the upper (associative) layers of the cortex, that they have the richest connections both with the upper parts of the brain stem and thalamic structures (Figure 15) and with all other cortical zones (Figure 16), and that they are thus superposed not only over the secondary zones of the motor cortex but also, in fact, over all the other formations of the brain. They thus possess bilateral connections both with the lower parts of the reticular formation, which modulates cortical tone, and also with the formations of the second brain unit which are responsible for the reception, analysis and storage of information, enabling the prefrontal zones to control both the general state of the cerebral cortex and the course of the fundamental forms of human mental activity.

In view of these two important functions of the frontal lobes it is perfectly logical to regard these structures as *tertiary zones* for the limbic system, on the one hand, and for the motor cortex on the other hand. These functions also enable us to understand the important role of the frontal lobes in the regulation of vigilance and in the control of the most complex forms of man's goal-linked activity. We shall now examine these two functions of the frontal lobes separately.

The function of the frontal lobes in the organization of behaviour has been studied closely by many workers. Their role in the organization of animal behaviour formed the subject of the classical investigation of Bekhterev (1905–7), Pavlov (1912–13; published 1949a; 1949b), Anokhin (1949), Bianchi (1895; 1921), Franz (1907), Jacobsen (1935), Malmo 1942), Pribram (1954–60), Rosvold (1956–9), Mishkin 1955–8) and others. The role of the frontal lobes in human behaviour has been analysed and investigated by Harlow (1968), Welt (1888), Khoroshko (1912; 1921), Feuchtwanger (1923), Kleist (1934), Brickner (1936), Rylander (1939), Hebb (1945, Halstead (1947), Denny-Brown (1951), Luria (1962; 1963; 1966a; 1966b), Luria and Homskaya (1963; 1966) and others. I shall now summarize briefly the results of our investigations.

The frontal lobes and regulation of states of activity

For any mental process to take place, a certain level of cortical tone is necessary and this cortical tone must be modified in accordance both with the task to be accomplished and the stage of the activity reached. The first important function of the frontal lobe is to regulate this state of activity.

I have mentioned above that each state of active expectancy arouses characteristic slow waves in the frontal regions of the brain, which Grey Walter has described as 'expectancy waves' (Figure 19) and that every active intellectual activity leads to the appearance of a large number of simultaneously working excited points (Figure 20). These facts are evidently closely connected with the activating role of speech, which formulates the problem or provides the special concentration necessary for some forms of intellectual activity.

It will naturally be expected that this *increase in cortical tone resulting from formulation of the problem* is disturbed in patients with a pathological lesion of the frontal cortex, and that a *disturbance of speech-based activation* is one of the principal results of a *frontal lobe lesion*.

This was the conclusion reached after long research by Homskaya and her collaborators (Homskaya, 1960; 1961; 1965; 1966a; 1972), Artemeva and Homskaya, 1966; Baranovskaya and Homskaya,

1966; Ioshpa and Homskaya, 1966; Simernitskaya and Homskaya, 1966; Simernitskaya, 1970). Let us briefly examine a few of their findings.

Any task associated with the appearance of an orienting reflex and requiring activation is known to evoke autonomic changes, manifested by constriction of the peripheral blood vessels and dilatation of the vessels of the head (Sokolov, 1958; Vinogradova, 1959a; 1959b), and a psychogalvanic reflex. This reflex continues until the subject becomes accustomed to the stimulus, and it disappears after interruption or successful performance of the task (Figure 53).

This appearance of autonomic components of the orienting reflex evoked by a spoken instruction is preserved in all patients with lesions of the posterior zones of the brain (Figure 54a); however, in patients with lesions of the prefrontal zones (and, in particular, the medial zones of the frontal cortex) it either becomes very unstable or it completely fails to arise (Figure 54b). This points to an important fact: *the frontal lobes participate in the regulation of the activation processes lying at the basis of voluntary attention.*

Similar facts are revealed by the use of *electrophysiological* methods. Under normal conditions the presentation of any complex task requiring increased attention arouses changes in the electrical activity of the brain which have been described as 'desynchronization' or 'depression of the alpha-rhythm'. In such cases the electrical waves with a frequency of 8–10 per second known as the alpha-rhythm are depressed whereas the faster waves are increased in amplitude.

These changes in the frequency spectrum of the electroencephalogram arising in response to any spoken instruction requiring increased attention (for example, in response to the command to count the number of signals, to look out for changes in signals, and so on) are manifested in every normal subject and also, to a certain extent, in every patient with a lesion of the posterior zones of the cortex (Figure 55a). However, as Baranovskaya and Homskaya (1966a) showed, these changes in the frequency spectrum of the EEG, which are still found in patients with lesions of the posterior zones of the brain (Figure 55b), either *are absent* in patients with lesions of the frontal zones of the brain or they are highly unstable and disappear rapidly (Figure 55c).

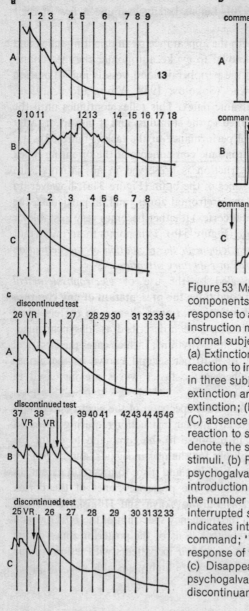

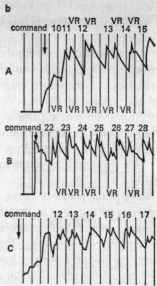

Figure 53 Manifestation of autonomic components of the orienting reflex in response to a corresponding spoken instruction mobilizing attention in normal subjects (after Homskaya). (a) Extinction of the psychogalvanic reaction to interrupted sounds (60 dB) in three subjects. Three types of extinction are shown: (A) rapid extinction; (B) prolonged extinction; (C) absence of a psychogalvanic reaction to sound. The numbers denote the serial numbers of the stimuli. (b) Restoration of arousal psychogalvanic reactions after introduction of the command to count the number of sounds in each interrupted stimulus. The arrow indicates introduction of the command; 'V.R.' denotes verbal response of the subject. (c) Disappearance of arousal psychogalvanic reactions after discontinuance of the test

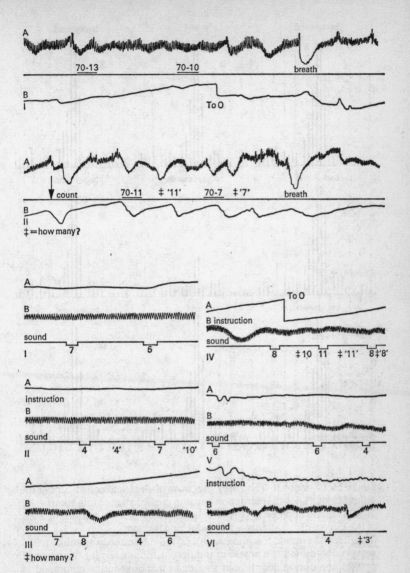

Figure 54 Regulation of autonomic components of the orienting reflex by the spoken command 'count the sounds' in patients with lesions of (A) the posterior and (B) the frontal zones of the brain (after Homskaya)

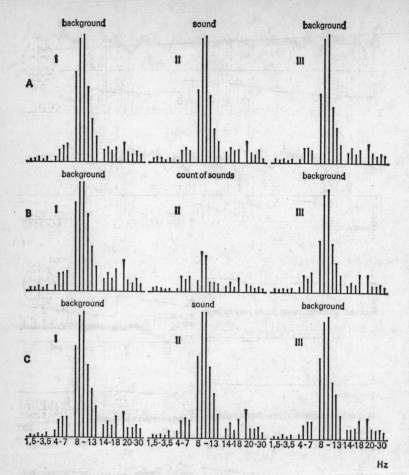

Figure 55 Changes in frequency spectrum of electrical activity under the influence of a spoken instruction causing mobilization of attention: (a) in a normal subject; (b) in patients with lesions of the posterior zones of the brain; (c) in patients with frontal lobe lesions (after Homskaya and Baranovskaya). (a) E E G frequency spectrum at rest (1) and during the action of indifferent sounds (2); (b) the same at rest (1) and during counting of sounds in response to the command (2) (c) changes in the frequency spectrum of the E E G relative to the background, taken at 100 per cent. Broken line: response to indifferent sounds; continuous line: response to informative sounds (action on a command to count the sounds)

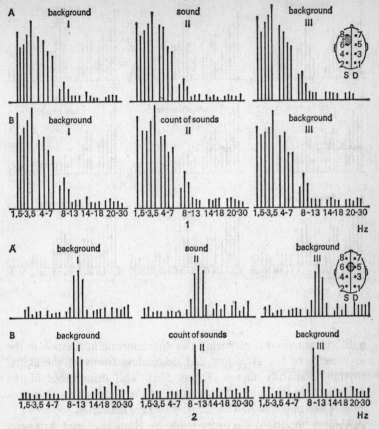

Figure 55 – continued

Electrophysiological studies in recent years have discovered yet another important and objective indicator of cortical activation. As Genkin (1962; 1963; 1964) has shown, the structure of the alpha-waves of a normal person, in a state of rest, fluctuates periodically: the relationship between the ascending and descending front of the alpha-waves varies (the length of the ascending front sometimes exceeds that of the descending front, sometimes is equal to it, sometimes is less), and these fluctuations are regular in character and follow each other in cycles lasting six to seven seconds. However, as soon as the subject's attention is activated (if, for example, he is given

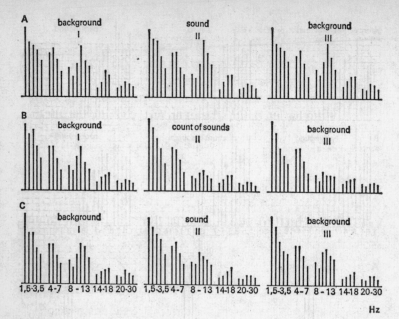

A background I | sound II | background III

B background I | count of sounds II | background III

C background I | sound II | background III

1,5-3,5 4-7 8 - 13 14-18 20-30   1,5-3,5 4-7 8 - 13 14-18 20-30   1,5-3,5 4-7 8 - 13 14-18 20-30

Hz

Figure 55 – continued

a difficult intellectual problem), this characteristic fluctuation in the asymmetry of the ascending and descending fronts of the alpha-rhythm is sharply altered (Figure 56a). This disturbance of the periodicity in the index of fluctuation of the alpha-waves thus provides a *new and objective indicator of cortical activation*.

A most important discovery made by Homskaya and Artemeva (Artemeva and Homskaya, 1966; Homskaya, 1972) was that this phenomenon of disturbance of asymmetry of the fronts of the alpha-waves under the influence of a spoken instruction evoking more intensive intellectual activity is preserved in patients with lesions of the posterior zones of the brain (Figure 56b), but either disappears completely or becomes unstable in patients with lesions of the frontal lobes (Figure 56c).

It now remains to give a brief description of the last indicator providing objective evidence of activation of cortical function. Physiological investigations have shown (Dawson, 1958a; Monnier, 1956; Jouvet and Courrion, 1958; Peimer, 1958) that the application

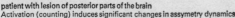

patient with lesion of posterior parts of the brain
Activation (counting) induces significant changes in assymetry dynamics

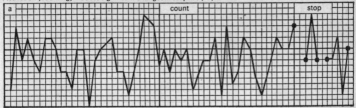

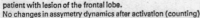

patient with lesion of the frontal lobe.
No changes in assymetry dynamics after activation (counting)

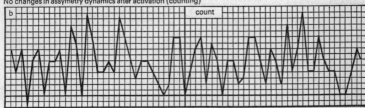

Figure 56 Changes in asymmetry of the ascending and descending fronts of the alpha-waves under the influence of an activating instruction mobilizing the subject's attention: (a) in a patient with lesion of the posterior part zones of the brain; (b) in a patient with lesions of the frontal lobes (after Homskaya and Artemeva)

of a stimulus evokes changes in electrical activity known as evoked potentials in the corresponding cortical zones and that these potentials are modified if the subject's attention is activated by a spoken command.

A new fact revealed by the work of Simernitskaya (Simernitskaya and Homskaya, 1966; Simernitskaya, 1970) is that these evoked potentials are considerably strengthened in normal conditions under the influence of a spoken command (for example, the command to wait for a given signal or to look out for changes in its nature); the same phenomenon is observed in patients with lesions of the posterior zones of the brain (Figure 57a); however, in patients with lesions of the frontal lobes this increase is either absent or is very unstable (Figure 57b).

In all the cases described above a *lesion of the frontal lobes disturbs only the higher, cortical forms of activation brought about by the aid*

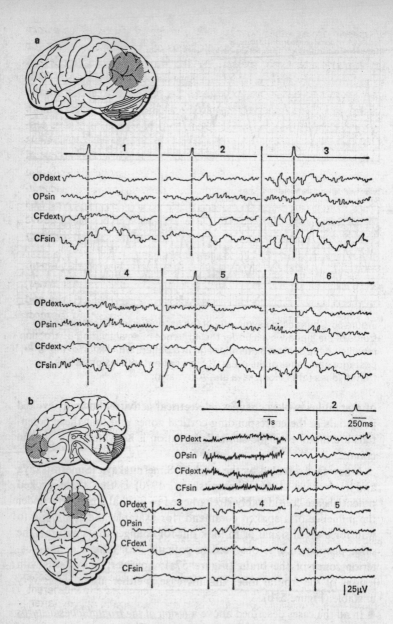

of speech or, in other words, *only the higher forms of voluntary attention are disturbed*; elementary forms of the orienting reflex (or involuntary attention), evoked by the direct effect of irrelevant stimuli, not only remain intact but may actually be enhanced. This fact can be clearly observed either by keeping careful watch on the behaviour of patients with frontal lobe lesions, who are much more easily distracted than normal subjects and cannot control this tendency, and also by analysis of the results of physiological experiments showing that both the autonomic and the electrophysiological indices of the orienting reflex, which disappear on the presentation of a spoken command, *remain intact in response to direct unconditioned stimuli* (for example, taking a breath, coughing, opening and closing the eyes and so on), and that the phenomena described above are thus connected with a *disturbance of only the higher forms of activation controlled with the aid of speech.*

We can summarize the facts just described. They show conclusively that the *frontal lobes (and, in particular, their medial zones) constitute the cortical apparatus regulating the state of activity and* that they thus play a decisive role in the maintenance of one of the most important conditions of *human conscious activity* – the *maintenance of the required cortical tone and modification of the state of waking in accordance with the subject's immediate tasks.*

The frontal lobes and regulation of movements and actions

Maintenance of the optimal cortical tone is absolutely essential for the basic condition of all forms of conscious activity, namely the

Figure 57 Changes in evoked potentials in response to a spoken instruction mobilizing active attention: (a) in patients with lesions of the posterior zones of the brain. Introduction of a spoken instruction leads to the gradual restoration of normal cortical responses, not only in the intact zones of the brain but even in the zone of the pathological focus; (b) in patients with lesions of the frontal lobes. Introduction of a spoken instruction causes no change in the character of bioelectrical activity: in response to both informative and indifferent stimuli the EP never exceed the level of the background activity (after Simernitskaya)

formation of plans and intentions that are stable enough to become dominant and to withstand any distracting or irrelevant stimulus.

The frontal lobes, which have such an important role in the regulation of the optimal cortical tone, therefore constitute an apparatus with the function of forming stable plans and intentions capable of controlling the subject's subsequent conscious behaviour. Observations on patients with sufficiently large lesions of the frontal lobes give clear evidence of this role.

The disturbance of plans and intentions in patients with massive lesions of the frontal lobes can be clearly seen by carefully observing their general behaviour. Patients with the largest frontal lobe lesions, associated with marked perifocal or general cerebral changes (for example, patients with massive tumours of the frontal lobes, accompanied by general hypertensive or toxic manifestations) usually lie completely passively, express no wishes or desires and make no requests; not even a state of hunger can rouse them to take the necessary action. The apathico-akinetico-abulic syndrome which clinicians have described as the most typical consequence of massive lesions of the frontal lobes reflects the maximal disturbance of the higher forms of activation of behaviour and it is the key to the understanding of dysfunction of these zones of the brain.

However, it must not be thought that the apathico-akinetico-abulic syndrome reflects a disturbance of *all* forms of behaviour. As experience shows, in such patients it is only the *higher forms of organization of conscious activity* that are significantly disturbed, and the more elementary levels of their activity remain unaffected. This is clearly revealed by observation of their *orienting reactions to irrelevant stimuli, unconnected with their intention*. Such elementary forms of responses as a rule not only are undisturbed, but sometimes they may actually be more brisk or even pathologically intensified.

Such patients cannot complete their tasks, cannot reply to questions and apparently do not pay proper attention to any one speaking to them. If, however, while the patient is being tested the door squeaks or the nurse comes into the ward, his eye will invariably turn in that direction, he will follow the nurse's movements, and sometimes he may actually reply involuntarily to her conversation with another patient. If the physician begins to question not himself, but his neighbour, the patient will at once join in this conversation, and experienced physicians know well that the best way of prompting such a patient's speech activity is by addressing his neighbour and starting a conversation with him. The patient will join in such a conversation much more easily than he will reply to direct questioning. This fact clearly shows that *massive lesions of the frontal lobes disturb only the most complex forms of regulation of conscious activity* and, in particular, *activity which is controlled by motives formulated with the aid of speech* (Luria, 1966a, 1966b; 1969a; 1969b).

Disturbance of the function of the frontal lobes may lead to the *disintegration of complex programmes of activity* and to their ready replacement either by *simpler and more basic forms of behaviour*, or by the repetition of inert stereotypes, neither relevant to the situation nor logical in character.

Suppose a patient with a massive frontal lobe lesion is asked to lift his hand. If his hand is resting on the bedclothes and thus ready to carry out the action, the required movement may be performed normally. In the case of a patient with a marked disturbance of active, voluntary behaviour he will very quickly cease to carry out his assigned programme: to begin with his hand will perform slow movements, but these will then become gradually smaller in amplitude, and while he continues to repeat: 'Yes, yes, lift your hand . . .,' he will soon cease to perform the required movement.

The disintegration of voluntary action is much more obvious if the command is given to the patient when his hand is *under the bedclothes*. In that case, the adequate performance of the action requires a more complex programme of movements, some of which are not contained in the instruction: the patient must *first* remove his hand from under the bedclothes, and *not until then* can he raise it. This complex programme is quite beyond the capacity of such a patient, and he repeats echolalically: 'Yes, yes . . . raise your hand . . .' but does not carry out the movement.

Very frequently actions required by a spoken command are not retained by the patient and are replaced by more habitual and more firmly established actions. One such patient, for instance, when asked to light a candle, struck a match correctly but instead of putting it to the candle which he held in his hand, he put the candle in his mouth and started to 'smoke' it like a cigarette. The new and relatively unstabilized action was thus replaced by the more firmly established inert stereotype. I have observed such disturbances of a complex action programme and its replacement by elementary, basic behaviour in many patients with a clearly defined 'frontal syndrome'. One patient, for example, on seeing the button operating a bell, was involuntarily drawn to it and pressed it, and when the nurse came in response to the bell, he was unable to say why he had done so. Another such patient, who had been given permission to leave the consulting room of the physician examining him, got up and, when he saw the open door of a cupboard, went into the cupboard, thus showing the same type of impulsive, stereotyped behaviour. A third patient with a similarly well-marked frontal syndrome, whom I send into the ward to fetch his cigarettes, began to carry out this instruction but when he met a group of patients coming towards him, turned round and then followed them, although he still clearly remembered the instruction which he had been given.

In all these patients the *verbal command remained in their memory, but it no longer controlled the initiated action and lost its regulating influence.* Such disturbances of an assigned programme of action often affected the behaviour of these patients in more complex and responsible situations. I shall never forget one patient with a marked frontal syndrome who, after being discharged from hospital, expressed the wish to go home but, while he was still some tens of kilometres away from home he followed the example of his companion and settled in a small town there in order to start work in a shoe factory. Hence, neither spoken instructions given to these patients nor their own intentions any longer provide a stable programme for their behaviour, and their regulatory function is lost.

It is easy to examine the intrinsic mechanisms of this disturbance of behaviour under experimental conditions. Suppose a patient with a massive frontal lesion and well-marked frontal syndrome (but with a less marked form of inactivity) is asked to lift his hand, reproducing the corresponding movement made by the physician examining him. This *imitative* or *echopraxic* action is performed by the patient without difficulty. If, however, the patient is given a conventional spoken command which clashes with the signal perceived directly, he has considerable difficulty in obeying the instruction. This occurs, for example, if such a patient receives a 'conflicting' instruction such as: 'when I raise my fist you must raise your finger'. In this case the patient who has to recode the directly perceived signal and to control his action not in accordance with the signal he perceives directly but with its conventional meaning, cannot obey the spoken command. Having raised his finger once he immediately begins to raise his fist echopraxically, thus replacing the action required by the command by an *echopraxic movement*. Characteristically in this case also the patient easily remembers and can repeat the spoken command, but it rapidly loses its controlling value and is replaced by the elementary imitative movement. A similar phenomenon can be seen if the patient is instructed to tap twice in response to one signal and to tap once in response to two signals or to give a long squeeze in response to a short signal and a short squeeze in response to a long signal. Observations (Homskaya, 1966b; Maruszewski, 1966) have shown that patients with even a relatively ill-defined frontal syndrome can carry out this instruction correctly only for a very short time and it is very quickly replaced by imitative (echopraxic) repetition of the directly perceived signal (Figure 58).

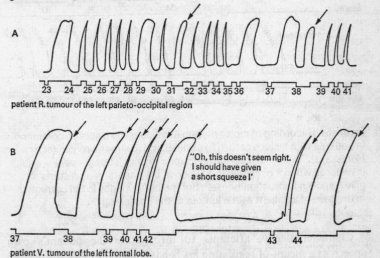

patient R. tumour of the left parieto-occipital region

patient V. tumour of the left frontal lobe.

Figure 58 Echopraxic character of motor responses of a patient with a massive tumour of the left frontal lobe (after Maruszewski). In response to a short signal the patient must squeeze slowly, and in response to a long signal he must squeeze rapidly. Instead of the response required, the movement matches the signal. In A that is possible but in B it becomes impossible and is replaced by echopraxic reaction

Frontal Lobes and Regulation of Mental Activity 201

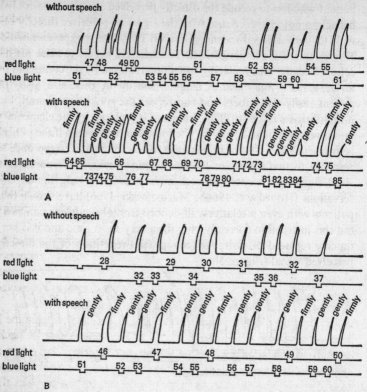

Figure 59 Recording of motor rhythm in response to a spoken command in patients with lesions of the (A) parietal and (B) frontal region (after Homskaya). The correct performance of a rhythm 'strong – weak – weak' is restored when a patient with a lesion of the parietal region starts to give a spoken instruction himself, but the performance is not corrected in the case of a patient with a tumour of the frontal region

Characteristically, attempts to incorporate the patient's own speech as a means of regulating his behaviour do not give the desired results. The patient either repeats the command correctly to himself, but does not subordinate his movement to it, or his own speech itself falls under the influence of the pathological inertia and the command given to the patient is disorganized.

An example of such a case is given in Figure 59, which shows that whereas a patient with a parietal lesion who has difficulty in reproducing rhythmic movements (pressing strongly once and weakly twice) can correct this defect successfully by giving the command himself (Figure 59a), a patient with a massive frontal lobe lesion cannot do so, and even though he repeats the command correctly, he continues to press inertly in exactly the same way (Figure 59b).

An example of the second case is shown in Figure 60. A patient with a massive lesion of the left frontal lobe, when instructed to tap out the rhythm 'strong – weak – weak' could not do so but instead tapped out a continuous rhythm. When he changed to giving the instruction himself, the same inertia began to show itself in his speech and the number of elements of the spoken command gradually increased ('strong – weak – weak', 'strong – weak – weak', 'strong – weak – weak – weak . . .' and so on).

This change from the level of conventional actions controlled by speech to the much more elementary levels of direct echopraxic responses or disturbances of the programme of action by an inert stereotype is a typical symptom of the disturbance of goal-directed behaviour in patients with massive lesions of the frontal lobes.

This inability of the patient to stick to an assigned programme is seen more clearly still if the actions take place against the background of previously established *stereotypes*. This is clearly seen if the patient is asked to draw pictures in response to a spoken command. In tests of this sort the patient often starts to carry out the instruction but is quickly distracted from it and replaces it by uncontrollable associations. I shall give only two examples to illustrate this disturbance of the carrying out of programmes typical of patients with a marked frontal syndrome.

The records of an experiment which I carried out in conjunction with Professor Zeigarnik as long ago as in 1941 are shown in Figure 61a.

A patient with a traumatic cyst, replacing both frontal lobes, was asked to draw three squares. He did so, but then drew a line around the remainder of the sheet, making an additional large square. The person carrying out the test at that point said to his companion in a quiet voice: 'Did you read today in the newspaper that a pact had been concluded?' Hearing this word, the patient at once wrote inside

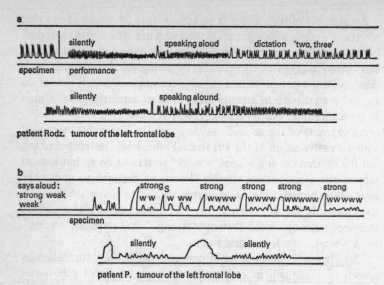

Figure 60 Disturbance of the regulatory influence of speech on the performance of motor rhythms in patients with extensive lesions of the frontal lobes. The patient is asked to reproduce the motor rhythm, one strong tap and two weak ones, silently and to the accompaniment of the speech reactions 'one, two, three' and 'strong, weak, weak'. (a) Saying the rhythm aloud ('one, two; one, two, three') does not lead to the desired effect. Dictation by the experimenter restores the motor rhythm. (b) Pathological inertia of the speech reactions during performance of motor rhythms (the number of repetitions of the auto-command 'weak' (W) is increased).When speech reactions are eliminated the motor rhythm disintegrates completely (after Knyazhev)

the large square the word 'Act No. ...'. The investigator then whispered to his companion: 'Look, this is exactly like in animals after extirpation of the frontal lobes ...'. On hearing the word 'animal' the patient wrote 'On animal breeding'. 'What is this patient's name?' – the experimenter asked his companion. The patient at once wrote in the square the name 'Ermolov'.

A similar example is illustrated in Figure 61b. A patient with a bilateral prefrontal tumour, a driver by occupation, was asked to draw two triangles and a minus sign. He did so, but drew the minus sign as a closed figure repeating the shape of the triangle. He was asked to draw a circle. He drew the circle, but at once drew a rect-

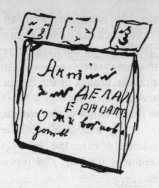

a

Patient Erm.   Injury to the frontal lobe with cyst formation

two triangles and a minus sign

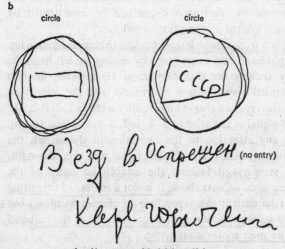

b

circle   circle

patient Vor.   tumor of the left frontal lobe

Figure 61 Disturbance of task completion programmes by patients with lesions of both frontal lobes

angle inside it and wrote the words: 'No entry', reproducing something firmly embedded in his past experience as a driver. Even when it was insisted that he draw only a circle, this did not have the required effect and he simply reproduced the same stereotype over again.

The inability of patients with massive lesions of the frontal lobes to carry out an assigned programme is evoked not only by the factors of 'basic behaviour', in which the performance of the programme is disturbed by direct impressions or by uncontrollable irrelevant associations. In almost the same number of cases the performance of a programme is disturbed in a different manner, and replaced by *uncontrollable floods of inert stereotypes.*

This fact indicates the responsible pathophysiological mechanism, namely pathological inertia of existing stereotypes. It explains the similarity between the symptoms of lesions of the prefrontal zones and lesions of the premotor area described above. The only significant difference is that, *whereas in lesions of the premotor zones the pathological inertia extends only to the effector components of the action,* and *performance of the programme as a whole is undisturbed, in massive lesions of the frontal lobes it extends to the scheme of the action itself, with the result that performance of the programme becomes impossible.* In its simplest forms this replacement of the assigned programme by inert stereotypes can be investigated by simple tests using a system of conditioned reflexes.

If a patient with a frontal lobe lesion is asked to respond to one tap by raising the right hand and to two taps by raising the left hand, he will easily begin to carry out this instruction. If, however, the two signals are presented several times alternately and the stereotype of alternation is then broken (for example, after a series 1–2, 1–2, 1–2 the order of the signal is changed to 1–2, 1–2, 2–1, 2–1 and so on), without paying any attention to the alteration in the signals the patient will continue to raise first the left hand, and then the right, reproducing in stereotyped fashion the established order of the movements. Here also, as tests show, it is not a matter of forgetting the instruction (the patient can reproduce its correct wording) but rather the *loss of its regulatory role* and replacement of the required programme by an inert motor stereotype.

The effects of such a lesion are seen most clearly in the *performance of graphic tests.* Examples of this type of disturbance of the carrying

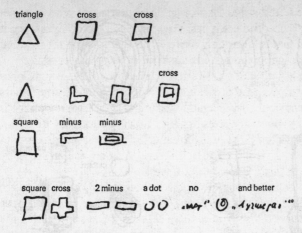

triangle   cross   cross

cross

square   minus   minus

square   cross   2 minus   a dot   no   and better

Patient K   Massive frontal injury

Figure 62 Disturbance of programme performance as a result of pathological inertia of previous stereotypes in a patient with a massive lesion of the frontal lobes

out of programmes are given in Figures 62 and 63.

The results obtained with one patient with a massive injury to the left frontal region, when instructed to draw certain objects, are shown in Figure 62. It is clear that the patient had no appreciable difficulty with the first drawing; sometimes he carried out the second task equally easily, although it was often impossible. However he was prevented from carrying out any subsequent tasks by the inert repetition of the established stereotype. Having once drawn a 'cross', the patient continued to draw it even when instructed to draw a 'circle', and the patient having drawn a 'circle' or 'square' he continued to repeat this action whatever the task given. Sometimes it is not the concrete figure, but a certain geometrical quality (for example, a 'closed' type of figure), which exhibits inert perseveration, and again the patient cannot perform the assigned programme correctly.

Characteristically in all these cases, by contrast with cases of deep-seated lesions of the premotor area involving the subcortical ganglia, there are no marked features of motor disinhibition or of uncontrolled superfluous strokes, and it is not *individual movements but the general forms of action* (for example, drawing closed geo-

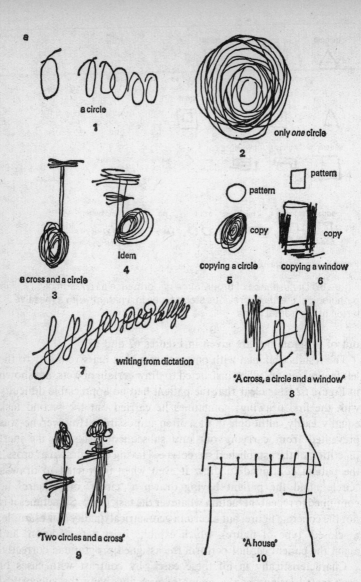

a

a circle
1

only *one* circle
2

a cross and a circle
3

idem
4

pattern

copy

copying a circle
5

pattern

copy

copying a window
6

writing from dictation
7

'A cross, a circle and a window'
8

'Two circles and a cross'
9

'A house'
10

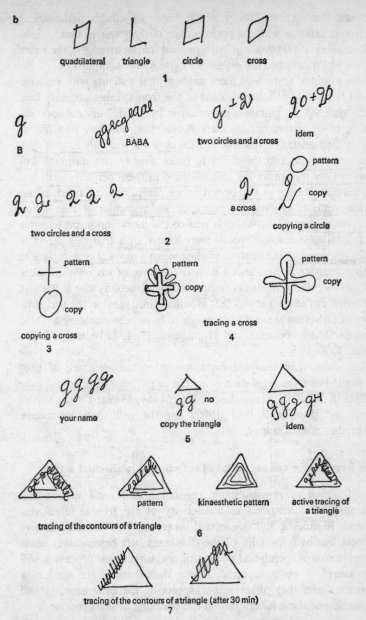

Figure 63 Two types of pathological inertia arising in cases of (a) deep lesions of the brain involving the basal motor ganglia, and (b) massive lesions of the lateral zones of the prefrontal region

metrical shapes, or writing) which begin to exhibit pathological inertia, interfering with the performance of the required task.

Examples of two types of pathological inertia arising in the cases I have just mentioned are given in Figure 63 for comparison.

The essential feature of these cases is that patients with massive (most frequently bilateral) lesions of the frontal lobes not only lose their assigned programme, replacing it by 'basic' or 'echopraxic' action or by pathologically inert stereotypes, but they also fail to notice their mistakes. In other words, *they lose not only control over their actions, but also the ability to check their results,* although frequently they remember the task assigned to them perfectly well.

This disturbance of the operation of comparing the result of an action with its original intention, or *disintegration of the 'action acceptor' function* (Anokhin) is one of the most important features of frontal lobe lesions. Special tests have shown that this defect is often restricted to the analysis of the patient's own actions. A patient with a massive frontal lesion who is unaware of his own mistakes will readily notice mistakes committed by somebody else if the test is carried out in such a way that identical 'mistakes' in the performance of an action are made to appear to have been made by a 'third person' (Luria, Pribram and Homskaya, 1964; Lebedinsky, 1966; Luria, 1970c).

The writer has analysed disturbances of the structure of programming and the regulation of action in patients with frontal lobe lesions in detail elsewhere (Luria, 1962; 1963; 1969a; 1969b; 1970c; Luria and Homskaya, 1963; 1966), and they will therefore receive no further attention here.

The frontal lobes and regulation of mnestic and intellectual actions

The function of programming, regulation and verification which has just been described as an activity of the frontal lobes also extends to mnestic and intellectual processes. The fact that massive frontal lesions (especially of the dominant, left hemisphere) cause disturbances of speech and of mnestic and intellectual processes, will not therefore be unexpected. These disturbances are similar in character and they affect some aspects of the programming and regulation of these functions and the checking of their course.

Frontal lesions do not disturb the phonetic lexical or logical-grammatical functions of speech as do the lesions I have already described. However, they give rise to a severe disturbance of a *different function of speech, namely its regulatory function*; the patient can no longer direct and control his behaviour with the aid of speech, either his own or that of another person.

The genesis of the regulatory function of speech and its disturbances in cases of abnormal development or pathological lesions of the frontal lobes have been discussed by the writer elsewhere (Luria, 1959b; 1960; 1963; 1969a; 1969b; 1970a; 1970b; Luria and Homskaya, 1963; 1966) and they will not be examined specially here.

Disturbances of a special kind are observed in the *mnestic activity* of patients with frontal lesions. Contrary to many of the views expressed in the literature, lesions of the frontal lobes do not cause primary disturbances of memory; this is apparent from the fact that firmly established stereotypes are preserved for a long time in patients with such lesions. However, in these cases another aspect of mnestic activity is substantially impaired: the ability to create *stable motives* of recall and to maintain the *active effort* required for voluntary recall, on the one hand, and the ability to *switch from one group of traces to another*, with the result that it is the process of recall and reproduction of material which is significantly impaired. It can thus be said that in frontal lobe lesions it is not the primary basis of the memory, but *complex mnestic activity as a whole* that is disturbed.

The basic features distinguishing the disturbances of mnestic activity in frontal lobe lesions are brought to light by simple tests of ability to learn by heart long series of spoken or written elements. As a rule the normal subject can fix such a mnestic problem firmly in his mind, make the necessary effort to memorize the particular series, and if he is unable to memorize the whole series at once, he makes a start so that with each repetition the number of elements which he reproduces grows steadily.

This does not happen with patients with frontal lesions. As a rule such a patient easily retains as many elements of the series presented as create a direct impression without the need for effort (from a series of ten words, four or five elements can be remembered in this way); however, despite frequent presentations of the complete series the number of words which he can reproduce does not increase but remains constantly at the level of four or five. If the process of memorizing is represented by a curve, with the number of repeated presentations plotted on the abscissa and the number of words reproduced each time along the ordinate, the graph for a patient with a frontal lobe lesion shows a distinctive plateau, characteristic of an inactive type of mnestic process (Figure 64).

Defects of mnestic activity in patients with frontal lobe lesions are seen more clearly in tests requiring the switching from reproduction of one group of traces to another group. For example, the patient may be asked to reproduce a short series of words (for example, house – forest – cat), and then a second similar series of words (for example, oak – night – table), after which he is asked to recall the first series. This test shows that the traces of the last series of words (oak – night – table) are so inert that the patient cannot revert to the first series, and in response to the request to recall it he begins inertly to reproduce the last series without any hesitation.

In patients with the most massive frontal lobe lesions the same defect is found also in the reproduction of phrases. For example, after such a patient had repeated the phrase ' the girl drinks tea' and then the phrase 'the boy hit the dog', and was asked to recall the first phrase he persisted in repeating 'the boy hit the dog' or 'the boy . . . drinks tea'. The number of these perseverations during attempts to reproduce the first structure after presentation of the second is more than twice as great in patients with frontal lobe lesions than in patients with lesions of the posterior zones of the brain.

I have investigated disturbances of this type in many cases (Luria *et al.*, 1970; Luria, 1973) and shall not therefore analyse them in detail here.

As a rule disturbances of the same character are observed in the *intellectual activity* of patients with frontal lobe lesions, ranging from the simplest and most direct forms to the most complex types of abstract, discursive activity. In all these cases the retention of a complex and consecutive programme for the intellectual act is disturbed. The patient either substitutes a series of impulsive, fragmentary guesses for true intellectual activity, or reproduces inert stereotypes instead of the adequate and adaptable programme of the intellectual act. I shall give a few examples to illustrate the character of the impairment of intellectual activity found in patients with frontal lesions.

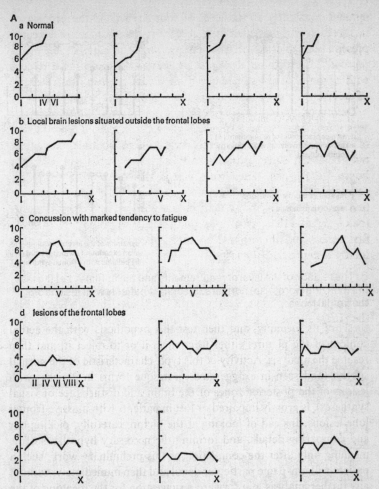

Figure 64 A: Memorizing curves showing learning of a series of ten words: (a) by a normal subject, and (b) by patients with lesions outside the frontal lobes, (c) by patients with concussion and easily fatigued, (d) by patients with lesions of the frontal lobes

The simplest form of intellectual operation based on visual perception is the analysis of the meaning of *thematic pictures*. To understand the meaning of such a picture the subject must distinguish its details, compare them with each other, formulate a definite hypo-

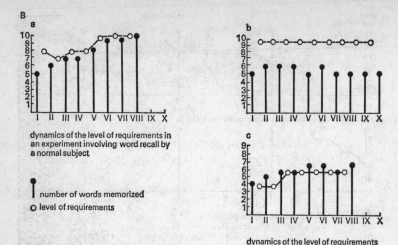

B

a

dynamics of the level of requirements in an experiment involving word recall by a normal subject

● number of words memorized
○ level of requirements

b

c

dynamics of the level of requirements in an experiment involving word recall by patients with a frontal syndrome

B: The relation of the level of requirements and the fulfilment of the task (memorizing words): (a) normal subjects; (b) patients with lesions of the frontal lobes

thesis of its meaning, and then test this hypothesis with the actual content of the picture, either to confirm it or to reject it, and then resume the analysis. Activity of this type, characteristic of the normal subject (and seen in exaggerated, grotesque forms in patients with lesions of the posterior zones of the brain and disturbance of visual syntheses), is grossly impaired or lost in patients with massive frontal lobe lesions. Instead of looking at the picture carefully, picking out and comparing details, and forming the necessary hypothesis of its meaning only after the completion of this preliminary work, such a patient will grasp one particular detail and then immediately, without any further analysis, put forward a suggestion for the meaning of the picture as a whole. If the picture is at all complex in composition, this impulsive hypothesis must of course be wrong, but the lack of effective verification by comparing the hypothesis with the actual information given by the picture prevents any misgivings regarding the validity of the hypothesis or, what is more, prevents the possibility of correction of mistaken ideas.

The example given in Figure 65 clearly illustrates what I have just said. A patient with a frontal lobe lesion is shown the picture of a

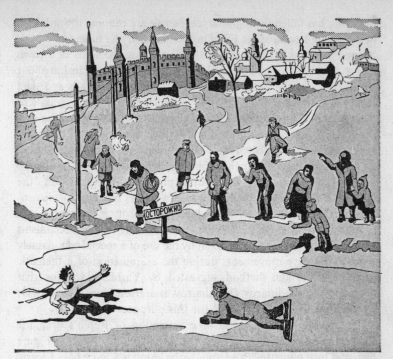

Figure 65 Thematic picture used to investigate disturbances of constructive thinking in patients with lesions of the frontal lobes

man who has fallen through the ice. People are running towards him in an attempt to save his life. On the ice, near the hole, is a notice 'danger'. In the background of the picture are the walls of a town and a church. Before the normal person reaches his conclusion about the meaning of the picture he first examines all its details and then makes his decision. The situation is quite different with a patient with a frontal lobe lesion. Instead of analysing the picture he sees the notice 'danger' and immediately concludes: 'the zoo' or 'high-voltage cables' or 'infected area'. Having seen the policeman running to save the drowning man, he immediately exclaims: 'war', while the walls of the town with the church prompt the explanation 'the Kremlin'. Analysis of the picture in this case is replaced by elementary guesswork, and organized intellectual activity is impossible.

An important step towards the understanding of the mechanisms of these disturbances can be taken by the use of a special test, namely by recording eye movements during the examination of a thematic picture. Either the method suggested by Yarbus (1965) or that developed by Vladimirov (Vladimirov and Homskaya, 1962; 1969; Vladimirov, 1972) can be used for this purpose.

The details of the process of examination of Repin's dramatic picture *Unexpected Return* by a normal person are shown in Figure 66a, and by a patient with a frontal lobe lesion in Figure 66b. Clearly each change in the problem presented to a normal subject changes the direction of his searches and his eye movements assume a different character. For instance, if he is asked about the age of the people represented in the picture, his eye fixes on their heads, if about how they are dressed, it fixes on their clothing, if asked whether the family is poor or well off, it fixes on the surroundings; and if asked how long the person returning home was imprisoned, the subject's eye actively begins to compare the ages of all the persons portrayed in the picture.

Nothing of the sort is observed when a patient with a massive frontal lesion examines the picture. To begin with he fixes on any point on it and immediately answers the question by the first guess which comes into his head, without attempting to deduce the answer from an analysis of the details of the picture. He therefore glances over the picture at random, and a change in the question put to him results in no change whatever in the direction of his fixation.

These observations indicate a *profound disturbance of the analysis of visual perception in massive lesions of the frontal lobes*, and the disintegration of the programme of analysis and synthesis can be seen as the basic mechanism of this disturbance.

Patients with frontal lesions show still greater disturbances in tests involving the *solution of verbal problems*, of two types in particular: the solution of arithmetical problems requiring the constant switching from one operation to another, and tests involving the solution of ordinary school exercises with a complex structure. The results obtained in both cases by tests on patients with frontal lesions are so interesting that we shall now consider each of them specially.

The most suitable method of investigating defects of arithmetical operations in patients with frontal lesions is by means of tests involving *long series of calculations*, typical examples of which are counting backwards from a hundred in sevens or in thirteens. In these cases, the diminuend is constantly changing, and the result obtained in one stage becomes the diminuend in the next. Add to this the fact that each operation frequently involves carrying over from the tens' column, and the breaking up of the number subtracted into its parts (when rounding off during the intermediate operations), and it will easily be seen how the correct performance of this exercise demands considerable mobility of the nervous processes.

The actual arithmetical operations present no special difficulty to patients with a frontal syndrome, which distinguishes them from patients with lesions of the parieto-occipital systems and disturbance of simultaneous syntheses. However, they are quite unable to switch from one type of calculation to another, and they are therefore readily distracted from performing the correct programme, which is either replaced by fragments of the necessary operations (for example, the typical mistake $93 - 7 = 84$, resulting from the omission of one of the intermediate operations: $7 = 3+4$; $93 - 3 = 90$; carry one from the tens' column (80) and transfer the remaining component 4 directly (84); or the constantly changing series of operations is replaced by an inert stereotype, so that the operation of counting backwards is converted into the inert repetition of the same final number ($100 - 7 = 93 \ldots 83 \ldots 73 \ldots 63 \ldots$ and so on).

Patients who replace the performance of a complex programme by

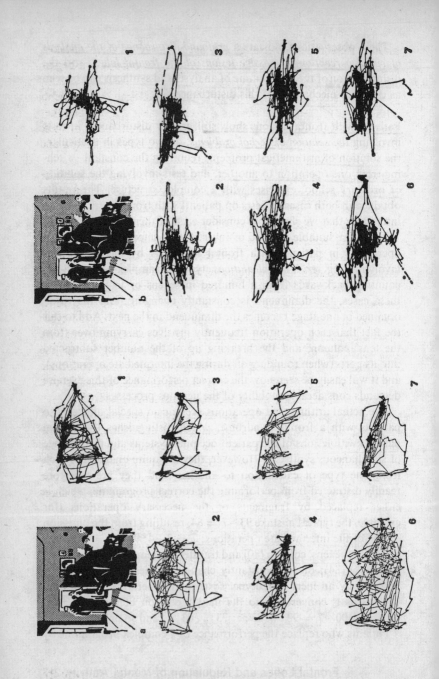

an inert stereotype characteristically are not aware of their mistakes, and they continue to reproduce the stereotype, once it has begun, without any attempt at correction.

The whole process of disturbance of intellectual activity of patients with lesions of the frontal lobes is even more clearly seen when they attempt to solve *complex problems*, and the characteristics of these defects have been fully examined by the writer elsewhere (Luria and Tsvetkova, 1967).

The process of solution of such problems, which we shall consider in detail, is a typical model of intellectual activity. The conditions of the problem are such that there is no ready answer to it, and the subject must first analyse the component elements of the conditions, formulate a definite strategy for the solution, carry out the operations required by this strategy, and then compare the results with the original conditions. It is this complex process of *formation and execution of a programme* which is beyond the power of a patient with a frontal lobe lesion. If the problem is simple and the method of its solution unambiguous (as, for example, in a problem of the type: 'Jack has three apples and Jill has four apples. How many apples have they together?'), its solution presents no difficulty. If however, the problem is more complex and a programme of action must be formed for its solution, and the necessary operation must be chosen from a number of possibilities, the situation is considerably altered.

As a rule, having read the conditions of the problem, the patient is unable to *repeat* them correctly, but usually omits the most important part of the problem, namely its final question, or replaces the question by inert reproduction of one of the conditions (for example, he is asked to repeat the problem 'There were eighteen books on two shelves, but they were not equally divided: there were twice as many

Figure 66 Eye movements during examination of Repin's picture
The Unexpected Visitor accompanied by different instructions:
(a) normal subject; (b) patient with massive lesion of the frontal lobes
(after Luria, Karpov, and Yarbus). (1) Specimen; (2) Free observation;
(3) after the question: 'is the family poor or rich?'; (4) 'how old are
the people in the picture?'; (5) 'what were they doing before the man
entered the room?'; (6) 'can you recall how the people were
dressed?'; (7) 'how were the people and furniture placed in the
room?'; (8) 'how long had the man been away from his family?'

books on one shelf as on the other. How many books were there on each shelf?' His version was 'There were eighteen books on two shelves, and twice as many on one as on the other. How many books were there on both shelves?'). This demonstrates the disintegration of the patient's retention of the problem itself.

However, even the correct repetition of the conditions of the problem does not enable a correct solution to be obtained. Having correctly repeated the conditions of the problem, the patient with a frontal lobe lesion cannot form the required programme (or strategy) for its solution, and instead of a logical, consecutive solution of the problem he substitutes fragmentary operations not subordinated to the general plan. For example, he begins to 'solve' the problem stated above with the words: 'Of course . . . eighteen books . . . on one shelf and twice as many . . . that means 36 . . . 36+18 = 54.' The attempt to arouse the patient's misgivings about the correctness of his 'solution' is ineffective. He does not compare his operations with the original conditions, he does not notice the contradiction between the original conditions and the results obtained, and he cannot, unaided, follow the course of consecutive performance of an intellectual act in conformity with a given programme.

The only way in which the patient can be helped to solve the problem, as Tsvetkova (1966a; 1966b; 1966c; 1972) has shown, is by analysing the necessary programme into a series of consecutive questions and by providing external supports for each component of the programme. However, even this method can be very difficult for a patient with a frontal lobe lesions, and the slightest attempt to contract this system of external supports leads once again to disintegration of the intellectual act (Tsvetkova, 1972).

Disturbance of the solution of complex problems is, of course, a most delicate test for the diagnosis of frontal lobe lesions, and the disintegration of intellectual activity of the type I have described reflects in the clearest manner possible the fundamental role played by the frontal lobes of the brain in the construction of human conscious activity.

Functional organization of the frontal lobes and alternative forms of the frontal syndrome

The frontal lobes are the most recent and, as Jackson (1874) called them, the 'least organized' structure of the cerebral cortex, implying by this term that they are the least differentiated part and their individual zones are the most capable of replacing one another. For these reasons, comparatively inextensive lesions of the prefrontal cortex can be compensated by neighbouring areas, and they may pursue an almost asymptomatic clinical course (Hebb, 1945; Hebb and Penfield, 1940).

That is why disturbances produced by a lesion of the frontal lobes are manifested most clearly in the case of massive, bilateral lesions complicated by disorganization of general brain activity (as, for example, when symptoms of general hypertension or toxic manifestations are present). However, this does not imply that lesions of all parts of the frontal lobe give rise to the same pattern of disturbances or that the frontal lobes constitute a single undifferentiated entity.

The functional organization of the frontal lobes and of their individual zones has been inadequately studied, and we can therefore examine only some of the most general features of those alternative forms of the frontal syndrome which arise in lesions of different parts of the frontal region.

First, we must clearly distinguish between the symptoms arising in lesions of the *lateral* (convex) and *mediobasal* zones of the frontal region. The *lateral zones of the frontal cortex* are very closely linked with the motor structures of the anterior parts of the brain; they possess the same vertical striation and they have intimate connections with the motor cortex. This explains why lesions in the lateral frontal zones, and in particular, in the *postfrontal* region, as a rule give rise to particularly marked disturbances of the organization of movements and actions, to disintegration of motor programmes, and to disturbance of the comparison of human motor behaviour with its original plan. For this reason, the motor perseverations, the pathological inertia of existing motor programmes, and the disturbances of regulation of external behaviour described above could be observed particularly clearly in patients with lesions of the lateral zones of the prefrontal and, in particular, the postfrontal region of the cortex.

All these disturbances are particularly pronounced in patients with lesions of the lateral zones of the left (dominant) frontal lobe which are closely connected with the cerebral organization of speech, and the disorganization of whose functions leads to particularly marked disintegration of *speech activity* itself and of these *behavioural acts* which are especially dependent upon the participation of speech for their regulation. I have already described some aspects of the disturbance of speech activity arising in lesions of the lateral zones of the left frontal lobe; it may take the form either of increased pathological inertia of the speech processes themselves, or the loss of their regulatory role (Luria, 1960; 1961; 1962; 1966a; 1966b; 1969c; Luria and Homskaya, 1963; 1966), or again, of a distinctive inactivity of the speech processes, occurring in lesions of the infero-lateral zones of the left frontal cortex and expressed as inability to make a spontaneous discursive statement, difficulty in expressing a thought in discursive speech, and a characteristic 'verbal adynamia', which I have described elsewhere (Luria, 1966a) under the name 'frontal dynamic aphasia'. Since I have analysed this particular form of speech disorder elsewhere in detail (Luria, 1947; 1966a; 1966b; Luria and Tsvetkova, 1968) I shall not pay special attention to it here.

We can say very little about the functions of the *right frontal lobe*, which has no direct connection with the speech organization of mental activity, and I would prefer to consider this problem when I discuss the functions of the right cerebral hemisphere as a whole.

The *basal (or orbital) and medial zones* of the frontal lobes have a completely different functional organization from the lateral zones, and their lesions give rise to highly distinctive symptoms. We must therefore take a close look at their functional organization and at the disturbances of mental activity arising in patients with lesions of these zones. Both the medial and basal zones of the human cortex are linked particularly closely with the structures of the reticular formation and limbic region (of which the medial zones of the frontal lobes form a part). They have no direct relationship to the motor cortex, the precentral gyrus or the premotor area. Clearly, therefore, even massive lesions of these zones of the frontal lobe are unaccompanied by any evidence of the de-automatization of movements, the pathological inertia of movements and actions, or even a disturbance of the completion of complex motor programmes. More than once I have been surprised when a patient with a massive lesion (haemorrhage, vascular spasm or tumour), disturbing the normal function of the basal and medial zones of the frontal lobe, showed no visible disturbance of praxis and no defect of the organization of his motor behaviour; Luria, 1969a; 1970; Luria, Konovalov and Podgornaya, 1970). However, absence of motor disorders is only a negative feature of the clinical pictures arising in lesions of the basal and medial zones of the frontal lobe. In recent years their positive characteristics have become much more widely known, and the symptoms arising in lesions of these zones have become much clearer.

The _basal (orbital)_ zones of the frontal cortex are very closely linked both with the structures of the first functional unit of the brain and also with certain parts of the archicortex (especially the amygdala and the structures of the 'visceral brain'). It is therefore a well-known clinical fact that a lesion of these zones leads not only to disturbances of olfaction and vision (because of its effect on the olfactory structures and optic tracts), but also to definite signs of _generalized disinhibition and gross changes in affective processes._ ✱

The phenomena of disinhibition arising in patients with lesions of the orbital cortex have been examined by Konorski (1961; Konorski and Lawicka, 1964) and Brutkowski (1966), and they have often been described. The affective disorders, in the form of lack of self-control, violent emotional outbursts and gross changes in character, arising in lesions of the orbital cortex are among the clearest symptoms of such lesions and they also have been well described in the past (Welt, 1888; Feuchtwanger, 1923; Kleist, 1934; Rylander, 1939).

I have observed that even the disturbances of intellectual activity in patients with lesions of the orbital zones of the frontal lobes are totally different in character from disturbances associated with lesions of their lateral zones; in the former it is rare to observe the adynamia of thought and the inertia of established stereotypes which I have described in patients with lesions of the lateral zones of the frontal region; their intellectual operations remain _potentially_ intact, although actually they are severely disturbed by this increased disinhibition of their mental processes, which leads to uncontrollable impulsiveness and fragmentation, so that they cannot carry out planned and organized intellectual activity (Luria and Tsvetkova, 1967).

A special syndrome is found in lesions of the *medial zones* of the frontal lobes. The study of this syndrome is still only in its infancy; it is found both in tumours of the medial zones of the frontal lobes (Luria, Homskaya, Blinkov and Critchley, 1967) and in patients with aneurysms of the anterior communicating artery, accompanied by spasm of both anterior cerebral arteries (Luria, Konovalov and Podgornaya, 1970), and it is a unique clinical picture.

The medial zones of the frontal lobes are part of the limbic region and, as I mentioned, they are linked particularly closely with the lower structures of the reticular formation, the thalamic nuclei, and the structures of the archencephalon. Naturally, therefore, lesions of these zones must give rise to particularly marked disturbances of cortical tone and, as Homskaya (1972) has shown, to marked disturbances of the regulatory and modulatory influences which the frontal cortex exerts, through its descending connections, on the structures of the reticular formation.

This explains why the first and most important consequence of a lesion of these brain zones is a *sharp decrease in cortical tone*, leading to *disturbance of the waking state* and sometimes to the appearance of *oneiroid states*, characteristic of lesions of the limbic region. A special feature of these states of diminished wakefulness arising in lesions of the medial zones of the frontal lobes is that they take place against the background of a *diminished critical faculty* characteristic of frontal lobe pathology or, in other words, against the background of a *disturbance of the action acceptor apparatus*, providing the essential control over the performance of conscious processes.

The principal symptom found in patients with lesions of the medial frontal zones is thus one which I have described as a *disturbance of the selectivity of mental processes* (Luria, Homskaya, Blinkov and Critchley, 1967), in which the patient is no longer clearly oriented relative to his surroundings or to his past, he utters uncontrollable confabulations, and his *consciousness* becomes unstable and is sometimes profoundly disturbed.

A second aspect of this syndrome is the gross *disturbance of memory* found in these patients, with a well-marked phenomenon of 'equalization of excitability' of traces, leading to a state of confusion and to the production of confabulations. These phenomena will be examined in detail in the next chapter.

It will be unnecessary to remind the reader that the functional organization of the human frontal lobes is one of the most complex problems in modern science, and so far only the first step has been taken in the analysis of the various syndromes which can arise in lesions of the corresponding parts of the brain. Nothing is more certain, therefore, than that the next decade will see a substantial increase in our knowledge of this complex region.

Part Three
Synthetic Mental Activities and their Cerebral Organization

I have already stated that the initial assumption on which this book is based is the view that psychological processes are not indivisible 'functions' or 'faculties', but complex functional systems based on the concerted working of a group of cerebral zones, each of which makes its own contribution to the construction of the complex psychological process.

We must now move on from this analytical part to the next, synthetic part in which we shall examine which brain system is responsible for a given form of concrete mental activity and how, at the present state of development of science, its cerebral organization can be represented.

We shall discuss the cerebral organization of perception, of movement and action, of attention, of memory and of speech in its various forms and, finally the cerebral organization of complex intellectual activity. We shall do so as briefly as possible bearing in mind that these chapters are no more than an introduction to the neuropsychological approach to the analysis of a series of very complicated problems of modern psychology.

Chapter 8
Perception

Psychological structure

The psychology of the nineteenth century regarded perception as a passive imprint made by external stimuli on the retina, and later in the visual cortex. Logically, therefore, the cerebral basis of visual sensation and perception must be the zones of the occipital cortex which receive the excitation generated in the retina, and in which structures absolutely identical (isomorphic) with the primary stimulation are formed.

This concept of isomorphism of the structure of excitation in the visual cortex with the structure of the peripheral excitation, and hence, with the structure of the object stimulating the eyes, assumed its clearest form in Gestalt psychology, the founders of which (Köhler, for example) devoted a large part of their lives to the vindication of this 'principle of isomorphism'.

Modern psychology attempts to analyse perception from quite different standpoints. It regards perception as an active process of searching for the corresponding information, distinguishing the essential features of an object, comparing the features with each other, creating appropriate hypotheses, and then comparing these hypotheses with the original data (Vygotsky, 1956; 1960; Bruner, 1957; Leontev, 1959; Zaporozhets, 1967; 1968). For this reason, besides receptor components, effector components are also essential to human perception, and whereas these effector, motor components take place step by step in the first stages of development, at subsequent levels of formation of perceptual function they begin to be carried out by 'short cuts', in a contracted form, of some 'inner actions' (Zaporozhets, 1967; 1968; Zinchenko *et al.*, 1962; Zinchenko and Vergiler, 1972).

The process of perception is thus evidently complex in character.

It begins with the *analysis* of the structure perceived, as received by the brain, into a large number of components or cues which are subsequently *coded* or *synthesized* and fitted into the corresponding *mobile systems*. This process of selection and synthesis of the corresponding features is *active* in character and takes place under the direct influence of the *tasks* which confront the subject. It takes place with the aid of ready-made *codes* (and in particular the *codes* of language), which serve to place the perceived feature into its proper system and to give it a *general or categorical character*; finally, it always incorporates a process of comparison of the effect with the original hypothesis or, in other words, a process of verification of the perceptual activity.

During the perception of familiar objects, firmly established in past experience, this process is naturally contracted and takes place by a series of short cuts, whereas during the perception of new and unfamiliar or complex visual objects, the process of perception remains full and uncontracted. Finally, it is essential to note that human perception is a complex process of coding of the perceived material, taking place with the close participation of speech, and that human perceptual activity thus never takes place without the direct participation of language. This has been demonstrated in many psychological investigations (Gelb and Goldstein, 1920; Vygotsky, 1934; Bruner, 1957), and it is therefore unnecessary to discuss these problems specially.

Cerebral organization

This complex character of perceptual activity naturally suggests that visual perception is not performed in its entirety by the structures of the occipital (visual) cortex, but that a complete 'working constellation' of brain zones is in fact involved, each zone playing its own role in the perceptual activity and making its own contribution to the formation of the perceptual process.

It is also evident that a lesion of each of these zones which participates in perceptual activity will disturb the complex system of visual perception as a whole, although the disturbance affects a different component each time, and thus follows a different course.

As we have seen already, human visual perception starts at the moment when excitation arising in the retina reaches the primary visual cortex, where these impulses, which are projected on the corresponding points of the cortex (in a strictly somatotopically organized pattern), are split up into a very large number of components. As I said earlier (part 2, ch. 3), this process of *visual analysis* can take place because the visual cortex contains a very large number of highly differentiated neurons, each of which responds to only one particular feature of the perceived object (Hubel and Wiesel, 1962; 1963).

Since lesions of the primary zones of the visual cortex never involve isolated neurons alone, but always extend over a certain area, the disturbances of visual perception in these cases are elementary and somatotopical in character, and are manifested either as *homonymous hemianopia* (the loss of the contralateral half of the visual field), as *quadrantic hemianopia* (loss of a particular sector of the visual field) or, finally, as the development of *scotomata* – the loss of isolated areas of the visual field corresponding to the affected areas of the primary visual cortex.

If the primary visual cortex is in a state of dysfunction in man (as occurs after injury to the occipital region accompanied by oedema) in the first stages vision may disappear completely, after which it may be restored. Although perception is unclear and 'blurred' in character at first, later it recovers completely.

It is a characteristic feature of all these types of disturbance (except in some special cases) that these elementary defects can be suitably compensated by movements of the eyes, and the person still remains able to work. The exceptions are those cases when lesions of the occipital cortex (either of the primary or the secondary zones) are superimposed on a background of inactivity or of unawareness of the subject's own defect (anosognosia) or when the defect stays unperceived and is not compensated, so that it assumes the character of fixed hemianopia or unilateral spatial agnosia (Holmes, 1919; Brain, 1941; Luria and Skorodumova, 1950; Hécaen *et al.*, 1956; Hécaen, 1969).

The second stage of the cerebral organization of visual perception requires the close participation of the *secondary zones* of the visual cortex. These constitute the chief system responsible for the formation of mobile *syntheses* of visually perceived elements, but are themselves under the regulating and modulating influence of other, non-visual zones of the cortex.

As we have seen, the secondary zones of the visual cortex consist largely of neurons of the upper cortical layers, possessing short axons and adapted for the formation of combinations and connections between the individual elements and the points of the cortex. They can thus produce the mobile syntheses of visual cues into which visual perception is analysed, and make the cues amenable to control.

A lesion of the secondary cortical zones naturally disturbs these visual syntheses, and the defect of perception arising in patients with lesions of these cortical zones assumes the form of disturbances of simultaneous visual syntheses, or of optic agnosia, in which each element of a visual structure is perceived sufficiently clearly, but the patient cannot synthesize the element into a single whole, so that he is unable to *recognize* objects or pictures of objects. We still know very little about the basic mechanisms of optic gnosis. However, one of its accessory mechanisms deserves mention.

The visual image formed in the retina is known to remain there for an extremely short time, and if the eye is completely stationary the image lasts not more than 1–1·5 seconds (Yarbus, 1965). It is thus essential not merely to bring about visual synthesis, but also to *stabilize the image* obtained as a result of the optic procedure. One way of doing this is by the formation of a *visual after-image*, which plays a very important role in image stabilization. Its physiological mechanisms have been studied in detail by Orbeli's school (Zimkina, 1957; Zimkin and Zimkina, 1953; Kaplan, 1949; Balonov, 1950).

A fact of the greatest importance is that this visual after-image, which normally lasts for twenty to thirty seconds and then gradually disappears, may *either fail to arise completely or may last for a very much shorter time* in patients with lesions of the occipital zones, but some degree of stabilization can be produced by the administration of caffeine (Zislina, 1955). This indicates that the visual cortex is responsible not only for the synthesis of visual impulses, but also for their *stabilization*. It thus performs a similar role to the one I mentioned when discussing the role of the temporal cortex in the stabilization of auditory stimuli (part 2, ch. 4).

It would be a mistake, however, to think that the secondary zones of the visual cortex are concerned only with the *effector* or *operative* part of perceptual activity. It is because this is not so that a lesion of the secondary visual zones interferes with or prevents the formation of visual syntheses, but does not deprive perceptual activity of its *controlled* and *purposive* character. A person with a lesion of the secondary visual zones can directly perceive only fragments of visual information, but he can still analyse the meaning of these fragments and he can compensate for his defects by reasoning. He actively looks for the solution to the problem of the nature of the picture he is shown, he puts forward various hypotheses, he compares them with the elements he actually perceives; he attempts to fit the cues he perceives into particular categories of meaning, and *codes* them. For this reason, since the patient can still hypothetically fit a cue into its proper category, but because he is unable to carry out the concrete synthesis of cues into a complete visual entity, his perception becomes excessively *generalized* ('this is . . . some sort of animal', 'this is . . . some sort of instrument'), becoming hyperintellectualized in character and lacking in concreteness.

A lesion of the secondary visual zones thus disturbs the *operation of visual syntheses*, but *leaves the whole structure of active perception intact*. The higher zones, bordering on the secondary zones of the visual cortex, make their own contribution to the structure of visual perception, and their lesions give the disturbance of visual perception certain special features of their own.

The individual components of the higher cerebral organization of visual perception are of special interest and merit separate consideration. Visual perception usually has its own *spatial organization*, and only in the simplest cases is this spatial organization elementary in character, so that all the spatial coordinates remain unambiguous. In many cases, however, this is not so and the figures perceived have a definite and, moveover, *asymmetrical* spatial position. These features are particularly conspicuous during the perception of a face-to-face situation, in which the words 'right' and 'left' have completely different (and often, vitally important) meanings. The same features are apparent in the perception of the position of the room in a flat, the object in a room, and so on. They are particularly conspicuous during the perception of geometrical structures and three-dimensional figures, when the incorporation of the directly perceived object into a system of fundamental *spatial coordinates* (the frontal, sagittal and horizontal planes) is vital to the correct course of perceptual activity.

An essential fact is that *spatial organization is not a function of the occipital* (*visual*) *cortex itself*, and that the participation of the *inferior parietal* (or parieto-occipital) zones of the brain is essential for it to happen.

It is these brain zones which give a role in spatial perception to the cortical zones of the *vestibular* and *kinaesthetic* (*haptic*) systems, in which the *right, master, hand* occupies a dominant position. The introduction of these non-visual components into complex visual perception introduces at the same time the possibility of spatial analysis: elements of three-dimensional spatial coordinates, on the one hand, and the asymmetrical assessment of the right and left sides of space on the other hand.

A lesion of the *inferior parietal* (or parieto-occipital) regions of the hemisphere thus leaves *visual* syntheses themselves intact, but the *spatial organization* of perception is disturbed. Accordingly, such patients cannot clearly perceive the spatial relationships between elements of a complex construction, they cannot distinguish right and left, they lose their way in surrounding space, they cannot tell the position of the hands of a clock, they confuse the countries on a map, and they cannot determine cardinal directions. I have already discussed these defects in the appropriate part of this book (part 2, ch. 5), to which the reader is referred.

A factor unique in visual perception is the possibility of *wide simultaneous synthesis*, enabling a *whole situation* to be perceived at the same time (for example, the simultaneous examination of a picture). There is good reason to suppose that this type of perception is not a function of the visual (occipital) cortex only, but requires the close participation of the *parieto-occipital* zones. These are apparently responsible for the 'conversion of the successive formation of a situation into simultaneous surveyability' and thus perform the condensed act of simultaneous comprehension of a complete optically perceived situation. This hypothesis is based on the fact that a lesion of the parieto-occipital cortex (most frequently of both hemispheres) causes the patient, who can still perceive individual objects, to be unable to perceive a *group* (sometimes even a *pair*) of objects, and, still less, to grasp a complete situation, such as a thematic picture, at once.

This disturbance is known as Bálint's simultaneous agnosia. It is always associated with a characteristic apraxia of fixation, resulting from the fact that the impaired 'wide visual sphere' cannot deal simultaneously with several excited points, so that the patient is unable to fix the centre of visual information by means of the central part of the retina. At the same time, he cannot perceive information at the periphery of the retina, and the coordinated eye movements, which are the first step in simultaneous perception of a complete visual situation, disappear. I have given a detailed analysis of this defect above (part 2, ch. 5), and will not, therefore, dwell further on it here.

The last type of disturbance of wide spatial perception is *unilateral spatial agnosia*. This differs from the ordinary homonymous hemianopia because patients with this disturbance, which usually arises in lesions of the parieto-occipital zones of the non-dominant (right) hemisphere, are unaware of the whole of the left side, in both the visual and the tactile spheres, and moreover, they are also unaware of their defects (Brain, 1941; Ajuriaguerra and Hécaen, 1960; Critchley, 1953; Piercy and Smith, 1962; Warrington *et al.*, 1966; Korchazhinskaya, 1971). This disturbance is a purely pathological fact, and although of undoubted interest in special neurology, it is only of limited importance to the understanding of the structure of normal human perception.

So far we have confined our attention almost completely to the analysis of the contribution of the occipital and parieto-occipital regions of the two hemispheres to the structure of visual perception, without devoting any particular attention to the relative roles of the dominant and non-dominant hemispheres in this activity. We must now rectify this omission.

The systems of the dominant, left hemisphere in right-handed individuals are intimately connected with speech, and through it, with all mental processes in whose organization speech plays an active part. At the same time, it is well known that speech participates directly in the formation of the most complex forms of perception, namely the coding of the perception of colours, shapes and objects into complex 'categories'. This problem has been studied in the past in connection with the analysis of colour perception (Gelb and Goldstein, 1920; Bruner, 1957), and it is of the utmost importance to the psychology of human perceptual activity. We shall therefore not be surprised to learn that the non-visual zones of the cortex directly concerned with speech can play an active role in the organization of visual perception, and that lesions of these zones can lead to substantial disturbances of visual perception.

The role of the 'speech zones' of the cortex in the structure of perception and in the genesis of disturbances of perception in lesions of the temporal and temporo-occipital cortex, leading to aphasia, have not yet been adequately studied. The investigations of Gelb and Goldstein (1920) are classical in this respect. These workers showed that speech disturbances can lead to loss of the ability to perceive colour categories, so that colours are not coded correctly. Elementary phenomena such as induction colour, which under normal circumstances are inhibited by the categorical perception of colour, become more clearly apparent. The later investigations of Goldstein (1944) are of great importance to this approach to visual perception and to the role of speech in it. Goldstein demonstrated the disturbance of the categorical character of perception of shapes in patients with brain lesions, and his pupil Hochheimer (1932) made what was perhaps the first attempt at a detailed approach to the analysis of the phenomena of optic agnosia on the basis of the role of speech in the construction of perceptual processes. Finally, a special place in this problem belongs to the classical (but, unfortunately, still unfinished) investigations of Pötzl, who in his important work on aphasia (Pötzl, 1928), from the beginning closely linked the analysis of the pathology of visual perception with speech disorders, and cites numerous facts to indicate how the 'wide visual sphere of the cortex' functions under the direct organizing influence of speech. Recently the concept of the role of speech in human perception and the characteristics of the cerebral mechanisms of perception which stem directly from this fact have again received careful attention, and the many investigations confirming this important conclusion have been summarized in several surveys (see, for example, Drew *et al.*, 1970).

Unfortunately, these investigations, laying the foundations of the approach to forms of perception in man, have not been adequately pursued during the subsequent development of neuropsychology, but there is no doubt that important facts will be obtained as the result of further work in this field of research.

Two factors, adequately confirmed by clinical experience, call for detailed comment. The first is the disturbance of *perception of letters and words* resulting from lesions of the left parieto-occipital region, and the second is the disturbance of the *emergence of visual ideas* observed in lesions of the temporo-occipital zones.

It will be obvious that the left (dominant) hemisphere, with its direct relationship to the organization of speech processes, must also participate in the perception of the symbols of written language (letters, words, numbers, punctuation marks). This is clear from the fact that *lesions of the parieto-occipital zones of the dominant left hemisphere can also lead to a disturbance of the perception of these symbols* even in the absence of any marked signs of object agnosia.

The optic alexia which, in some cases, assumes the character of a disturbance of the visual perception of the individual letters (literal alexia), and in other cases of inability to combine visually perceived letters into whole words and a disturbance of the visual perception of words (verbal alexia), has been studied and described in detail. Very often these phenomena are accompanied by a disturbance of the visual perception of numbers or of musical notation, and they are always produced by a lesion of the parieto-occipital zones of the dominant hemisphere. In some cases congenital malformations of this region are manifested by inborn defects which prevent learning to read (congenital word-blindness); this is a special section of neuropsychology which has also received considerable study. In other cases a disturbance of the recognition of letters is found in lesions of the occipital and parieto-occipital zones of the dominant left hemisphere, so that when the patient looks at letters and drawings he perceives their spatial arrangement indistinctly and does not recognize the meaning of written letters and words (literal and verbal optic alexia). This syndrome has often been described and is well known in clinical practice (Dejerine, 1914; Pötzl, 1928; Benton, 1965; Money, 1962; Hécaen, Ajuriaguerra and Angelergues, 1957; Hoff, Gloning and Gloning, 1962; Gloning *et al.*, 1966; Weigl, 1964; Benson and Geschwind, 1969; Zurif and Carson, 1970).

So far I have described defects of the direct reception of visual information resulting from certain brain lesions. However, it is well known that perceptual activity is not confined to the processes of visual perception, but necessarily includes the *active formation of visual images corresponding to a single word meaning.* This process, an aspect of perceptual activity which has not yet been adequately studied, merits our special attention.

Under normal conditions the visual image, which is bright and approaching eidetic in some places but dull and indistinct in others, is readily evoked by a simple word denoting the corresponding object; with time, it undergoes certain changes, either being converted into a more generalized form, or exhibiting more clearly defined distinctive features (Soloviev, 1966). Cases of the complete absence of visual images evokable by words denoting objects are unknown under normal conditions.

However, complete inability to form a visual image of an object denoted by a word, despite adequate preservation of the visually perceived object is a familiar condition in brain pathology. As we have seen, lesions of the temporo-occipital lobes of the left hemisphere frequently result in the subject understanding the meaning of a word, although the word does not arouse a distinct visual image. The patient's attempts to draw the object denoted by a word are in sharp contrast to the ease with which he can copy such a drawing. I have already given examples (Figure 39) of this type of dissociation, and will not therefore discuss it further.

We still know very little about the role of the right hemisphere in the formation of perception despite what can be learned from the nature of the disturbances of visual perception produced by its lesions.

Although Jackson (1874) ascribed a special function to the right hemisphere in perceptual activity, and despite the fact that some workers (for example, Sperry, 1968) have pointed to its role in the preservation of speech perception, we still have very few reliable facts to point unequivocally to a specific role of the right hemisphere in perception.

Within the last decade, work has been published (Hécaen and Angelergues, 1963; Piercy and Smith, 1962; Kok, 1967) which shows that the parieto-occipital zones of the right hemisphere evidently play an important role in the most direct forms of perception and, in particular, in those forms in which the contribution of speech is minimal.

For instance, it has been shown that a lesion of the right occipital region leads to a disturbance of the recognition of faces, or to prosopagnosia, far more frequently than a lesion of the left occipital region (Hoff and Pötzl, 1937; Faust, 1947; Bodamer, 1947; Chlenov and Bein, 1958; Hécaen and Angelergues, 1963; Bornstein, 1962; Kok, 1967). Disturbances of direct forms of visual and visuo-spatial perception in lesions of the right hemisphere have also been described by various workers, who have drawn attention to the occurrence in such cases of constructional spatial apraxia, disturbance of the ability to draw, and so on (Paterson and Zangwill, 1945; Hécaen, Ajuria-guerra and Massonet, 1951; Ettlinger, Warrington and Zangwill, 1957; Piercy, Hécaen and Ajuriaguerra, 1960; Warrington *et al.*, 1966; Hécaen and Assal, 1970).

Finally, I must mention one more phenomenon which evidently provides some information about the role of structures of the right hemisphere in perception. Perception of an object is always asso-ciated with its *recognition* or, in other words, its inclusion in a system of familiar associations. As I have said, this process of recognition may be disturbed if visual syntheses are impaired and if the subject, although he perceives the individual cues, is unable to synthesize them into a single visually perceived entity.

However, in some cases the process of direct visual synthesis is unimpaired and the patient can still clearly see an object or picture shown to him, yet he is unable to relate it to his past experience or, in other words, he cannot recognize it. This disability was described originally by Lissauer (1898) under the name associative mental blindness, which he distinguished from the optic agnosia (or apper-ceptive mental blindness) already described.

The mechanisms lying at the base of the associative mental blind-ness have not yet been explained, although some results suggest that the underlying defect may be a disturbance of the systems of connec-tions of the visual and non-visual cortex (Geschwind, 1965). How-ever, I have frequently observed one form of this disturbance in patients with lesions of the parieto-occipital zones of the *right* (non-dominant) hemisphere. This type of disturbance more closely resembled paragnosia than true optic agnosia, for although the patient could still see an object or picture of it clearly, either he could not relate it to his personal experience (for example, as I have already said, when looking at a picture of a group of soldiers on a tank, he said: 'This is my family, my father, sisters and children'), or he assessed its meaning on the basis of irrelevant associations;

for example, one such patient interpreted the picture of a boy who had broken a window and had been caught by the owner of the house as follows: 'Someone from the Buryat Republic has won a competition (!), and they are presenting him with a cup.'

Such cases demonstrate a unique type of disturbance of visual perception which is evidently based on the uncontrollable emergence of irrelevant associations, and which, as a rule, is associated with the patient's unawareness of his own defects (or anosognosia), characteristic of a lesion of the right hemisphere.

Nevertheless, the facts available concerning the role of the right hemisphere in perception are still grossly inadequate, and we can only hope that in the future there will be information which will shed more light on this role.

We must now briefly examine the last of the problems which I have mentioned, one which occupies a special place in the cerebral organization of perception. I refer to the role of the *frontal lobes* in this context.

Perception, as I have said before, *is an active process* which includes the search for the most important elements of information, their comparison with each other, the creation of a hypothesis concerning the meaning of the information as a whole, and the verification of this hypothesis by comparing it with the original features of the object perceived. The more complex the object perceived, and the less familiar it is, the more detailed this perceptual activity will be. Both the direction and character of these perceptual searches vary with the nature of the perceptual task, as is clearly shown by eye movements recorded during the examination of a complex object. It is this *active* character of the process which is *dependent on the role of the frontal lobes* in perception. This can be seen by analysing the disturbances of perceptual activity found in patients with lesions of the frontal lobes.

Patients with massive lesions of the frontal lobes show no noticeable disturbances of direct visual perception. They readily perceive and recognize simple pictures, letters or numbers, and they read simple words or even elementary sentences without difficulty. However, the situation changes if they are required to exhibit active perceptual activity. This happens when the object is shown to them under unusual conditions, and work must be done in order to inhibit the first, incorrect impression which immediately arises. This may also happen when the patient must actively distinguish the required figure against a homogeneous background, or again, if interpretation of the meaning of a complex picture requires active analytical work, with the identification of the essential items of information followed by their comparison and synthesis.

The first case is the simplest. In order to reveal such a disturbance of visual perception, all that is necessary is to show the patient with a massive frontal lobe lesion either a picture drawn in a stylistic fashion, or a picture in an unusual position, or finally, a picture capable of being perceived in several different ways. In all these cases it will be clear that the patient with a massive frontal lesion replaces the adequate evaluation of the object by a *direct impression*, which he fails to correct. In many such cases I have seen how a patient with a frontal lobe lesion perceives an upturned hat as a plate, a cartridge as a clock, a leather strap as a loaf of bread, a telephone as a petrol can, a tie as a bird, a ship as a pigeon with a swollen neck, a cup and saucer as a statue, and so on. A considerable obstacle to correct perception in these patients is the *pathological inertia* of an image once it has appeared. This prevents the change to a new image, and thus interferes with normal perception. An example of this disturbance of perception by an inert stereotype is shown in Figure 67.

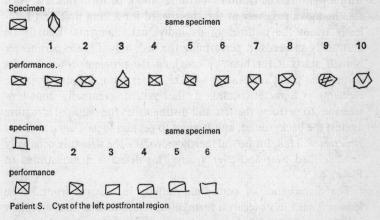

Patient S. Cyst of the left postfrontal region

Figure 67 Effect of pathological inertia on perception of patients with a massive frontal syndrome

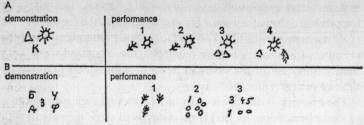

Patient S   Cyst of the left postfrontal region

Figure 67 – continued

The second type of disturbance of active perception in a patient with a frontal lobe lesion can be observed if a patient with a well-marked frontal syndrome is required to *actively distinguish a given figure against a homogeneous background.* Probably the best method to use for this purpose is the one which was suggested some years ago by Révault d'Allones (1923), in which the subject must distinguish a white cross with a black centre, or some other such shape, against the background of a chessboard.

The normal subject can do this without difficulty, thereby demonstrating the high mobility of his perception and the ease with which he can reconstruct the perceptible visual field. However, a patient with a well-marked frontal syndrome cannot perform this test. As a rule he looks passively at the chessboard for a long time and helplessly traces the outlines of its individual fragments. Usually he eventually succeeds in performing the task only if the experimenter himself starts it for him, by breaking the problem down into its component parts and tracing with his finger around the appropriate elements. Characteristically, if the patient eventually somehow manages to perform the test and distinguishes the required structure against the background, any attempt to get him to *pick out a different structure* will fail, for he will inertly reproduce the structure originally distinguished over and over again. This defect is demonstrated in Figure 68.

The disturbance of perceptual activity in massive frontal lobe lesions is seen in its clearest form, however, in tests of the *perception of complex optic structures* and, in particular, tests involving the interpretation of *thematic pictures*, the final assessment of which requires active analysis, the comparison of details, the production of hypotheses, and their subsequent verification (see part 2, ch. 7).

All these stages of active perception are most severely disturbed in patients with a massive lesion of the *frontal lobes*, and careful observation will show how in such patients the normally complex structure of perceptual activity is replaced by simple impulsive conclusions, based either on the perception of individual details or on formal verbal answers, without any preceding analysis of the presented material. This severe disturbance of active perception in patients with massive brain lesions is seen particularly clearly in tests in which the *eye movements* of these patients *are recorded*. These tests show that patients with frontal lobe lesions easily follow an object moving along a standard trajectory, but they have considerable difficulty in *actively transferring their fixation from one point to another* (Luria and Homskaya, 1962).

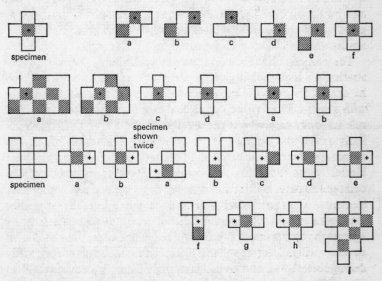

Figure 68 Distinguishing a given structure from a homogeneous background by a patient with an extensive frontal lesion. Patient Sar. (tumour of the left frontal lobe with cyst formation). The diagrams show the trajectory of the movements of the patient's finger during his attempt to distinguish the required figure from a chessboard. The cross (+) marks the square which was indicated each time by the experimenter beforehand

This defect is seen still more clearly during the examination of a thematic picture when the perceptual tasks are constantly changing. We saw above that whereas recording of the eye movements of normal subjects under these conditions clearly reflects the dynamics of the active perceptual process, the eye movements of patients with massive frontal lobe lesions remain chaotic or, sometimes, inertly stereotyped (Figure 66), thus reflecting the fact that their perceptual activity easily loses its active, searching character (Luria, Karpov and Yarbus, 1965; Karpov, Luria and Yarbus, 1968).

The material described above shows that the process of visual perception is in fact a *complex functional system* based on the *concerted working of a whole group of cortical zones*, and that each of these zones makes its own contribution to the structure of active perception.

Chapter 9
Movement and Action

Psychological structure

Classical psychology approached human voluntary movement and action as manifestations of an act of volition, and considered that they resulted either from an 'effort of will' or an 'ideo-motor representation' which automatically evoked a movement. Such an idea, of course, actually prevented an approach to the study of voluntary movements and made them inaccessible to scientific, deterministic analysis. This idealistic approach, divorcing the study of human voluntary movement from science, was therefore very quickly forced to give way to the opposite approach which, although at one time it showed some progressive tendencies, nevertheless led to the same dead end as the voluntaristic idea of a 'free act of will' as the cause of voluntary movement.

This approach, basically mechanistic, was based on the idea that voluntary movements or conscious actions are only apparent, and in reality are nothing more than obligatory responses to external stimuli. Although this view was a logical one at the time when Sechenov wrote his famous *Reflexes of the Brain* and was justified by the reaction against the 'psychological aberration' and those who supported an open indeterminism, it had the result, however, that real research into human voluntary activity was abandoned for more than half a century.

The view that voluntary movement and actions are reflex in origin took away everything specific from these important causes of human activity and replaced their study by approaches which could be justified only in relation either to relatively simple, inborn programmes of behaviour, triggered by the most elementary signals operating like the 'innate releasing mechanisms' (IRM) of the ethologists (Lorenz,

1950; Tinbergen, 1957), or to such artificially formed models as conditioned reflexes. Despite the great success of this scheme, which appeared to a whole generation of psychologists (those of the behaviourist school, for example) to be the only scientific approach to behaviour, the concept of voluntary movement and action as an innate or conditioned reflex was unacceptable on two counts.

First, by removing all movements and actions from the influence of *past experience*, it in fact closed its eyes to those forms of behaviour which are controlled, not by the past, but by the *future*, which are constructed as the putting into effect of intentions, plans or programmes, and which, as it can easily be seen, constitute the greater part of all specifically human forms of activity. Second, the view of voluntary movement and actions as simply the efferent components of a reflex arc was unacceptable because, as the eminent Soviet physiologist Bernstein showed, human movements are so variable, and they possess such an unlimited degree of freedom that it would be impossible to find a formula from which human voluntary movements could be derived from efferent impulses alone (Bernstein, 1947). Hence, neither the idealistic nor the mechanistic concepts of voluntary movement in fact made any significant advance on the dualistic ideas of Descartes, for whom the movements of animals were reflex-like or mechanistic, while the movements of man were determined by some mental principle or by free will, releasing the same reflex mechanisms.

A radical change was necessary to the basic ideas of voluntary movement and action, in order to *preserve the distinctive feature* of these higher conscious forms of activity, but at the same time to make them accessible to truly *scientific, deterministic analysis*. The first step in this direction was taken by Vygotsky (1956; 1960), who introduced into psychology the concept that the source of voluntary movement and action lies, not within the organism, not in the direct influence of past experience, but in *man's social history*: in that work activity in society which marks the origin of human history and in that communication between child and adult which was the basis of voluntary movement and purposive action in ontogeny.

Vygotsky considered that any attempt to seek 'biological roots' of voluntary action were doomed to failure. He considered that its true source lies in the period of communication between the child and adult when 'function was shared between two people'; when the adult gave the child the spoken instruction 'take the cup!' or 'here is the ball!' and the child obeyed the instruction, took the thing which was named, or fixed it with his eye.

In the next stages of development, the child who had previously obeyed the adult's instruction had now learned to speak and could *give himself spoken instructions* (to begin with, external, detailed instructions, but later internal and contracted in form) and he began to *subordinate his own behaviour to these instructions*. Characteristically, at this stage *the function previously shared between two persons became a method of organization of the higher forms of active behaviour* which are social in origin, dependent on speech in their structure, and voluntary in their course. This meant that voluntary movements and action were freed from the history which had always surrounded them both in idealistic and in 'positive' biological investigations, and that these specifically human forms of active behaviour could be a true object for scientific investigation.

I shall not dwell in any more detail on the basic theoretical arguments concerning the genesis of higher forms of conscious human activity, which have often been published elsewhere (Vygotsky, 1934; 1956; 1960; Vygotsky and Luria, 1930; Leontiev, 1959), or on a detailed account of the dramatic history of the formation of voluntary activity and the regulating function of speech, on which much has also been written (Luria, 1956; 1957; 1958a; 1961; 1966a; 1969a; 1969b; 1970c), and I shall now turn to the second source of modern views regarding the psychophysiological structure of voluntary movement and action.

Although modern psychologists, notably Vygotsky, have formulated the basic principles of psychological analysis of movement and conscious action, it was the work of contemporary physiologists, and especially of Bernstein (1947; 1957; 1966; 1967), which made possible this constructive approach to the study of their basic mechanisms. Having demonstrated the 'intrinsic uncontrollability of movements purely by efferent impulses', Bernstein then had the task of creating not only a *scheme* for the *construction* of motor acts, but also a theory of the *levels* of movement construction which, together with innate, elementary synergisms, would also include the most complex and specifically human forms of activity. The starting point for Bernstein's theory of the structure of movement was the proposition regarding the dominant role of *afferent systems*, which differ in character at each level and which lead to different types of movement and action.

I shall not discuss in detail the elementary levels of movement regulating the fundamental processes of homeostasis or the level of inborn synergisms which occupy a leading place in the lower vertebrates, but will merely mention the principal features of construction of the highest forms of specifically human voluntary movement and action.

The initial component of human voluntary movement and actions is the *intention* or *motor task* which, in man, is hardly ever a simple, direct response to an external stimulus (only the simplest forms of firmly established, habitual actions still remain in this category), but always creates a '*model of the future need*', a scheme of what must take place and of what the subject must achieve or, to use Bernstein's term, the 'Soll – Wert'.

This motor task, or model of the future need, is *constant* or *invariant*, and it demands an equally *constant, invariant* result. For instance, if the motor task is to go up to a cupboard and to take a tumbler, or to hammer a nail, the fulfilment of these acts is the constant, invariant result by which the action is completed. However, it would be a mistake to imagine that the invariant motor task creates an equally constant and invariant programme for the fulfilment of the required action. It is a most important fact that the *invariant motor task is fulfilled not by a constant, fixed set, but by a varying set of movements which, however, lead to the constant, invariant effect.* This thesis applies both to elementary and to the most complex motor systems.

As I have mentioned, in the act of breathing the *invariant task*, that of bringing oxygen to the alveoli of the lung, can be accomplished with the aid of widely *different methods*: movements of the diaphragm regulating the entry of air, movements of the intercostal muscles, expanding and contracting the chest, and sometimes, if both these methods are impossible, movements of air swallowing; the effect of all these widely different methods is always the invariant *result* of the set problem. The same situation is found in the performance of complex, purposive movements. In order to take down a tumbler from a cupboard, the subject must approach or reach up to the tumbler, grasp it with his right or left hand, move it towards him by simple movements or, perhaps, with the aid of a ruler – different and widely varying movements which ultimately, however, lead to the same constant effect. This variation in the methods of performance of the movement (or of the 'motor innervation') is not accidental, but is *essential, in principle*, for the normal course of an active movement and for its successful accomplishment.

As Bernstein showed, human movements are based on a system of articulations possessing an infinite degree of freedom, and on the constantly changing tone of the muscles. This makes it absolutely essential to have a constant, *plastic succession of innervations* corresponding to the changing position of the limbs and to the changing state of the muscular system at each moment. It is this factor which introduces the mobile, variative character of the motor innervations as the basic conditions for fulfilment of the constant, invariant result of the movement. All these factors fully explain why it is that, in the performance of a voluntary movement or action, although the motor task preserves its regulatory role, the highest responsibility is transferred *from efferent to afferent impulses*. In other words this responsibility is transferred to those *afferent syntheses* which provide information on the position of the moving limb in space and on the state of the muscular system, which take into consideration the difference between the future requirement ('Soll – Wert') and the position of the moving organ in the present ('Ist – Wert'), and which obtain the coefficient of this difference (δW). According to Bernstein, this is the basic factor determining the structure of movement.

The system of constant afferent information, forming the necessary basis for the fulfilment of the *operative* or *executive* part of the movement, cannot itself be simple and homogeneous: it must inevitably incorporate analysis of the *visuo-spatial coordinates* in which the movement takes place, a system of *kinaesthetic signals* indicating the position of the locomotor apparatus, information regarding the general *muscle tone*, states of equilibrium, and so on. The motor act can follow its proper course only if such a system of *afferent syntheses* exists. A constant supply of afferent information is essential for the successful performance of the last component of every voluntary movement: the *checking* of its course and *correction* of any mistakes made. This checking of the course of an action and correction of any mistakes are accomplished with the aid of the constant *comparison between the action as it is performed and the original intention*, and with the aid of an apparatus described by some workers as a 'feedback', by others (Anokhin) as the 'action acceptor', or (Miller, Pribram and Galanter) as the T-O-T-E (Test-Operant-Test-Exit) system. This constant inspection system, continually analysing the feedback signals and comparing them with the original plan, is the last, but an absolutely essential component, of the voluntary movement, and without it the performance of the required task is extremely unlikely to succeed.

The scheme outlined above, summarizing the modern psychological and physiological approach to the structure of movement, is of course only a beginning and a sign pointing the way to future research. However, it demonstrates the complexity of the voluntary *motor act* and provides important guidance for research into its cerebral organization.

Cerebral organization

The views regarding the structure of voluntary movement and actions described above naturally make nonsense of any search for the localization of the physiological mechanisms of the motor act in any one brain zone (for example, in the precentral gyrus), and, as I have done in other cases, they compel an examination of the *role of each brain zone in the construction of the complex motor act*.

The foundation for construction of voluntary movement or conscious action is the *frontal lobe system* which, as we have seen, not merely maintains and controls the general tone of the cortex, but, with the aid of internal speech and under the influence of afferent impulses reaching them from other parts of the cortex, formulates the *intention* or *motor task*, ensures its preservation and also its *regulatory role*, enables the performance of the action *programme*, and keeps a constant *watch* over its course.

I have dealt at length with the disturbances of the organization of activity which arise in lesions of the frontal lobe (part 2, ch. 7), and will not discuss them further here. I shall merely recall that the essential feature of massive frontal lobe lesions is the patient's inability to formulate intentions or motor tasks, so that he remains completely passive where the situation demands an appropriate plan of action, and if such a plan is given to him from outside as a verbal instruction, he can memorize the instruction but is unable to convert it into a factor actually controlling its movements. I would also remind the reader that frontal lobe lesions lead to inability to preserve and retain an *action programme* and to its easy replacement by any *direct reactions* arising uncontrollably in response to every stimulus (in some cases assuming the character of unsuppressable orienting reflexes, and in others of impulsive responses to direct impressions or 'echo-praxic' movements), or to the eruption of *inert stereotypes*, replacing a purposive action by the perseveration of previous motor acts. Finally, massive frontal lobe lesions disturb to a marked degree the process of comparing the result of action with the original motor task (and sometimes completely prevent it), so that the patient is no longer aware of his mistakes and he can no longer keep a constant *check* over the course of his action.

A *frontal lobe* lesion, although producing no primary defect in the structure of the executive (operative) component of the motor act, nevertheless *disturbs the structure of a programmed, goal-directed activity*, and thus makes *voluntary movement and purposive action impossible*. Other parts of the brain, responsible for the *executive, operative* aspect of movement, make a different contribution to its structure. These parts of the brain are much more varied, and a lesion of any one zone disturbs the normal course of movement in its own characteristic way. Every movement takes place in *a three-dimensional system of coordinates* which, for some types of movement (elementary motor synergisms), is relatively unimportant, whereas for others (locomotion, hitting a target, constructional activity) it plays an important or even decisive role. Analysis of the basic spatial coordinates and their preservation as the framework within which voluntary movements and actions are performed are associated with the active function of the *parieto-occipital zones* of the brain, which include the central structures of the visual, vestibular, kinaesthetic, and motor systems and which form the *highest level of spatial organization of movements.*

A lesion of these brain zones does not therefore disturb the formation of intentions or motor tasks, the formation of an action programme, or the checking of its course, or in other words, it does not lead to *disintegration of the system of goal-directed activity*, but it gives rise to important disturbances of the *structure of movements in space*. I have already discussed the disturbances of spatial orientation, the loss of direction in space, and the symptoms of 'constructional apraxia' which arise in patients with such lesions. It will also be clear that patients who are unable to perform an elementary action requiring the performance of movements within a system of definite spatial coordinates can still carry out types of movements and actions which do not require this spatial coordination (such as beating time) and are clearly aware of their difficulties in the performance of spatially organized actions, so that in the attempt to compensate their defects they introduce logical analysis, they use auxiliary logical schemes, and so on. I shall not analyse in detail all the methods by which such patients attempt to compensate their defects in the spatial organization of movement, for they have been examined elsewhere (Luria and Tsvetkova, 1965a; 1965b; Tsvetkova, 1972). I would merely draw attention to the highly specific character of the motor disorders which arise on the basis of disturbances of the central apparatus for spatial analyses and syntheses.

I have also mentioned that the second, hardly less important, condition for the performance of movement is *integrity of its kinaesthetic afferentation*. Only if a constant flow of kinaesthetic impulses arrives from the motor system can definite information be obtained about the position of the joints and the state and tone of the muscles, so that the efferent impulses can reach their correct destination and the required set of motor impulses can be found and maintained. These functions are the responsibility of the *postcentral zones of the brain*, the cortical apparatus for kinaesthetic analysis and synthesis, and as we have seen above (part 2, ch. 6), lesions of these brain zones can impair the findings of the required set of motor impulses and disturb postural praxis. The fact that, depending on the extent of these lesions, the disturbance of the normal course of movement of these patients may assume different forms ranging from 'afferent paresis' to 'afferent motor ataxia and apraxia', although the motor disorders are of the same *character*, demonstrates convincingly the contribution of the postcentral cortical zones to the structure of movement and the conditions for motor activity which they provide.

The third condition for the normal course of movement is constant regulation of *muscle tone*, on the one hand, and a sufficiently rapid and smooth *changeover* from one system of motor innervations to another, with the formation of complete *kinaesthetic melodies* in the final stages of development of skilled movement. The control of any coordinated movement requires constant changes in tone, and if this tone does not change but remains at the same level or is increased, coordinated movements will be impossible. Neurologists are well aware that a pathological change in the activity of the basal ganglia (the striopallidary system) usually leads to gross disturbances of tone, giving rise to the picture of parkinsonism, and making normal movements impossible.

However, the subcortical motor structures are under the constant inhibitory and modulatory influence of the cortex and, in particular, of the *premotor zones*, which can inhibit excessively long excitation of the basal ganglia and which are themselves an important system organizing consecutive chains of movement which take place over a period of time. For these reasons, although the premotor cortex does not participate in isolated human movements, it becomes an essential apparatus for the organization of *series of movements*, by making possible the denervation of components of the motor action once they have been completed, and by ensuring the smooth transition to the next component, the *premotor zones constitute the important cerebral apparatus for 'kinetic melodies' or skilled movements*.

This role of the premotor cortex in the organization of movement can easily be appreciated by observing the disturbances of movement in patients with lesions of these zones. In such cases there is a distinctive dissociation of motor functions: the performance of individual postural movements of placing the hands in a certain position in space still remains possible, constructional praxis is undisturbed, but complex, serially organized movements are impaired, for each successive component of a complex motor act requires its own special innervation and its own special denervating impulses, so that the 'kinaesthetic melody' or skilled movement disintegrates into its components.

I have described (part 2, ch. 6) some of the features of this disturbance of the successive organization of movement and indicated the difficulties in the transition from one component to another and the superfluous perseveration of motor elements in cases where a brain lesion lies deep in the premotor zones and disturbs their regulatory role over the basal ganglia; this problem will not therefore be discussed further here. It remains for me to mention another brain structure whose role in the organization of movement cannot be ignored.

Human movements are performed only comparatively rarely by only *one* hand. As a rule they require the coordinated participation of *both* hands, and this coordination has different degrees of complexity. In some cases, the simplest, it takes the form of equal, allied movements in which both hands simultaneously perform the same actions. However, these most elementary cases are relatively rare and they occur only in acts such as swimming or during gymnastic exercises. In other cases, the great majority, the movements of the two hands are coordinated in a more complex fashion, in which the master (right) hand performs the principal action and the subordinate (left) hand merely provides the optimal conditions under which the right hand can work, playing the role of a provider of the motor background. This form of coordination, pointing to the concerted working of both hemispheres, has been closely studied by several investigators (Ananev, 1959). Finally, the most complex types of movement of the two hands are those which are mutually opposite, or reciprocally coordinated in character, when flexion of one hand is accompanied by simultaneous extension of the other.

All these forms of coordinated organization of the movements of both hands can take place only with the close participation of the *anterior zones of the corpus callosum*, the fibres of which connect symmetrical points of the premotor and motor cortex and thus enable these mutually coordinated movements to be performed. It is because of this role of the anterior zones of the corpus callosum in movement coordination (and, in particular, in reciprocal coordination, requiring strict cortical control) that in all patients with a lesion of the anterior part of the corpus callosum whom I have examined, coordinated movements of each hand in isolation were intact, but the *smooth performance of mutually coordinated movements of both hands was impaired* and the most complex forms of reciprocal coordination were completely impossible. The reader is referred elsewhere (Luria, 1962; 1966a; 1966b; 1969a; 1969c) for a discussion of this problem.

Everything I have said about the cerebral organization of voluntary movements and actions is, of course, simply a first step towards the solution of this very difficult problem. However, the general principles of the cerebral organization of voluntary movements and conscious actions are at last beginning to be clarified.

The facts I have described above show without a shadow of doubt that human voluntary movements and actions are complex functional systems, carried out by an equally complex dynamic 'constellation' of concertedly working brain zones, each of which makes its own contribution to the structure of the complex movements. For this reason, a lesion of one of these zones, by blocking one component of this functional system, disturbs the normal organization of the functional system as a whole and leads to the appearance of motor defects.

However, these disturbances of voluntary movement and conscious action differ in character from one case to another, for whereas lesions of some cortical zones disturb the motor plan, cause disintegration of motor programmes, disturb the regulation and verification of the movement, and thus cause the *whole structure of activity to collapse*, lesions of other brain zones disturb only the various *effector* mechanisms of the movements and actions, giving rise to defects of motor *operations*.

For these reasons it is not sufficient simply to state that movements and actions are disturbed. Instead, a careful study of the *structure* of their disturbance in lesions of different parts of the brain is absolutely essential both for the analysis of the pathology of movement in local brain lesions and also for conclusions to be drawn regarding the complex and dynamic cerebral organization of motor acts.

Chapter 10
Attention

Psychological structure

Any organized human mental activity possesses some degree of directivity and *selectivity*. Of the many stimuli which reach us, we respond to only those few which are particularly strong or which appear particularly important and correspond to our interests, intentions or immediate tasks. From the large number of possible movements we choose only those which enable us to reach our immediate goal or to perform a necessary act; and from the large number of traces or their connections stored in our memory, we also select only those few which correspond to our immediate task and enable us to perform some necessary intellectual operations.

In all these cases the likelihood that particular stimuli will reach our consciousness, that particular movements will arise in our behaviour, or that particular traces will spring up in our memory can vary very considerably. The circle of possible sensations, movements or memory traces is narrowed, the probability of appearance of certain impressions, movements or memory traces becomes unequal and selective: some of them (essential or necessary) begin to dominate, while others (inessential or unnecessary) are inhibited.

The directivity and selectivity of mental processes, the basis on which they are organized, is usually termed *attention* in psychology. By this term we imply the factor responsible for picking out the essential elements for mental activity, or the process which keeps a close watch on the precise and organized course of mental activity.

Although the facts concerning attention have been described without any substantial change throughout the history of psychology, starting with the classical publication of Müller (1873) and continuing by the work of Titchener (1908) to the present day, highly conflicting opinions have been expressed by psychologists on the nature of attention.

An extreme position was occupied by the supporters of Gestalt psychology, one of whom (Rubin) actually published a paper entitled 'The non-existence of attention', in which he argued that the selectivity and direction of attention are purely the result of the structural organization of the perceived field, and that the laws governing attention are thus in fact nothing more than the structural laws of visual perception.

The opposite position was held by the supporters of extreme idealism, who drew a sharp line between direct perception and attention and who saw attention as the manifestation of a specific mental factor. Wundt regarded it as the manifestation of active will or apperception, and the French psychologist Révault d'Allones (1923) described it by the term 'schématisation'. In their view, human attention does not arise directly in the process of sensory perception, but is determined entirely by ideal forces which are mental in character and which are described by some workers as the subject's 'set', and by others as his 'creative activity'.

It will be obvious that these widely different approaches to the act of attention and to the facts of the selectivity of mental processes make any scientific solution to the problem of their cerebral mechanisms almost impossible, for whereas psychologists who support the first of these views naturally deny any need for seeking special structures or systems of attention and are perfectly satisfied by pointing to the structural character of excitation taking place in the receptor zones of the cortex, those psychologists who occupy extremely idealistic positions have in general considered it unnecessary to seek any material basis for this fundamentally mental act.

Before any adequate analysis of the cerebral mechanisms of attention could be made, it was necessary to take a completely fresh look at the classical views of this process and to interpret the phenomena of attention from essentially different positions.

This was done firstly, by the introduction into psychology of the new, historial principle of analysis of complex forms of mental activity, associated above all with the work of Vygotsky and his collaborators; and secondly by the examination of physiological facts which provide a new approach to the mechanism governing the selective course of neurophysiological processes. The main task of this new, historical approach to attention was to bridge the gap which had always existed in psychology between elementary, involuntary forms of attention, on the one hand, and the higher, voluntary forms of attention on the other.

It is well known to psychologists that those features of the most elementary, involuntary attention of the type which is attracted by the most powerful or biologically significant stimuli can be observed very early on, during the first few months of the child's development. They consist of turning the eyes, and then the head towards this stimulus, the cessation of all other, irrelevant forms of activity, and the occurrence of a clearly defined group of respiratory, cardiovascular and psychogalvanic responses which Bekhterev called the 'concentration reaction' and Pavlov the 'orienting reflex'. Definite signs of this reaction, distinguishing the most powerful or the most biologically meaningful stimulus and giving behaviour its organized character, could be observed in a child of only a few weeks, at first in the form of an arousal reaction, and later, when the child was awake, initially as fixation of the external stimulus, and later as an active search for it, so that the reaction itself could be defined in precise physiological indices (Polikanina, 1966; Fonarev, 1969). Some investigators have succeeded in observing individual fragments of these features in the newborn infant, especially in the form of a very interesting sign – the cessation of rhythmic sucking movements on presentation of photic stimuli (Bronstein, Itina *et al.*, 1958). Signs of the orienting reaction – this most elementary form of attention – were grouped very early into a definite complex, making their objective study feasible.

Besides this turning of the eyes and head towards the corresponding stimulus, the complex also included autonomic responses: a psycholgalvanic reflex, changes in the respiration rate, and constriction of the peripheral blood vessels (in the finger, for example) while the blood vessels in the head are dilated. Later, as the electrical activity of the cortex matures, these are joined by other phenomena well known in electrophysiology: inhibition of the alpha-rhythm (or desynchronization), or strengthening of the evoked potentials in response to presentation of the corresponding stimulus. This whole complex of autonomic features of the orienting reaction has been studied in great detail by Sokolov, Vinogradova, and their collaborators (Sokolov, 1963; Sokolov *et al.*, 1959; Vinogradova, 1958; 1959a; 1959b). Their investigations have shown that the manifestations of the orienting reaction precede the specific response (for example, constriction of the blood vessels in response to cold and their dilatation in response to warmth) and they are among the essential conditions for the formation of a conditional reflex, which will be slow to develop if the conditioning takes place in the absence of an orienting reflex.

Autonomic or electrophysiological indices of the orienting reaction have definite structural and dynamic features which are manifested as soon as the stimulus is changed (and what is particularly interesting this change need not necessarily be an increase, but it can be a decrease in strength or even the omission of the preceding stimulus), and which are gradually extinguished if the same stimulus continues to be repeated over and over again with the development of habituation. Examples of the manifestations of the orienting reaction as vascular and psychogalvanic responses and as depression of the alpharhythm are illustrated in Figure 69 (Sokolov and Vinogradova), while the manifestation of an orienting reaction to an acoustic stimulus in the form of increased amplitude of the evoked potentials is shown in Figure 70 (Farber and Fried, 1971).

An essential feature of the orienting reaction distinguishing it from the general 'arousal reaction' is that it may be *highly directive and selective in character*. Sokolov, for example, observed that after extinction of the autonomic and electrophysiological components of the orienting reaction to an acoustic stimulus, all other sounds which differed from it continued to evoke orienting reflexes. He accordingly concluded that the phenomenon of habituation, or extinction of the orienting reaction, is highly selective. Consequently, orienting reflexes appear on the slightest sign of mismatching between the 'neuronal model of the stimulus' and the newly presented stimulus (Sokolov, 1960). Hence from the outset, the *orienting reaction may be highly selective in character*, thus creating the basis for *directive and selective, organized behaviour*.

Naturally it will be asked: how can this highly complex form of voluntary attention, manifested as the ability of the subject to verify his own behaviour and which psychologists in the classical period

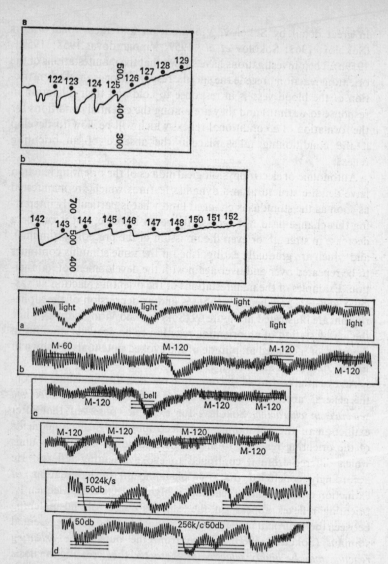

Figure 69 (a) Psychogalvanic and (b) vascular components of the orienting reflex and their participation in the habituation process (after Sokolov and Vinogradova). (a) The numbers mean signals. The subject has to pay attention to signals (to count them). After signals 125 and 146 the signal is eliminated

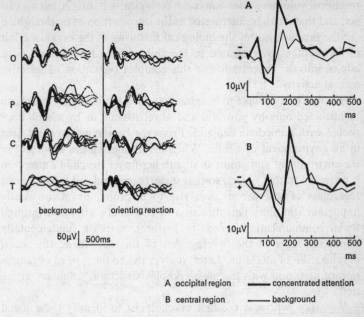

Figure 70 Effect of expectancy on the strengthening of evoked potentials
(after Farber and Fried)

interpreted as a special form of manifestation of mental life having
no roots in biological spheres of activity, arise from these elementary
orienting reactions which physiologists have regarded as a type of
inborn reflex? Does this higher form of attention have its roots in,
and can it be interpreted from the same scientific, deterministic
standpoint, as the forms of elementary, involuntary attention we
have just described?

It is only very recently that a scientific approach to the solution of
these problems, as proposed originally by the leading Soviet psychologist Vygotsky, has secured a firm place in psychology. This approach
differs radically from the typical approach of classical psychology,
and for the first time it provides a scientific key to the understanding
of these complex forms of attention, while, at the same time, it
traces its origin from completely different roots. It consists essentially
of the recognition of the fact that, unlike the elementary orienting

reactions, voluntary attention is not biological in its origin, but a *social* act, and that it can be interpreted as the introduction of factors which are the product, not of the biological maturing of the organism, but of forms of activity created in the child during his relations with adults, into the organization of this complex regulation of selective mental activity.

It would be a mistake to imagine that the attention of the infant can be attracted only by powerful and novel stimuli, or by stimuli connected with immediate demand. From the beginning the child lives in an environment of adults. When his mother names an object in the environment and points to it with her finger the child's attention is attracted to that object, so that it starts to stand out from the rest regardless of whether it gives rise to a strong, novel, or vitally important stimulus. This direction of the child's attention through social communication, words or gestures, marks a fundamentally important stage in the development of this new form, the social organization of attention. Later, it gives rise to the type of organization of attention with the most complex structure, voluntary attention.

Vygotsky, who was the first psychologist to identify these social roots of the higher forms of attention, expressed his views in the principle which I have already cited.

In the early stages of development the complex psychological function *was shared between two persons*: the adult *triggered* the psychological process by naming the object or by pointing to it; the child *responded* to this signal and picked out the named object either by fixing it with his eye or by holding it with his hand. In the subsequent stages of development this socially organized process becomes reorganized. The child himself learns to speak. He can now name the object *himself*, and by naming the object himself he distinguishes it from the rest of the environment, and thus directs his attention to it. The function which hitherto was shared between two people now becomes a method of *internal organization of the psychological process*. From an external, socially organized attention develops the *child's voluntary attention*, which in this stage is an internal, self-regulating process.

This identification of the social roots of the higher forms of voluntary attention, which Vygotsky first recognized, is of decisive importance: it bridged the gap between the elementary forms of involuntary attention and the higher forms of voluntary attention, thus preserving their unity, and maintaining a common, scientific and deterministic approach to a form of attention which psychologists in the past had usually placed in the category of 'mental', so that this most complex form of attention became completely accessible to scientific analysis. Of course these higher forms of voluntary attention do not become possible immediately. Long study has shown that the reverse is the case: the formation of voluntary attention has a long and dramatic history, and the child acquires an efficient and stable, socially-organized attention only shortly before he is due to start school.

Observations have shown that the child does not immediately develop the ability to obey even a direct, simple verbal instruction directing his attention to a certain object. The simple arousing (or 'impulsive') action of a verbal instruction can be observed in a child by the end of the first or beginning of the second year of life: I have already stated that in response to the mother's simple question – 'where is the doll?' or 'where is the cup?' the young infant directs his fixation towards the object named and reaches out for it. However, this takes place only in the most simple conditions, namely when there are no distracting objects in the external field of vision.

As soon as this test is repeated under different conditions, and the child is instructed to 'give the doll', while at the same time another distracting or unfamiliar toy, such as a fish or bird, is placed alongside it, a different result will be obtained. In this case the child's fixation at first wanders between all these objects, and it frequently rests not on the doll which has been named, but on the brightly coloured or new bird or fish which happens to be near; the child reaches for the new, brightly coloured or distracting object and gives it instead. At this stage of development (roughly one year six months to two years four months) a spoken instruction cannot yet overcome factors of involuntary attention competing with it, and victory in this struggle goes to the factors of the direct field of vision. The direct orienting response to a new, informative or distracting stimulus, formed in the early stages of development, easily suppresses the higher, social form of attention which has only just begun to appear. Not until four and half to five years of age is this ability to obey a spoken instruction strong enough to evoke a dominant connection, so that the child is easily able to eliminate the influence of all irrelevant, distracting factors, although signs of instability of higher forms of attention evoked by a spoken instruction may still continue to appear for a considerable time longer.

I shall not attempt to examine in detail the further course of formation of this higher type of internal, voluntary attention, which by school age has become established as a stable form of selective behaviour, subordinated not only to the audible speech of an adult, but also to the child's own internal speech, nor shall I describe the successive stages through which this type of attention passes during its formation in ontogeny; this has been done elsewhere (Vygotsky, 1956; Luria, 1961; 1969b) and it does not fall within the scope of this book.

Characteristically, by the time the child goes to school the forms of selective behaviour organized with the participation of speech may have developed to such an extent that they can significantly change not only the course of movement and actions, but also the organization of sensory processes. One example will suffice to illustrate this statement.

At the end of the 1950s, Homskaya (unpublished investigation) observed the following fact which clearly indicates the influence of speech on the increased precision of sensory processes. A child who had just started school was instructed to make a certain movement in response to a pale pink colour but to make no movement in response to a darker shade of pink. With an increase in the speed of presentation of the cues the subject's performance fell off sharply, and mistakes occurred, sometimes as many as 50 per cent. If, however, the test was carried out so that the child was instructed to evaluate the shades in words at the same time (by saying 'pale' or 'dark'), and to give the appropriate response at the same time, the accuracy of discrimination between the shades was considerably increased, with a consequent decrease in the number of mistakes. The inclusion of the child's own speech enabled the differential features to be distinguished, made sensitivity more selective, and made the responses much more stable. Other published investigations by Homskaya (1958) have shed light on some of the internal mechanisms of this organizing influence of the child's own speech and point to a new approach to the analysis of its role in the structure of the higher forms of voluntary attention.

Physiological indicators of attention

The process of attention can be observed not only during organized, selective behaviour. It is also reflected in precise physiological indices, which can be used to study the stability of attention.

When I analysed the work of the first functional unit of the brain – the unit responsible for cortical tone–I pointed out that any phenomenon of arousal is accompanied by a whole group of symptoms which indicate a general increase in the level of preparedness or tone of the organism. These include the familiar changes in cardiac activity and respiration, constriction of the peripheral blood vessels, the appearance of a psychogalvanic reflex, and the occurrence of desynchronization phenomena (depression of the alpha-rhythm) which are observed whenever attention is attracted by a stimulus or by some form of activity.

As the result of recent work it is necessary to supplement this list of well-known phenomena with others: changes in the slow potential of the electroencephalogram now generally known by the term 'expectancy waves' introduced by Grey Walter, the appearance of numerous synchronously functioning cortical points (Livanov, 1962; Livanov *et al.*, 1967) and, finally, changes in the normal periodic alternation of slow waves and in the relationship between the ascending and descending fronts of the alpha-waves, first described by Genkin (1962; 1963; 1964).

All these phenomena are *generalized* in character and they take the form of activation, regardless of whether it is evoked by the change from sleep to waking, by an elementary change in intensity, or by the novelty or attractiveness of the stimulus, or by a verbal instruction. They can therefore be regarded as signs of a change in the *general background of the subject's attention*. However, besides these signs there are others of a different type, revealing the specialized forms of activation or of directed, selective attention. First on the list for our consideration are changes in cortical evoked potentials.

The phenomenon of evoked potentials, first invstigated by Adrian (1936), Jouvet (1956), Hernández-Peón (1961; 1966), Dawson (1958a; 1958b; Dawson *et al.*, 1959), Peimer (1958) and many others, is essentially as follows. Presentation of a special (visual, acoustic,

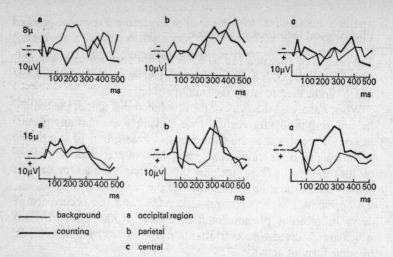

_____ background   a   occipital region

_____ counting   b   parietal

                c   central

Figure 71 Increase in amplitude of evoked potentials during an effort of active attention (after Farber and Fried)

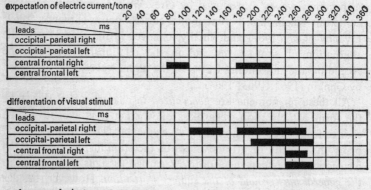

Figure 72 Spread of significant changes in evoked potentials to various cortical zones during activation of selective attention (after Simernitskaya)

266 Synthetic Mental Activities

tactile or nociceptive) stimulus evokes an electrical response (evoked potential) in the corresponding (occipital, temporal and central) regions of the cortex. A particularly important feature for our purpose here is that the structure of these changes varies substantially depending on the intensity of the stimulus and on the subject's activity; a change (increase in amplitude) of the evoked potentials may arise as the direct response to a sensory stimulus in the first phase of the evoked potential (after a latent period of 30–50 ms), while changes induced by more complex activity, such as by the analysis of information, arise in the late stages of the evoked potentials (after a latent period of 150–250 ms).

The phenomenon of evoked potentials can be used not only to indicate a direct response to a specific sensory stimulus, but also to record objectively changes in the reception and analysis of information arising through the *mobilization of active attention*.

Evoked potentials can be studied as an objective indicator of attention in two ways. First, a comparison can be made between the way in which the evoked potential changes during the distraction of attention by an irrelevant stimulus, and how it is increased when attention to the relevant stimulus is strengthened. Tests of the first type were included in the classical investigations of Hernández-Peón (1956; 1960; 1969), who showed that potentials evoked by an acoustic stimulus in a cat are sharply inhibited on the presentation of the sight or smell of a mouse. Tests of the second type have been carried out mainly on man; evoked potentials obtained in response to the usual presentation of sensory stimuli were compared with evoked potentials obtained during *active expectancy* of these stimuli (after a warning instruction), or when the analysis of these stimuli was complicated by the presentation of the instruction: 'Count the number of stimuli', 'Distinguish between changes in the tone or intensity of the stimulus', and so on. The results obtained by various workers under these conditions (Lindsley, 1960; 1961; Peimer, 1958; 1966; Simernitskaya, 1970; Tecce, 1970) showed that the attraction of attention by *active expectancy* or *complication of the task* leads to an appreciable *increase in amplitude of the evoked potential*, and comparison of such tests with those undertaken under 'background' conditions, in which the sensory stimuli were presented without any preliminary instruction, clearly showed that this increase in amplitude of the evoked potentials (and especially in their second, late phase) is a definite and *objective sign of voluntary attention*.

Another characteristic fact is that this feature of a lasting increase in amplitude of the evoked potentials under the influence of a spoken instruction, mobilizing attention, is ill-defined in the child before and on just reaching school age, but becomes definite and stable in character in the later stages of development of the schoolchild. This is illustrated in Figure 71.

However, with the use of the evoked-potentials method it is possible to make a much more detailed analysis of the cerebral mechanisms of the physiological processes lying at the basis of voluntary attention.

Investigations have shown that a change of task (such as giving an instruction to look carefully for a change in the stimulus) not only increased the amplitude of the evoked potential, but also led to its spread to *other cortical zones* lying outside the cortical nucleus of the particular analyser, i.e. the primary sensory area, so that it could be detected even in distant parts of the cortex.

This phenomenon is demonstrated most clearly by the graphs, which I have taken from an investigation undertaken by Simernitskaya in our laboratory (Figure 72). This graph shows that whereas direct presentation of the stimulus gives rise after a delay of about 80–100 ms to evoked potentials restricted to the corresponding primary sensory zones, a preliminary instruction to expect the stimulus or to look out for changes in its intensity or character, increasing the load on differential attention, caused significant changes in potentials to begin to appear after 200–250 ms in other, distant regions of the cortex, including the frontal cortex. The great importance of these experiments to the detailed analysis of cortical systems participating in processing involving higher forms of active attention will be obvious.

These objective electrophysiological studies not only provide an insight into intimate mechanisms of complex types of attention, but they also enable the principal stages of their formation to be studied. This opportunity has been presented by a number of recent investigations, notably those of Farber and her collaborators (Farber, 1969; Farber and Fried, 1971; Fried, 1970). These investigations showed that whereas an *immediate orienting reaction* leads to a per-

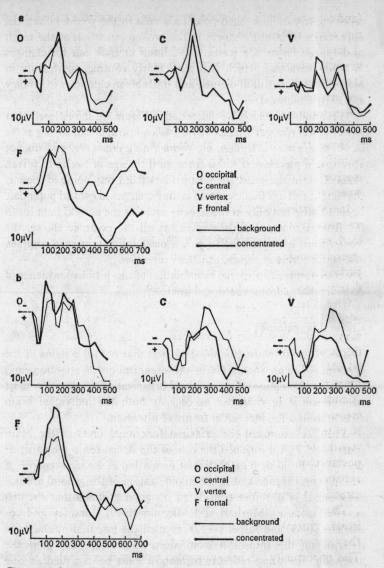

Figure 73 Spread of changes in evoked potentials to different cortical zones during mobilization of active attention in children of various ages. Changes in evoked potentials under the influence of a spoken instruction to assess different visual stimuli: (a) in a child aged seven years; (b) in a youth aged fourteen years (after Farber and Fried).

ceptible increase in evoked potentials even in the young infant, the appearance of lasting changes in the evoked potentials as the result of a *spoken instruction* (count the stimuli or look out for changes in their character), which is a particularly conspicuous feature in older children, is still ill-defined and unstable in character in infancy and early childhood.

These findings, which are illustrated in Figure 73, show clearly that *physiological changes produced by a spoken instruction and lying at the basis of voluntary attention, are formed only gradually*, and do not appear in a precise and stable form until the age of twelve to fifteen years. One of the most significant facts from our point of view is that it is at this age that clear and lasting changes in evoked potentials begin to arise not only in the sensory areas of the cortex, but also in the frontal zones, at a time when, as all the evidence shows, the *frontal zones* are beginning to play a more intimate part in complex and stable forms of *higher, voluntary attention*.

Let us now make a special examination of this problem, which is of considerable neuropsychological interest.

Cerebral organization

The facts we have just examined suggest that not all systems of the forebrain play an equal role in the organization of attention, and that our examination of the cerebral organization of attention must be differential in character as regards both the individual brain structures and the individual forms of attention.

When we examined the principal functional units of the brain (part 1, ch. 2), I mentioned the role of the structures in the superior part of the brain stem and reticular formation in the maintenance of waking cortical tone and in the manifestation of the general arousal reaction. It is therefore considered on good grounds that the discoveries made by Moruzzi and Magoun (1949), Lindsley and coworkers (1949) and Jasper (1957) revealed the essential mechanisms determining the transition from sleep to waking, and that the ascending activating reticular formation must be regarded as one of the most important systems ensuring the most generalized and elementary forms of attention.

These hypotheses have been confirmed not only by numerous well-known experiments with animals, in which division of the reticular formation of the brain stem induced sleep, while its stimulation induced increased vigilance and sharpened sensation (see the survey of this material by Lindsley, 1960), but also by clinical observations in which lesions of the upper part of the brain stem and the walls of the third ventricle lead to the onset of sleep or to an oneiroid, drowsy state, and that cortical tone in these cases is sharply reduced, and the waking, selective state of consciousness profoundly disturbed.

However, the mechanisms of the superior brain stem and ascending activating reticular formation are responsible for only one, the most elementary, condition of attention – the generalized state of waking.

Any complex form of attention, involuntary or, more especially, voluntary, requires the provision of other conditions, namely the possibility of *selective recognition of a particular stimulus* and inhibition of responses to irrelevant stimuli, of no importance in the current situation. This contribution to the organization of attention is made by other brain structures located at a higher level: in the *limbic cortex* and in the *frontal region*. Let us examine the relevant facts for each case separately.

The role of structures of the old cortex or limbic region (hippocampus, amygdala) and the connective systems of the caudate body has recently attracted the close attention of investigators. Studies at the single unit level, as I have pointed out, have clearly shown that neurons not responding to modally-specific stimuli, but apparently comparing old and new stimuli and enabling a response to be made to *new* stimuli or to their properties, while responses to old, habitual stimuli are extinguished, occupy an important place in these particular structures (Vinogradova, 1969; 1970a; 1970b). That is why hippocampal structures, intimately concerned in the mechanisms of inhibition of irrelevant stimuli and of habituation to stimuli repeated over long periods of time, at an early stage began to be regarded as essential components of the inhibitory or 'filtering' system, of necessity participating in selective responses to specific stimuli and forming a part of the system of inborn orienting reflexes and instinctive behaviour. For this reason the hippocampus, and later the caudate body began to be regarded as essential structures for the elimination of responses to irrelevant stimuli and enabled the organism to behave in a strictly selective manner (Grastyan, 1961; Douglas and Pribra̍m, 1966; Vinogradova, 1969; 1970a, 1970b), and that a lesion of these structures was a source of the breakdown of selectivity of behaviour, which is in fact more a disturbance of selective attention than a defect of memory. These views regarding the role of the limbic region and, in particular, hippocampal structures in the organization of behaviour correspond also to changes in behaviour and in the state of consciousness observed in patients with lesions of this region which are manifested either in the clinical picture or in the results of special electrophysiological tests.

Clinically, the patients of this group, with tumours deep in the midline, do not exhibit disturbances of gnosis and praxis, speech or formally logical processes. The whole pathology of their behaviour amounts to instability of their selective responses, marked fatiguability, and the rapid transition to unselective responses to different stimuli.

In relatively mild cases, this lesion is manifested by increased distractability, the rapid termination of goal-directed activity, the ready eruption of irrelevant associations, and well-defined disturbances of memory; we shall discuss these again. In more severe cases (massive tumours affecting the walls of the third ventricle and the limbic region) this syndrome is more severe in character and begins to manifest itself as a drowsy, oneiroid state in which the patient loses the distinction between present and past, becomes confused, and starts to confabulate. In both cases, irrelevant stimuli are at once woven into their train of thought and the structure of their consciousness becomes completely confused instead of organized directive and selective. Such a patient may declare that he is not in hospital, but at home or at work (sometimes in both places at once), or he may say that he is in some vague, temporary place (for example, at a railway station); he may say that his relatives are with him in that place, or he may take the physician for one of his acquaintances at work; he may show other signs of gross disturbances of consciousness which are particularly obvious if the anterior zones of the limbic region are involved in the pathological process, and if his awareness that the selective course of his mental processes is impaired (Luria, Homskaya, Blinkov and Critchley, 1967). These phenomena are confirmed by the electroencephalographic changes in cortical activity arising in such cases.

The clinical facts described above were to some extent explained by the results of recent electrophysiological tests on patients with massive diencephalic lesions or tumours of the walls of the third ventricle and adjacent zones of the limbic region. These investigations (Latash, 1968; Filippycheva and Faller, 1970) showed that the autonomic and electrophysiological components of the orienting reflex are severely depressed in these patients, and even repeated stimuli begin to evoke only very weak and rapidly disappearing responses; this clearly results from a deficiency of those non-specific brain-stem influences which under normal conditions maintain the appropriate level of cortical tone.

The law of strength, according to which strong stimuli evoke strong, and weak stimuli evoke weak responses, no longer applies; stimuli of different intensity begin to evoke equal responses, and sometimes a stimulus produces not depression, but paradoxical exaltation of the alpha-rhythms. The process of habituation to a new stimulus, which is clearly observed when the cortex is in a normal state, also undergoes profound changes and the electrophysiological components of the orienting reflex are either absent altogether or become inextinguishable. At the same time these investigations show that in this group of patients distortions of the normal process of excitation may take place, a feature which brings us directly to the explanation of the mechanisms of the mental disturbances I have just described.

However, an essential feature of all these cases is that *all these signs of a primary disturbance of directive and selective attention* may to some extent be compensated in time by the *introduction of a verbal instruction* or, in other words, by the incorporation of intact higher structural levels of the process into the system. Usually this compensation is only temporary in character, and the selectivity of the electrophysiological processes is quickly lost; *however, this potential integrity of the higher, voluntary forms of attention* in the presence of a primary disturbance of its elementary forms is an important sign distinguishing these patients from those with lesions in other situations.

The *frontal lobes* of the brain have an altogether different role in the organization of attention. In the classical investigations on animals, as I have already mentioned (part 2, ch. 7), it was often held that the frontal lobes are directly concerned with the preservation of memory traces, and that this is manifested by the disturbance of delayed responses in animals after extirpation of the frontal cortex. However, as I have already stated, this fact has received a completely different interpretation as a result of later work. It was shown (Malmo, 1942; Pribram, 1959b; 1963a; Weiskrantz, 1968) that an animal cannot perform delayed responses correctly after extirpation of its frontal lobes not only because it cannot retain the previous traces, but rather because it begins to be distracted constantly by irrelevant stimuli, and it cannot inhibit these inadequate responses. That is why, as these workers showed, the removal of all irrelevant stimuli (for example, by placing the animal in complete darkness or by carrying out the experiment after administration of tranquillizers, lowering the general cortical tone) led to the restoration of normal delayed responses. The essential role of the frontal lobes in the inhibition of responses to irrelevant stimuli and in the preservation of goal-directed, programmed behaviour, has also been demonstrated by the experiments of Konorski and Lawicka (1964), Brutkowski (1964; 1966) and others. Because of the disturbance of these inhibitory mechanisms, extirpation of the frontal lobes in these animals always led to severe forms of disturbance of goal-directed, directive and selective behaviour and to disinhibition of impulsive responses to irrelevant stimuli. The changes in animal behaviour which were described in the classical works of Bianchi (1895; 1921; Jacobsen (1935), Anokhin (1949), and Pribram (1954; 1958b) clearly demonstrate this primary source of the disturbance of their activity.

A wealth of information regarding the disturbances of selective behaviour and, above all, of the *higher forms of attention* is given by clinical studies of patients with frontal lobe lesions.

By contrast with patients with lesions of the superior part of the brain stem and the limbic region, in patients with massive lesions of the frontal lobes the elementary forms of involuntary attention or of impulsive orienting reactions to irrelevant stimuli may not only be preserved, but may also be pathologically enhanced. Conversely, *all attempts to induce stable voluntary attention in these patients with the aid of spoken instructions* are ineffective.

Inability to concentrate on an instruction and to inhibit responses to irrelevant stimuli becomes apparent even during the first clinical observations of patients with massive frontal lobe lesions. Usually these patients begin to perform the task set, but as soon as a stranger enters the ward, or the person in the next bed whispers to the nurse, the patient ceases to perform the task and transfers his gaze to the newcomer or joins in the conversation with his neighbour. It is therefore best to investigate such a patient by starting to carry out the test on his neighbour; in such cases the patient will involuntarily join in the conversation and thereby exhibit the involuntary activity which would be difficult to induce by directly instructing the patient himself.

This increased distractability of patients with massive frontal lobe lesions is the cause of those profound disturbances of his goal-directed behaviour which I have described above (part 2, ch. 7) and to which I shall turn again when discussing disturbances of thinking in frontal lobe lesions.

The profound disturbances of voluntary attention or of higher forms of verification of activity, associated with the revival of elementary forms of the orienting reflex, create a picture of behavioural disturbances which I have so often seen in patients with frontal lesions.

As a result of psychophysiological investigations undertaken during the last few years, we can now distinguish the mechanisms lying at the basis of the disturbance of these higher forms of attention. Grey Walter (see part 2, ch. 7) established the fact that the expectation of a stimulus evokes specific slow potentials in the human frontal lobes, which he describes as 'expectancy waves', and these waves subsequently spread to other areas of the brain (Figure 19). At the same time, Livanov and his collaborators found that intellectual stress gives rise to a sharp increase in the number of synchronously working points in the frontal cortex (Figure 20).

These phenomena unequivocally indicate that the human frontal lobes participate in the activation induced by a spoken instruction and are a part of the brain system directly involved in the processes associated with the higher forms of active attention. The fact that the frontal lobes have so many connections with the reticular formation provides a morphological and physiological basis for the participation of the frontal lobes in these higher forms of activation.

All these facts provide an explanation of some of the fundamental results obtained by psychophysiological tests on patients with frontal lobe lesions discovered in the course of many years of careful research by Homskaya and her collaborators (Homskaya, 1960; 1965; 1966a; 1966b; 1969; 1972; Luria and Homskaya, 1970; Artemeva, 1965; Artemeva and Homskaya, 1966; Baranovskaya and Homskaya, 1966; Baranovskaya, 1968; Simernitskaya, 1970; Simernitskaya and Homskaya, 1966).

As I have stated, lesions of the superior parts of the brain stem and limbic system may disturb the primary basis of attention, the orienting reaction, which either may be unstable and easily extinguished, or may cease to be suppressed by habituation factors. However, it is characteristic that in these cases the attraction of attention to a stimulus with the aid of a verbal instruction can compensate for its defects and strengthen the electrophysiological and autonomic components of attention. The same sort of situation can be observed in patients with lesions of the posterior zones of the brain, in whom pathological states of the cortex may lead to instability of the physiological basis of attention, but in whom, however, the receipt of a verbal instruction immediately raises the tone of attention and compensates for the defect. The diligent efforts to compensate for the defect which can be observed in all patients of this type during rehabilitative training, and which demand special concentration and the stability of voluntary attention, illustrate this situation.

It is a very different matter with patients with massive frontal lobe lesions. As I have already mentioned, the elementary orienting reflexes of these patients are frequently pathologically enhanced, and this interferes with their purposive and steadfast performance of the task.

A different picture is found in these patients if the stability of their responses to excessively presented stimuli is tested. Many patients of this group in such cases exhibit gross instability of attention, so that after a few presentations of the same stimuli, the autonomic and electrophysiological components of their orienting reflex disappear.

However, there is another difference between patients with frontal lobe lesions and those with local lesions in the posterior zones of the brain: whereas in the latter the mobilizing of special attention by means of an additional instruction, which has the effect of increasing activity (for example, the instruction 'count the stimuli', or 'look out for changes in them' and so on) at once restores the extinguished symptoms of the orienting reflex and stabilizes the attention, in patients with frontal lesions this does not happen, and an *instruction which should increase the patient's activity in fact produces no consistent changes.*

The same pattern is seen in other indices of the activation process which, under normal conditions, arises in response to stimuli mobilizing attention. Whereas under normal conditions the repeated presentation of a stimulus leads to extinction of the vascular orienting reflex, as soon as the subject is instructed to direct his attention to changes in the quality or intensity of the stimulus, or to count the number of stimuli, the vascular components of the orienting reflex are immediately restored and they persist for a long period of time. This does not happen in patients with massive lesions of the frontal lobes, for although their vascular responses to repeated stimuli are rapidly extinguished, a verbal instruction which, under normal circumstances, would mobilize attention, in this case has no effect and the plethysmographic curve remains unchanged.

Whereas under normal conditions the first presentation of a stimulus evokes distinct changes in the electrophysiological responses of the brain, in the form of depression of the alpha-rhythm and augmentation of the fast components of the electroencephalogram, and whereas repeated presentation of stimuli leads to the development of 'habituation' and to the disappearance of these responses, as soon as the subject receives an instruction which raises his attention to these stimuli, the electrophysiological components of the orienting reflex are restored and stable in character for a long time. There is a partial change in the composition of this activation reaction in both the alpha and beta bands. This role of attention in stabilizing the phenomena of activation, which remains intact in patients with lesions of the posterior zones of the brain, is absent in patients with massive frontal lobe lesions, for even though they may still continue to carry out the instruction given them, they do so without any appreciable mobilization of attention, and the electrophysiological signs reflecting the elevation and stabilization of the background of activity against which these responses take place are not restored. Often under these conditions the activation reaction becomes reversed in sign (Homskaya, 1972).

Finally, whereas under normal conditions stimulation of a particular modality leads to the appearance of evoked potentials in the corresponding cortical zones, in these patients the preliminary instruction to expect the stimulus or to look out for differences between the stimuli causes a marked increase in the amplitude of the evoked potentials and to their spread to other zones of the cortex over a wide area. These phenomena, which have been described in detail by many writers, persist in patients with lesions of the posterior zones, but are absent in patients with massive frontal lesions, in whom, as in other subjects, the stimulus evokes a definite response, specific for that particular modality, in the form of an evoked potential, but the intensity of this potential remained unchanged despite the instruction which must have raised the level of attention or distorted the character of the evoked potentials.

The facts I have described above are illustrated very clearly in Figures 53–7.

These results suggest that the *frontal lobes play an important role in raising the level of vigilance of a subject* when performing a task, and they thus *participate decisively in the higher forms of attention*. This fact, of great importance to the study of the cerebral mechanisms of complex forms of attention, has been studied in detail by Homskaya and her co-workers, whose comparative observations on patients with different types of frontal lobe lesions have not only fully confirmed the proposition expressed above, but have filled in many of its details.

They found that this phenomenon of loss of activation as a result of a spoken instruction was seen particularly clearly in patients with massive and bilateral frontal lesions affecting the *medial portions* of the frontal lobes. It occurred in patients whose behaviour was marked by the features of inactivity, distractability, and a profound disturbance of the selectivity of their mental processes, and also occasionally in patients with almost no clinical manifestations of a change of behaviour that were detectable on external observation.

Patients with lesions of the lateral portions of the frontal lobes exhibited a rather different picture. Activation arising through the direct influence of stimuli was sufficiently well marked in these patients and was quickly extinguished; however, these features of activation could be strengthened and stabilized by verbal instruction only after its frequent repetition, and in these cases the activation was very unstable and quickly disappeared, making further frequent repetition of the instruction necessary for its reappearance.

These observations showed that the mechanism of the higher forms of activation is either completely disturbed in patients with frontal lobe lesions, or it loses its stable and generalized character, and that the frontal lobes, and especially their medial zones (which are particularly closely connected with the descending tracts of the reticular formation and with the limbic region), play a decisive role in this process of raising the general level of background activity.

The great importance of these investigations (described by Homskaya, 1972) in the study of the cerebral mechanisms of the higher forms of attention and the great contribution they have made to our views of the organization of the dynamics of human intentions and complex forms of human conscious activity are evident.

Chapter 11
Memory

Psychological structure

For a long time the study of the cerebral organization of memory was one of the least explored fields of psychophysiology, and it is only in the last decade that interest has appreciably awakened. However, despite this fact, the cerebral organization of complex forms of mnestic activity still remains a new and largely unopened chapter of neuropsychological science.

The reasons for this situation are the oversimplified views of memory held by the great majority of physiologists, and the total failure to appreciate the complex structure of mnestic processes which psychologists have studied only in the last twenty or thirty years.

An attempt to summarize everything known about the nature and the material substrate of memory at the beginning of this century will make it clear how little there was of scientific value. On the one hand there were the views of Richard Semon and Karl Eward Hering, who considered that memory, or the ability to retain traces, is a 'universal property of matter', the truth of which cannot be denied, but which is much too general and tells us nothing. On the other hand, there were the well-known views of Henri Bergson (1896), that there are two types of memory – bodily memory and mental memory – and that whereas the former is a natural phenomenon, of the same sort Semon and Hering wrote about, the second must be regarded as a manifestation of 'free will', able through a mental effort of will to evoke individual traces of past experience.

Comparatively little was added to the discussion of the nature and physiological basis of memory as a result of the morphological and physiological studies undertaken in the first forty years of this century. Painstaking morphological investigations of the nerve cell and connections produced nothing more than the general assertion that the retention of traces of previous excitation is evidently the result of the possession of a synaptic system (Ramon-y-Cajal, 1909–11), and that it must evidently consist of biochemical processes connected with the balance between acetylcholine and cholinesterase, substances with an important role in synaptic transmission of impulses (de Robertis, 1964; Eccles, 1957–64). Research into the physiology of the conditioned reflex, entirely devoted to processes concerned with the fixation of experience, established nothing more than some basic physiological factors of what was very conventionally described as 'opening the pathways' and 'the reinforcement of conditioned connections', but in fact contributed nothing of substance to the elucidation of the nature of memory. Equally unproductive were the investigations of learning conducted by the American behaviourists, for despite the fact that there are many thousands of publications on this subject, the nature of memory still remains completely unknown. It was facts such as these that led the American psychologist Lashley, in his well-known paper 'In Search of the Engram' (1950), to the pessimistic conclusion that the material nature of memory is just as much an enigma as it was many decades ago.

The quest for a solution to the problem of the material basis of memory took a new turn as a result of the work of Hydén (1960; 1962; 1964), who showed that retention of a trace from previous excitation is associated with a lasting change in the structure of ribonucleic acid and who found a lasting increase in the RNA/DNA content in nuclei subjected to intensive excitation. Hydén's work initiated a flood of intensive research, increasing yearly in quantity, and it led to the hypothesis which has now gained wide acceptance that RNA/DNA molecules are the carriers of memory, that they play the decisive role both in the transmission of inherited traces and in the retention of traces from previous experience during the life of the individual. It has even been concluded from this hypothesis that information arising in one individual can be transmitted by a humoral mechanism to a second individual, and the extensively publicized (although not finally authenticated) experiments of McConnell, Jacobson and Kimble (1970) have recently raised the hopes that the material substrate of memory will soon be discovered.

Other investigations display the hitherto unsuspected role, not of the nerve cell itself, but of the surrounding *glia*, in the retention of traces of previous excitation. It was shown that processes of excitation arising in the neuron and in the glia not only have different latent periods (several hundred times longer in the glia than in the neurons), but are reciprocally related, so that at the moment of excitation the RNA level in the neurons rises while that of the surrounding glia falls, whereas in the after-period (evidently connected with trace retention) it falls sharply in the neurons but rises equally sharply and remains high for a long time in the glia. The hypothesis that the glia is concerned in the retention of memory traces is unquestionably one of the most important discoveries in modern neurophysiology and it must shed considerable light on the intimate mechanisms of memory.

The last observations which I cannot fail to mention were obtained as the result of electron-microscopic investigations on nerve cells engaged in the process of storing excitation. The movements of the tiny vesicles which accompanies this process, in conjunction with changes in the membranes during trace formation (de Robertis, 1964; Eccles, 1957; 1961a; 1961b), have also revealed new aspects of this process and they must evidently be regarded as important components of the intimate mechanisms of excitation and trace formation.

Research at the cellular and subcellular (molecular) level into the mechanisms of trace processes have undoubtedly yielded important facts concerned with the intimate biochemical and morphophysiological mechanisms of memory. However, they have done nothing to answer the question of which brain zones actually contribute to the processes of memory, and which aspects of mnestic activity are the responsibility of particular brain systems.

To find the answer to these questions, two decisive steps had to be taken. Firstly, it was necessary to abandon the too generalized and diffuse concept of trace processes for more precise psychological concepts of the actual *structure of mnestic activity*. Secondly, instead of investigating trace processes at the cellular molecular level, it was necessary to study the actual cerebral *architectonics of memory processes* or, in other words, to analyse the *contribution which each brain zone makes to the organization of human mnestic processes*.

Attempts to find the answers to these questions have been made, on the one hand by psychologists, and on the other hand by neurologists and neuropsychologists, and during the last twenty years the structure of mnestic processes has been the subject of a whole series of investigations which have substantially enriched our previous ideas.

I shall now attempt to summarize these investigations briefly before turning to the main subject of this chapter; analysis of the role of the human brain structures in the organization of mnestic processes.

Classical psychology regarded memory either as a process of direct imprinting of traces in consciousness, or of imprinting the single-valued associative connections formed by individual impressions with each other. This oversimplified view does not satisfy modern investigators.

Recent work (Norman, 1966; 1968; Norman and Rumelhart, 1970; Wickelgren, 1970; Kintsch, 1970a; 1970b; Miller, 1969; Kubie, 1969; Posner, 1963; 1967; 1969; Shiffrin, 1970; Reitman, 1970) has shown that memorizing is a complex process consisting of a series of successive stages, differing in their psychological structure, in the 'volume' of traces capable of fixation, and in the duration of their storage, and extending over a period of time.

It has been suggested (Sperling, 1960; 1963; Sperling and Spellman, 1970; Morton, 1969; 1970) that the process of memorizing begins with the imprinting of sensory cues (if it is a question of verbal traces, the phonetic features of a word heard). These cues are multiple in character, and the imprinting naturally picks out only some of them, making an appropriate selection, which occurs at this stage (Norman and Rumelhart, 1970; Wickelgren, 1970; Sperling and Spellman, 1970). Some writers have pointed out that this stage of imprinting is very narrow in its scope and very short in the duration of the imprinted traces, and they describe it as 'ultrashort memory' (Broadbent, 1970); however, they point out that traces of stimuli received in this period can be greatly extended in volume in cases of visual stimuli (Sperling, 1960; 1963).

The next stage in the mnestic process is considered by many authorities to be the transfer of stimuli to the stage of the *image memory*: stimuli perceived are converted into visual images. However, this conversion is never a simple conversion of a single-valued sensory stimulus into a visual image, but it presupposes the selection of an appropriate image from many possible ones and it can be interpreted as the distinctive processing or coding of stimuli received (Kintsch, 1970a; 1970b; Shiffrin, 1970; Reitman, 1970; Posner, 1969). However, this stage is regarded by most workers as merely *intermediate*, and one which is quickly followed by the last stage, the complex *coding of traces* or their inclusion into a *system of categories*.

Careful analysis of this network of categories into which the trace of virtually every stimulus imprinted by the subject (or every piece of information received by him) is included, constitutes the central object of many investigations of mnestic processes published in recent years. Some of these are purely psychological or a combination of psychological and logical in character (Norman and Rumelhart, 1970; Wickelgren, 1970; Kintsch, 1970a; 1970b; Posner, 1963; 1969), some have the character of attempts to construct complex models of memory based on ideas regarding the role of this coding (Reitman, 1970; Feigenbaum, 1970), and others again are based on an analysis of psycholinguistic data (Miller, 1969; Morton, 1969; 1970). All, however, unanimously agree that the systems of connections into which traces of information reaching the subject are introduced are *coded with respect to different signs*, and consequently they form *multidimensional matrices* from which the subject must *choose* each time the system which, at that particular moment, will form the basis for coding. This approach to memory processes naturally shows that, far from being a simple and passive process, *recall is complex and active in nature*. A person wishing to recall a certain item of information exhibits a certain recall strategy, choosing the necessary means, distinguishing the important and inhibiting the unimportant signs, selecting, depending on the purpose of the task, the sensory or logical components of the imprinted material and fitting them into appropriate systems (Kintsch, 1970a; 1970b; Shiffrin, 1970; Posner, 1963; 1969; Reitman, 1970). This approach approximates the process of recall to a *complex and active investigative activity*, it enables the subject to use the activities of language (Miller, 1969; Morton, 1969; 1970), and, in the opinion of most investigators, it constitutes the essential link in the transition from *short-term* to *long-term* memory (Miller, 1969).

The problem of *forgetting* is closely linked with that of remembering, and it has attracted the same close attention. What causes the *disappearance of memory traces* or, as it is usually called, forgetting?

A generation ago the answer to this question seemed relatively simple. Ever since the classical investigation of Ebbinghaus (1885) investigators have classically accepted the view that with the passage of time every trace left by every stimulus becomes obliterated, and that tests carried out several hours or days after the original imprinting of the trace disclose this natural process of forgetting.

In the last decade the view that forgetting is the natural result of the gradual extinction or decay of the trace has been put forward by a number of workers (Brown, 1958; 1964; Conrad, 1960a; 1960b). However, this hypothesis has been questioned. Objections to it were that sometimes, with the passage of time, not decay but, on the contrary, enhanced reproduction of traces can be observed, and in psychology this has received the special name of 'reminiscence'. Another fact not in agreement with the simple theory of trace decay as the mechanism of forgetting was that frequently subjects make mistakes in their recalling from memory before the lapse of the appropriate time. Finally, an important fact which could not be reconciled with the view that forgetting is simply trace decay was the very strong influence of any irrelevant activity, taking place between the moment of imprinting and the moment of recall, which greatly strengthened the forgetting process.

As a result of these developments the previous views regarding forgetting as a passive process were revised. At the beginning of the present century, Müller and Pilzecker (1900) postulated that forgetting is the result of *inhibitory influences of irrelevant or interfering actions on the traces*, rather than the result of their gradual decay. This hypothesis was supported by other leading authorities (Robinson, 1920; Skaggs, 1925; McGeoch, 1932; Melton and Irvin, 1940; Melton and von Lackum, 1941; Smirnov, 1966; Underwood, 1957; Underwood and Postman; 1960; 1962; Postman, 1961a; 1961b; 1963; 1967; Keppel, 1968) who had made a careful study of the inhibitory effect of preceding and succeeding events on traces. The phenomena of 'proactive' and 'retroactive' inhibition, which came to be regarded as essential factors in forgetting, found a firm foothold in the literature and the theory that forgetting is largely a *regulator of irrelevant, interfering actions*, inhibiting the normal recall of previously imprinted traces became the predominantly held theory of mnestic processes.

These complex views on the structure of mnestic processes formulated by psychologists all over the world were confirmed by investigations by Soviet psychologists which began in the 1930s and subsequently expanded rapidly.

By the end of the 1920s, Soviet investigators (Vygotsky, Leontiev, and others) were pointing out the fact that memory is elementary and direct in man only in relatively rare cases, and that as a rule the process of recall is based on a system of intermediate aids, and is thus indirect in character. Various special techniques were suggested for the objective study of the formation of this intermediary (or, as we now call it, coding) of the material to be recalled, and these have now been adequately described (Leontiev, 1931). These techniques have revealed the stages through which this process of coding of the memorized material passes through a child's development.

Meanwhile, in another series of investigations (Smirnov, 1948; 1966) the role of active logical organization in the process of active recalling of material was analysed in detail, and the vast storehouse of codes available to the normal adult person for recalling the categorized material was demonstrated. Finally, in special investigations, Soviet psychologists (Zinchenko, 1961) made a detailed study of the process of involuntary recall and examined the role of the actual task presented to the subject, determining the direction of attention and the selection of material for recall, in this process.

All these investigations showed clearly that recall is a *complex, active process* or, in other words, a special form of complex and active *mnestic activity*. This mnestic activity is determined by special *motives* and by the *task* of recalling the appropriate material; it uses a certain strategy and appropriate *methods* or *codes*, which increase the volume of recallable material, increase the time during which it can be retained, and sometimes – as special tests have shown – abolish the inhibitory action of irrelevant, interfering agents which, as has been mentioned, lies at the basis of forgetting.

All these investigations, describing the complex and rich psychological structure of human mnestic processes, shed considerable light on the cerebral mechanisms which we must seek when we undertake the neuropsychological investigation of memory. Naturally the process of strictly directed, selective recall requires *optimal cortical tone* or a state of total vigilance, without which any selective mental processes would be impossible. Naturally, also, the process of active recall requires that the subject has a stable *intention*, and if the intention is absent, or if it is unstable, recall will be impossible. In addition the complex process of receipt and coding of incoming information, already described as consisting of a series of successive stages, requires complete integrity of the cortical zones of the corresponding analysers, which must be able to break up the incoming information into elementary, modally-specific (visual, auditory or tactile) cues, select the relevant cues and, finally, assemble them without hindrance into integral, dynamic structures.

Last of all, the transition from the most elementary (sensory) stage of reception and imprinting of information to the more complex stages of its organization into images and, finally, to the still more complex stages of its coding into certain organized systems of categories, requires integrity of the highest secondary and tertiary cortical zones. Some of these zones are concerned with the synthesis of a successive series of incoming stimuli into successive or simultaneous structures, while others are concerned with the organization of these traces with the aid of the codes of language.

In man, therefore, this highly organized process of recall is based on a complete system of concertedly working systems in the cortex and subjacent structures, and each of these systems makes its own specific contribution to the organization of mnestic processes. It is therefore reasonable to expect that the destruction or even a pathological state of any one of these systems must lead to a disturbance of the course of mnestic processes and that the character of this disturbance will vary depending on which brain system is affected.

We can use these ideas regarding the structure of human memory (which are incomparably more complex than those put forward after the classical investigations of last century, and also those which have lately begun to reappear in biological literature), as the basis for analysis of the results of neuropsychological investigations into the cerebral organization of mnestic processes.

Just as I have done in the preceding chapters, my method will be to analyse changes taking place in mnestic processes in patients with localized lesions in different parts of the brain, and then to use the results of this analysis to attempt to describe the structure of these changes.

I shall discuss these problems briefly as the reader will find a much more complete analysis of these data in my book *Neuropsychology of Memory* (1973).

Primary (non-specific) forms of memory

We have seen that each fundamental condition for the imprinting of traces is *maintenance of the necessary cortical tone*. Lowering of this tone is the principal factor preventing selective imprinting and retention of traces and *disturbing general, involuntary and modally-non-specific memory*. Clearly, therefore, steps which have been taken to reveal the physiological mechanisms providing the fundamental conditions for maintenance of optimal cortical tone are also important steps towards the elucidation of the *physiological basis of general ability to imprint and retain selective systems of traces* or, in other words, to explain the cerebral mechanisms of elementary, general memory.

I stated earlier that the first steps in this direction were taken by Bekhterev (1900), who first postulated that lesions of the medial zones of the temporal region may lead to disturbances of memory, and by Grünthal (1939) who showed that a lesion of the mamillary bodies, the relay nuclei for fibres running from the hippocampus in the 'circle of Papez', gives rise to severe disturbances of memory.

Not until much later, as the result of the work of Scoville, Milner, and Penfield (Scoville, 1954; Scoville and Milner, 1957; Penfield and Milner, 1958; Milner, 1958; 1962; 1966; 1968; 1969; 1970), was it shown that bilateral lesions of the hippocampus do not inter-was it shown that bilateral lesions of the hippocampus do not interfere with higher gnostic processes but substantially disturb the patient's general ability to imprint traces of current experience, and lead to disturbances of memory similar to the classical Korsakov's syndrome.

These discoveries have received a twofold explanation by morphological and physiological investigations. On the one hand, morphological and physiological studies of the brain-stem and thalamic portions of the reticular formation and their tracts have shown that the limbic zones of the brain and, in particular the hippocampus, are structures with an essential role in the modulation of cortical tone, and that a lesion of these zones of the archicortex must lead to a lowering of cortical tone and, hence, to a disturbance of the selective imprinting of traces. On the other hand, recent studies at the neuronal level have shown that many neurons of the hippocampus and connected nuclei do not respond to modally-specific stimuli of any sort, but serve to compare present stimuli with traces of past experience; they react to every change in the stimuli and thus play to some extent the role both of 'attention neurons' and of 'memory neurons'.

These findings suggest that our best approach to the study of the cerebral systems responsible for the *general function of retention of traces*, the first and most elementary form of memory, will be to study the functions of the reticular formation and its superior levels bordering on the hippocampus and the 'circle of Papez'. This hypothesis is fully confirmed by analysis of the available clinical material.

As I have stated (part 1, ch. 2), definite evidence of the participation of the medial zones of the cortex (especially the hippocampus) and connected structures between mnestic processes is given by the disturbances of memory found in patients with the corresponding lesions. Patients with relatively mild forms of dysfunction of these brain zones, such as may be found, for example, in connection with pituitary tumours affecting the limbic structures secondarily, exhibit definite disturbances of memory which are such that the patients themselves complain about them and they can be detected by objective testing. In patients with massive lesions of the medial zones of the brain, involving the structures of the 'circle of Papez' (bilateral lesions of the hippocampus and mamillary bodies) these disturbances may be severe in character, so that the patient is completely unable to retain traces of current experience, and it may often lead to gross disorientation in space and time and with respect to current events. These disturbances of memory are marked by three distinct features.

Firstly, they are evidently not confined to any particular sphere or to any one modality, and they are therefore of a general or *modally-*

non-specific character, so that they may be observed in all forms of the patient's behaviour (the forgetting of intentions, the forgetting of recently completed actions, and so on).

Secondly, they are exhibited equally in the elementary, unpremeditated imprinting of traces, and in special mnestic activity, so that their character is not one of a special disturbance of the mnestic task or the mnestic methods, but of *primary defects of trace retention*. This is clear from the fact that some of these patients, those with the mildest forms of memory disturbance, may actually resort to aids, for example to writing down their intentions, in order to compensate for their defects. This is a characteristic feature of patients with bilateral lesions of the hippocampus described by Milner (1958; 1966).

Finally we come to the third feature, and one which clearly distinguishes disturbances of memory resulting from lesions of the deep zones of the brain involving the medial zones of the cortex. In mild cases it takes the form of relatively slight degrees of forgetfulness, but in patients with massive brain lesions it may actually lead to severe *disturbances of consciousness*, which are never found in patients with local lesions of the lateral zones of the cortex. As I have already mentioned, in the severest cases these patients had no idea where they were, they could not estimate the time correctly, they had completely lost their bearings, and they exhibited those symptoms of confusion which are frequently seen in psychiatric patients but which are relatively rare in patients with local brain lesions.

The features described above show clearly that a lesion of the deep zones of the brain leads to *primary disturbances of memory* which are completely unconnected with special defects of gnostic (analytical and synthetic) activity, and that consequently the *deep zones of the brain, neighbouring on the reticular formation of the upper part of the brain stem and including the limbic structures, are directly concerned not only with the maintenance of optimal cortical tone, but also with creation of the necessary conditions for retention of traces of direct experience.*

My recent experimental investigations, (Luria, 1971; Luria, Konovalov, and Podgornaya, 1970; Popova, 1964; Kiyashchenko, 1969; Luria, 1973) have enabled further progress to be made in the description of these primary memory disorders resulting from deep brain lesions, and in the identification of the physiological mechanisms lying at the basis of these disturbances and the levels and spheres in which they are exhibited.

Without repeating what has been said already (part 2, ch. 8), I should mention the most important results of these investigations. The first attempt to find the chief manifestations and the physiological mechanisms of the primary disturbances of memory in patients with the lesions described did not yield the anticipated results. Even patients with massive disturbances of memory, bordering on Korsakov's syndrome, were frequently able to reproduce series of five or six words dictated to them, and in this respect they did not differ significantly from normal subjects. This fact suggested that the defect manifested as a disturbance of memory in this group of cases is evidently not in the *retention* of incoming information (except, perhaps, within relatively narrow limits).

Further investigations showed that short series of imprinted elements can be *retained* by these patients for a short time (one to two minutes, sometimes longer), unless this time interval is filled by some other, interfering activity. This means that the observed defects could not be due to ordinary *weakness of traces*, leading to their rapid, spontaneous extinction. The observation in these patients of the disappearance of traces after a longer time interval was not convincing, because no experimenter can be quite certain that interfering agencies were not at work in the course of these intervals. Significant results were obtained in tests in which the experimenter set out to determine to what degree traces formed in patients with the disturbances of memory described above were able to counteract interfering and distracting factors.

The reasons motivating these experiments were, firstly, the fact that as a rule any information given to such a patient, or any action he performed, immediately disappeared from his memory when he was distracted by another stimulus or another activity, and secondly, the theory was supported by a number of writers (Melton, 1963; 1970; Underwood, 1945; 1957; Underwood and Postman, 1960; Postman, 1954; 1969), that traces once formed are normally retained for a long time, and that the disability is based more on inhibition of these traces by interfering agencies than by trace decay.

To test the hypothesis that the pathological state of the brain in general, and the lowered cortical tone resulting from disturbance of the normal activating influences of the brain-stem reticular formation on the cortex in particular, lead to *pathological inhibition of established traces*, a series of experiments was carried out, the results of which are analysed in detail elsewhere (Luria, 1971; 1973; Luria, Konovalov and Podgornaya, 1970; Kiyashchenko, 1969). In the first of these experiments, after verification that traces of the given series (words, sentences, pictures, actions) were retained after a pause of a certain duration, unoccupied by any type of irrelevant activity (an empty pause'), the experiment was repeated, except the pause was filled by some form of interfering activity (counting, for example), after which the subject was again instructed to reproduce the series memorized previously. In the second experiment, the subject was first instructed to memorize one (very short) series of two or three words, sentences or pictures, after which he was instructed to memorize a second similar series, and he was then asked which series he had memorized first.

Both these series of experiments gave unexpectedly clear results. Whereas in the case of a normal subject the change to a different, interfering activity had no significant effect on recall of the first series, and memorizing the second short series of elements did not prevent the recall of the series memorized first, in patients with lesions of the deep zones of the brain and a syndrome of general (primary) disturbance of memory, these two tests gave quite different results. Whereas such a patient easily retained a series of three or four words, after distraction by interfering activity (counting, for example), he was completely unable to recall the series retained previously, or he could recall only isolated residual fragments of it. If, after memorizing a group of two or three words, the patient was instructed to memorize a second, similar group, he could not recall the first group, and its traces appeared to be completely obliterated.

In cases of severe disturbances of memory in patients with deep-seated brain lesions affecting the limbic region (hippocampus) and the thalamic nuclei, the required effect could not be obtained even by repeating the test many times over. Although such a patient could easily remember a series of five to six words, even after an 'empty' interval of one and a half to two minutes, he could not recall a first series of two or three words if followed by a second, similar series ('homogeneous interference'), even if the test were repeated six to eight times.

An example of this defect is given below:

Series 1 is House forest cat
Series 2 is Night needle pie

	What was series 1?	*What was series 2?*
1	I don't remember ...	night ... pie ... No I don't remember
2	I don't remember ...	cat ... pie
3	House, needle ...	I don't remember
4	House, needle ...	Pie ... cat ...
5	I don't remember ...	Cat ... pie ... and so on.

Characteristically, these results, so clearly indicating an increased inhibitability of traces by irrelevant, interfering actions, were seen not only in the recall of series of words, but in *any other activity* (memorizing series of pictures, movements, or even organized groups such as sentences or anecdotes), and that *pathologically increased inhibitability of traces was of a general, modality-non-specific character.*

Even clearer results were obtained in the experiments to test the recall of the first series of words (sentences, pictures or actions) after memorizing a second similar series. The *retroactive inhibition* produced by the second group of words on the first in these cases was so strong that the first group of traces either disappeared completely from the patient's memory, or was reproduced with a well-marked loss of selectivity, reflected in the fact that the patient mixed traces of the first and second groups or, to use the expression applied to such cases, *contaminated* them.

Just as in the tests described above, this increased inhibitability of traces and loss of their selectivity were exhibited *regardless of modality*, and most important of all, were *not abolished by organization of the traces into semantic structures.*

For instance, after memorizing the sentence 'Apple trees were growing in the garden beyond the high fence' followed by the second sentence 'The hunter killed a wolf at the edge of the forest', a patient with a marked disturbance of memory resulting from a deep brain lesion either could not recall the first sentence at all, or he mixed (contaminated) it with elements from the second sentence, and reproduced something like 'The hunter killed a wolf at the edge of the garden' or 'Apple trees grew at the edge of the forest'. The same results were found during reproduction of a first anecdote after the second had been read to him, for under these conditions the patient usually completely forgot the substance of the first anecdote.

The increased inhibitability of traces by interfering actions was found to be so severe in patients with the largest lesions that the performance of even the simplest *action* was entirely forgotten after the patient had performed a second similar action. In many cases, if the patient drew a figure and then drew a second figure, he not only forgot what figure he had drawn first, but he actually refused to admit that he had in fact drawn the first figure when it was shown to him. A characteristic feature is the frequent repetition of the experiment usually led to no improvement in the results. This fact showed that the *pathologically increased mutual inhibition of traces is the basic physiological factor in primary disturbances of memory observed in deep brain lesions.*

Conclusions can be drawn from the results I have just described on the basic physiological mechanisms of the primary, modally-non-specific disturbances of memory we have been considering. However, the facts from which the level of these disturbances can be judged are no less interesting. As I have pointed out, patients with relatively mild disturbances of the functions of the medial zones of the brain (for example, those that arise in pituitary tumours extending beyond the sella turcica and affecting the structures of the limbic region) exhibit this increased inhibitability of traces only at the level of the retention of series of isolated traces (words, pictures) when interfering stimuli are in action. The retention of organized series of traces (sentences, anecdotes), as well as the retention of more elementary sensorimotor traces, remain intact in these cases and are not exposed to the inhibitory influence of interfering agencies.

A different picture can be seen in patients with massive lesions of the deep zones of the brain (situated in the midline) leading to gross disorders of memory. In these cases, the *primary mnestic disorders extend both to the more elementary levels and also to more highly organized series of traces*, and the memory disturbances become more general in character. This fact can be demonstrated by a series of tests.

If what Uznadze described as a 'fixed haptic set' is produced in a normal subject (or in a patient with mild forms of disturbance of non-specific memory), for example by instructing him to touch a larger ball several times with his right hand and a smaller ball with his left hand, and then giving him two balls of equal sizes, so that by contrast the left ball appears larger, it will be found that this illusion (known as a 'fixed set') can be produced in the subject and retained for a relatively long time despite the intervention of irrelevant, interfering stimuli. The same result is found if patients with mild disturbances of memory resulting from, for example, pituitary tumours are tested (Kiyashchenko, 1969).

However, if the test is carried out on patients with gross disturbances of primary memory resulting from massive lesions of the deep zones of the brain, different results are obtained. The fixed set is well retained if the intervening time is not occupied by irrelevant stimuli, but the moment this interval is filled by irrelevant activity, the set is immediately lost (Kiyashchenko, 1969). This fact shows that the pathological mutual inhibition of traces in these cases extends *not only to mnestic activity*, but to *all other traces* which were not the special object of premeditated memorizing.

The same result can be observed if Konorski's test is carried out. In this test the subject is presented with a certain stimulus (for example, a geometrical shape of a particular colour), and after an interval of a half to two minutes this is accompanied by the presentation of another figure, either identical, or different in shape or colour. The normal subject, or the patient with only mild disturbances of memory, easily retains the image of the first figure and can state whether it is identical with or different from the second figure either after an 'empty' interval or after an interval occupied by irrelevant activity.

On the other hand, if this test is carried out on patients with massive, deep brain lesions and with gross disturbances of memory, it can be successfully performed only if the interval between the first and second stimuli is not filled by irrelevant activity; as soon as any interfering activity is introduced into this interval, the image of the first figure disappears and the patient can no longer compare the two (Kiyaschhenko, 1969).

These facts, however, are not the only differences found between patients with mild, non-specific disturbances of memory and those with severe forms arising as the result of massive deep brain lesions. An important difference between the two degrees of disturbance of primary, non-specific memory is that whereas in *mild* disturbances the change to retention of organized (semantic) mnestic groups *can be used to compensate the defect*, in patients with *massive disturbances of memory* of the same type, not even this change to organized (semantic) mnestic groups can free the patient from the inhibitory influence of interfering agencies, so that the *memory disturbances easily become converted into disturbances of consciousness*.

These facts show that massive, deep brain lesions prevent the corresponding coding of the material to be memorized, and thus give rise to disturbances of primary memory which render Bühner's law (according to which thoughts can be committed to memory incomparably more firmly than isolated elements) inapplicable. This demonstrates the essential role of these brain structures in the most severe mnestic disorders and it obliterates the dividing line between disturbances of memory and disorders of consciousness which these lesions produce. All these findings are described in sufficient detail and with proper documentation in reports of special investigations by Kiyashchenko (1969) and Pham Ming Hac (1971), and in my book *The Neuropsychology of Memory* (vol. 1, 1973; vol. 2, in preparation).

We shall not discuss the severest forms of disturbance of logical memory, when lesions of the deep zones of the brain are complicated by the additional presence of lesions of the frontal lobes. In these cases, carefully studied elsewhere (Luria, 1971; 1973; Luria, Konovalov, Podgornaya, 1970) the whole system of mnestic activity is severely deranged, the patient becomes unable to control his memory of the data he had to retain, and his memory of a series of words, phrases or paragraphs becomes open to a series of extra-context factors (stereotypes, immediate impressions, outside associations).

Modality-specific forms of memory

Disturbances of memory exhibited in patients with lesions of the lateral cortical zones, or in other words, with lesions of the *second* and *third functional units* of the brain, differ fundamentally in character from the memory disorders found in patients with lesions of the first functional brain unit. The principal feature of the disturbances now to be described is that they are never global and they *never lead to general disorders of consciousness*. As a rule they have the character either of a disturbance of the mnestic basis of individual *modality-specific operations*, retaining their close connection with defects of some aspects of gnostic processes, or of specific dynamic disorders, leading to the disturbance of the structure of goal-directed activity. Let us examine these disturbances separately.

Specific disturbances of *audio-verbal memory*, which I have mentioned earlier (part 2, ch. 4), are a typical feature of lesions of the *temporal cortex* of the left (dominant) hemisphere.

Investigations (Luria,; 1947; 1970a; Bein, 1947; Klimkovsky, 1966) have shown that in no patient so far observed has a local lesion of the left temporal cortex ever given rise to a general disturbance of memory or consciousness similar to those described in patients with deep brain lesions, or to the inactivity of mnestic processes which I shall describe in my analysis of the disorders of mnestic activity in lesions of the frontal lobes. It is only in cases where the lesion extended to deep (medial) zones of the temporal lobe, involved the right temporal region, and was accompanied by marked general cerebral changes, that features of disorientation and confusion typical of the deep brain lesions I have just described could be observed. A lesion of the lateral zones of the left temporal region led to a disturbance mainly of complex forms of acoustic gnosis, giving rise to defects of phonemic hearing; these lesions resulted in highly specific disturbances of *audio-verbal memory* which have already been mentioned.

In patients with the most massive lesions these phenomena were well-marked; in the case of lesions of the middle zones of the temporal region they were exhibited particularly clearly and the patient could no longer retain lengthy series of sounds or words. This symptom, described in detail by Klimkovsky (1966) is the chief feature of *acoustico-mnestic aphasia*. Characteristically this symptom occurred in a particularly marked form as a defect of retention of a series of spoken sounds and words; however, it was also manifested as difficulty in retaining groups of musical notes and rhythmic structures (Klimkovsky, 1966), although there was no difficulty in the retention of a series of visual images or a series of movements (Luria and Rapoport, 1962; Luria, 1971; Pham Ming Hac 1971).

The essential basis of these defects could be either increased inhibitability of audio-verbal traces or the levelling of excitability of the cortical area for audible speech, as the result of which some elements of an audio-verbal series either are inhibited by others, or begin to arise with equal probability to irrelevant traces (Luria, Sokolov and Klimkovsky, 1967a; 1967b). Finally, the other characteristic feature of these defects of audio-verbal memory is that they can be overcome if the elements of the audio-verbal series are given to the patient at relatively long intervals, so that the action of the dynamic factors mentioned earlier can to some extent be overcome (Tsvetkova, 1969).

All the defects of memory already described arising in lesions of the left temporal region were thus closely connected with hearing processes and with speech, or in other words they were strictly *modality-specific* in character and were *not disturbances of active mnestic activity*, and the patient could still exert himself and attempt in various ways to compensate his defects.

We still know very little about the nature of memory defects arising in lesions of the lateral zones of the *right* temporal region, but there is no doubt that they also are modality-specific in character in their own way, possibly on account of the longer time required for consolidation of traces (Simernitskaya, unpublished investigation).

Memory disturbances arising in lesions of the *left parietal* (*or parieto-occipital*) *region possess quite different features*. It is in these cases, as I have described (part 2, ch. 5), that the patient develops difficulty with *simultaneous syntheses*, and the disturbance of his mnestic processes is a direct continuation of these gnostic disorders. Investigations by Phan Ming Hac (1971) have shown that disturbances of retention of simple shapes (or sounds) can remain unaffected in these cases, but visual structures incorporating simultaneous (spatial) relationships are difficult not only to distinguish, but also to retain in the memory. As a rule long training in direct imprinting of these relationships does not give the desired results.

As I mentioned, the symptom of disturbance of recalling the names of objects, known in clinical practice as amnestic aphasia, which arises in lesions of this region of the cortex, may in all probability be explained in the same way as the result of the 'levelling of excitability' of individual systems due to the pathologically changed dynamics of these cortical zones. Arising as it does against the background of a disturbance of these simultaneous syntheses, this disturbance leads to the equally likely recalling of different systems of verbal traces (phonetically, morphologically, or lexically similar), and it is manifested very clearly in the phenomena of literal and verbal paraphasias which are observed in these cases (Lotmar, 1919; 1935; Sapir, 1929; Bein, 1947; Luria, 1971; 1972).

The defects of memory observed in these cases are characteristically highly specific, for they affect the operations of *memorizing* and *recalling* but are *never transformed into a disturbance of the structure of mnestic activity as a whole*, so that the patient is still able to make effort to compensate his defects (Luria, 1948; 1963; Bein, 1947; 1964; Tsvetkova, 1970).

I shall not dwell here on the highly specific phenomena of disturbance of recall of visual images in response to a spoken name which are found in lesions of the left temporo-occipital region which have been discussed (part 2, ch. 4), but will go on at once to examine mnestic defects associated with lesions of the *frontal lobes*.

The basic condition for voluntary recall is preservation of *mnestic activity* or, in other words, of motives for recall, a mnestic task, and a system of active search for methods to assist in the performance of this task and in the comparison of the results with the original intention. These components of mnestic activity are intact in patients with lesions of the temporal and occipital regions I have just described, in whom the operative component of the mnestic act or the mnestic operations are disturbed, but *active mnestic activity is never affected*.

The completely opposite picture arises in patients with massive lesions of the frontal lobes, interfering with the normal working of the left frontal lobe or of both frontal lobes. Analysis of the functional organization of the frontal lobes and of their role in the structure of active behaviour (part 2, ch. 5) revealed that a lesion of the frontal lobe leads to gross disturbances of the formation of intentions and plans, disturbance of the formation of behaviour programmes, and disturbance of the regulation of mental activity and the verification of its course and results. In other words, while leaving the operative part intact, it leads to a *profound disturbance of the whole structure of human conscious activity*. Clearly these disturbances are bound to cause the disintegration of *mnestic activity* as a special case of human conscious activity as a whole.

Observations show that patients with massive lesions of the lateral zones of the prefrontal region cannot form a stable and active intention to memorize incoming information even though their general orientation and ability to retain traces or visual impressions remains unimpaired. Also, they cannot make active attempts to find ways or means of assisting memorizing.

The mnestic activity of such a patient, in whom this component is disturbed, is converted into *passive imprinting* of the presented material, as is easily seen if such a patient is instructed to learn by heart a series of words or pictures. The observer will note that the learning process is converted in such a patient into the simple, stereotyped repetition of a group of elements he has managed to retain, that there is no increase in the number of components retained (a typical feature of passive memorizing) and the 'learning curve' climbs to a plateau and stays there, a clear sign of the passive character of learning (Figure 64). This passive character of all (including mnestic) activity of patients with a lesion of the prefrontal zones is also reflected in the following fact. If, while learning a presented series, the normal subject is instructed to take note of the result and, depending on that result, to change his 'level of pretension' (by stating how many elements he would remember after the next presentation of the same series), there is a steady rise in the level of the pretension. In a patient with a severe frontal syndrome, however, it does not rise and the level of pretension becomes nothing more than the inert repetition of the same number over and over again. This result clearly reflects the absence of a mobile system of intentions, controlling mnestic activity, in such patients (Zeigarnik, 1961; 1968; Luria, 1963; 1966a, 1966b, 1970a).

The inability to take active steps to find aids to memorizing can be demonstrated in patients of this group by tests involving assisted memorizing (Leontiev, 1931). Whereas a normal subject, when instructed to use aids for memorizing, actively seeks and produces auxiliary connections, and begins to use them, so that his memorizing becomes converted into an *active*, *aided process*, the patient with a marked frontal syndrome is unable do this, and tests show that he neither uses aids suggested to him nor, still more, actively produces them (Zeigarnik, 1961; 1968; Bondareva, 1969).

The distinctive nature of disturbances of mnestic processes in massive frontal lesions is clearly revealed by special tests to study memorizing processes when the subject is exposed to the inhibitory influence of interfering activity.

Whereas, as we have seen, any brain lesion (regardless of its locality) leads to *pathologically increased inhibitability of traces by irrelevant, interfering agents*, in patients with massive frontal lobe lesions this inhibitory influence of interfering agents assumes the special character of *pathological inertia of recently established traces*, which prevents the patient from recalling previously imprinted traces if he has subsequently to reproduce another, analogous group of stimuli. In such cases the patient with a massive frontal syndrome will inertly repeat the last group of traces. This pathological inertia prevents him from reviving the traces of previously imprinted series. It is interesting to note that this pathological inertia is clearly apparent during the reproduction not only of a series of isolated elements, but also of *whole organized structures*. For instance, if after repeating the sentence 'Apple trees grew in the garden' he is asked to repeat the sentence 'The hunter killed a wolf on the edge of the forest', in response to the request to recall both sentences he will inertly repeat 'The hunter killed a wolf at the edge of the forest'. In response to further questioning he will state that the two sentences 'differed in meaning' or 'differed in intonation', but that both consisted of the same inertly frozen sentence 'the hunter killed a wolf' (Luria, 1971; 1972; Akbarova and Pham Ming Hac, unpublished investigations).

If the pathological focus lies in the lateral zones of the prefrontal cortex (predominantly the left), the disturbances of the patient's mnestic activity will be of the character just described; if, however, the focus spreads to the *medial zones of the frontal lobes*, a syndrome of mnestic disorders is produced in which the disturbances of active mnestic activity and pathological inertia of existing traces will be combined with the phenomena of *lowering of cortical tone* and disturbance of primary memory, which I described previously, so that the patient's syndrome will be one of severe disturbance of orientation in space and loss of the selectivity of mnestic processes (I have described this syndrome elsewhere: Luria, Konovalov and Podgornaya, 1970; Luria 1973), progressing from the severest disorders of memory to equally severe global disturbances of consciousness.

The differences between memory disturbances caused by lesions in different parts of the brain are thus readily apparent. These observations help us to take an important step towards the better understanding of this complex psychological process.

Chapter 12
Speech

Historical

Although the facts relating to the cerebral organization of memory have been accumulated entirely during the last fifteen to twenty years, our knowledge of the cerebral organization of speech processes is based on experience gained over more than a century. When Broca, in 1861, expressed the view that *motor* speech is 'localized' in the posterior zones of the third left frontal gyrus, and when in 1873 Wernicke linked the posterior third of the superior left temporal gyrus with the function of *sensory* speech, the first important steps were taken toward a scientific understanding of the cerebral organization of speech activity. These two discoveries, of decisive importance at the time they were made, initiated many subsequent investigations in an attempt to determine which cortical zones participate in the organization of speech and which forms of disturbance of speech activity arise in lesions in various parts of the brain.

Despite the accumulation of much clinical material and the intensity with which the research was conducted, as will be clear from the fact that by 1914 Monakow was able to list about 1500 publications on aphasia, attempts to describe the actual cerebral mechanisms of speech activity came up against substantial difficulties. Perhaps the greatest difficulty was the fact that the investigators were hindered by a lack of available morphological and physiological data and by insufficiently mature psychological concepts of speech, and they attempted to explain their clinical findings from the standpoint of the very imperfect psychological theories accepted at each corresponding period.

The effects of this handicap were seen from the earliest stages of creation of the theory of cerebral organization of speech and speech disorders, when the clinical facts discovered were described in terms of the *associationism* which dominated the second half of the nineteenth century. It was this system of ideas which made it necessary to seek a cerebral substrate for 'sensory speech' and 'motor speech' and for various types of connections between them. That is why, in the first stage, well-known and naïve schemes (such as Lichtheim's scheme) were produced. According to this scheme, speech processes are localized in a system of connections running from the 'sensory speech centre' to the 'centre for concepts', and thence to the 'motor speech centre', and disturbances of speech may have the character of 'subcortical sensory aphasia', 'cortical sensory aphasia', 'amnestic aphasia', 'subcortical motor aphasia', 'cortical motor aphasia', 'conduction aphasia' and 'transcortical' motor or sensory aphasia.

These attempts to compare hypothetical associationist schemes of speech structure directly with equally hypothetical anatomical schemes were successful only on paper. They did not lead to the description of actual clinical pictures of speech disorders, they directed searches for the cerebral basis of speech along the wrong lines, and they made no attempt to analyse the pathology of speech activity on the basis of the analysis of the physiological mechanisms of speech disturbances. Naturally, therefore, by the beginning of the present century the classical associationist schemes of the cerebral organization of speech and speech disturbances had reached an acute crisis which led to the introduction of fresh approaches, starting from completely different standpoints, but unfortunately they were no more successful than their predecessors.

This time, clinicians, despairing of the classical associationist approach sought aid from another psychological concept which was fashionable at that time – an idealistic concept. According to this 'noetic' concept, speech processes are a manifestation of *mental* activity – an 'abstract or categorical function' (Kassirer) or an 'abstract mental act' (Külpe). These processes, while retaining their mental character, have no direct relationship to any particular part of the brain, but are merely incorporated into the work of the brain as a whole rather than formed by its individual systems.

Naturally, therefore, neurologists attempting to explain the pathology of speech from these standpoints regarded aphasia purely as a disturbance of 'intellectual schemes' (van Woerkom, 1925), or of abstract sets (Goldstein, 1925; 1948). Abandoning all attempts to localize these disturbances in particular brain zones, they limited themselves to the highly conventional correlation of these disturbances with 'the brain as a whole', at best correlating a disturbance of these higher mental forms of speech activity with the *mass* of brain substance damaged.

These theories, the gift of the idealistic philosophy of the twentieth century, did not make much of an impression in clinical practice and they were quickly replaced by others. The new theories were based on attempts to compare forms of speech disorders arising in local brain lesions with *linguistic* rather than psychological data. Perhaps the most lucid of these attempts was that made by the famous English neurologist Henry Head (1926) to establish a theory of aphasia based on linguistic analysis of speech disturbances arising in local brain lesions and the comparison of these *linguistic forms* of aphasia with the *localization* of the brain lesion.

Thus there arose the concepts of nominative, syntactic and semantic aphasia, which were correlated, with some approximation, with lesions of particular zones of the cortex. The merit of this theory was that Head, for the first time, pointed out the need for linguistic analysis of the speech structures which are disturbed in the various local brain lesions. However, his mistake was to try to correlate particular linguistic structures directly with particular brain areas, thus repeating the now meaningless attempt to correlate simplified psychological schemes directly with narrowly localized brain zones, which had already been shown to be worthless even a generation before Head. That is why Head's attempts, despite the great clinical authority of their founder and the brilliant clinical descriptions of the cases, contributed only a little to the theory of aphasia and had virtually no influence on the subsequent study of the forms of mechanism of disturbance of speech processes in local brain lesions.

Psychological structure of speech

We have seen that attempts to compare simplified psychological schemes and complex linguistic structures directly with particular zones of the cerebral cortex were unproductive. It is now perfectly clear that a way out of this impasse must be found, and that the essential conditions for its discovery are, first, a sufficiently precise view of the *psychological structure of speech processes* and their individual components, and secondly, a properly directed search for the *physiological conditions* essential for the normal organization of these components of the complex speech structure. Let us look at each of these conditions in detail before going on to examine the possible cerebral organization of speech activity.

First of all, views on the structure of the |word|-this essential part of the language and speech have been substantially revised. We do not now suppose a word is an image of a certain object, property or action; nor do we think a word is merely an association of an image and a conditional acoustic complex. This new knowledge gives us a new approach. We now conceive a word as a *complex multidimensional matrix* of different cues and connections (acoustic, morphological, lexical and semantic) and we know that in different states one of these connections is predominant. We have even found an objective method of evaluating the kind of connections predominant in different states, and we are able to qualify and even to measure these connections on 'semantic fields' (Luria and Vinogradova, 1959, 1971). This has opened new ways for studying the psychological structure and neuropsychological forms of the organization of this basic component of our speech.

Now we can take a further step. Modern psychology regards speech as a special *means of communication* using *language* for the transmission of information. It regards speech as a complex and specifically *organized form of conscious activity* involving the participation of the subject formulating the spoken expression and of the subject receiving it. Correspondingly, it distinguishes two forms and two mechanisms of speech activity.

First, there is *expressive* speech, which begins with the motive or general idea of the expression, which is coded into a speech scheme and put into operation with the aid of internal speech; finally, these schemes are converted into narrative speech, based on a 'generative' grammar. Second, there is *impressive* speech, taking the opposite course from perception of a flow of speech received from another source and followed by attempts to *decode* it; this is done by analysis of the perceived spoken expression, the identification of its significant elements and their reduction to a certain *speech scheme*; this is converted by means of the same *internal speech* into the *general idea* of the scheme running through the expression, and finally the *motive* lying behind it is decoded.

Such speech activity (whether expressive or impressive) is clearly a highly complex psychological structure incorporating several different components. The general characteristics of speech activity, as a special form of social communication, represent only one aspect of this process. However, there are other aspects of speech: as a *tool for intellectual activity*, and finally, as a method of *regulating* or organizing human mental processes.

Speech, based on the *word*, the basic unit of language, and on the sentence (or syntagma, or combination of words) as the basic unit of narrative expression, automatically uses these historically formed facilities, firstly, as a method of *analysis and generalization of incoming information* and secondly, as a method of *formulating decisions and drawing conclusions*. That is why speech, a means of communication, has at the same time also become a mechanism of *intellectual activity* – a method for use in operations of *abstraction* and *generalization* and a basis for *categorical thinking*.

By distinguishing certain features, by fixing the *intentions* and formulating *programmes* of activity, speech becomes at the same time a method of regulating behaviour and setting the course of mental processes, as I have already described. It is only by taking all these aspects into consideration that a proper approach can be made to the analysis of human speech activity, as it has been studied by psychologists in the last decades (Vygotsky, 1934; 1956; 1960; Luria, 1947; 1956; 1958b; 1961; 1966a; 1970a).

functions
1.
a)
b)
b).

The facts I have just described constitute the chief characteristics of speech activity and its chief functions. However, human speech, using language as its principal tool, also has its executive or operative aspect, and a careful analysis of the components of this operative aspect of the organization of speech processes will be just as important for our purpose as analysis of the structure of speech activity as a whole.

The first component of this operative or executive organization of speech is the mechanism of its *phasic* or *acoustic* aspect. This mechanism includes the *acoustic analysis* of the flow of speech, converting a continuous flow of sounds into discrete units or *phonemes*, each of which is based on the isolation of useful sounds playing a decisive role in the discrimination of meaning, and which differ in each language. I have already discussed the psychological characteristics of these phonemes (part 2, ch. 4), and I shall not repeat them here. They include the discovery of the necessary *articulatory cues*, enabling the required phoneme to be pronounced, and converting it into the unit of expressive speech – the *articuleme*. This structure has also been discussed (part 2, ch. 6) in the appropriate context of my investigation.

The phasic (acoustic) aspect of speech is only the first component in the organization of the executive function of the speech process. The next component is the lexical-semantic organization of the speech act, using mastery of the lexical-morphological code of language to enable images or concepts to be converted into their verbal equivalents, which in itself is composed of the radical symbolization (or objective categorization) of speech and the function of its generalization or 'signification', or in other words the function of incorporating whatever has to be designated into a concrete system of connections based on morphological or semantic criteria. The formation of such a network of morphological groups (constan*cy*, legitima*cy*, pira*cy* or hesitan*cy*; strange*ness*, happi*ness*, forgive*ness* or eager*ness*, and so on) or of semantic groups (hospital, school, police station, in accordance with the principle of 'public institutions', or headmaster, matron, inspector, on the principle of the person directing the staff of an institution) illustrates only special examples of the highly *complex semantic categories* into which every word constituting the generalized unit of speech is included.

Words are only the basic unit of the executive (operative) aspect of the speech process. The next component in its organization is the *sentence* or expression, which can vary in complexity and which can be converted into connected, *narrative speech*. This expression is not so much a process of categorical generalization, which is a quality of individual words, as a process of *transition from thought to speech*, or a coding of an original plan into an expanded system of sentences, based on objective syntactical codes of language and incorporating the internal speech which, with its condensed and predicative structure, is the essential link of any narrative expression (Vygotsky, 1934; 1956).

I have listed only the chief components of the structure of the complex speech process. Its analysis has recently been the subject of many psychological and psycholinguistic investigations; I have summarized these elsewhere (Luria, 1966–70), and will not therefore consider them here in detail. Nevertheless, a brief outline of speech activity and the identification of the principal components of speech are absolutely essential for the purpose of this book. The reason is that in patients with lesions of *different parts of the brain* this complex structure of speech activity may suffer *damage to its various components*, resulting in *various forms of speech defects*. Careful analysis of the different forms of speech disturbances, with a study of their direct physiological causes and their connections with the localization of the pathological focus, may thus provide what is a difficult, yet the only reliable, means of solving the problem of the cerebral organization of speech activity.

We can now turn to the facts at our disposal when we try to solve this complex problem. I have analysed this material in detail elsewhere (Luria, 1947; 1948; 1963; 1966a; 1966b; 1970a; 1972), and shall therefore only summarize it here.

Impressive (receptive) speech

I shall begin my analysis of the cerebral organization of speech with the most elementary mechanisms of impressive speech. The first condition for the decoding of incoming speech is the isolation of precise spoken sounds or *phonemes* from the flow of speech reaching the subject. I pointed out earlier (part 2, ch. 4) that the *secondary zones of the temporal* (*auditory*) *cortex* of the left hemisphere play the decisive role in this process. With their powerful system of connections with the postcentral (kinaesthetic) and inferior zones of the premotor cortex (Figure 35), the postero-superior zones of the left temporal region are particularly adapted for the isolation and identification of the fundamental phonemic characteristics or, in other words, for highly specialized acoustic analysis. It is this physiological function (and not the 'sensory image of words' postulated by Wernicke) which is the direct contribution of this cortical region to the structure of speech processes.

A lesion of these zones naturally interferes with the identification of these phonemic characteristics, disturbs the highly specialized verbal hearing and leads to the development of the familiar picture of temporal or 'acoustico-gnostic' aphasia.

The disturbance of phonemic hearing as a direct result of a lesion of the superior temporal zones of the left hemisphere (Wernicke's area) is a typical case of the removal of an essential condition for the operative aspect of impressive speech. It leaves the patient's intention to analyse the meaning of the perceived words intact, it does not destroy active attempts to decode audible speech, but it makes these attempts unsuccessful as the result of a disturbance of the fundamental condition essential for the performance of this task. While leaving the patient's fundamental intellectual activity intact (as is clear from the fact that his written arithmetic and visual constructive activity remain normal), it completely prevents those forms of intellectual activity which depend on speech formulation and integrity of the intermediate speech operations. That is why, as we shall see again, the patient's understanding of the *general meaning* of what is said to him may remain intact in such cases, as a result of his guesses about its context and his study of the general intonation of audible speech, whereas the precise and concrete understanding of the meaning of the words is almost completely impossible.

I have already mentioned the secondary (systemic) consequences of such a disturbance and will not dwell on them again in particular. However, a disturbance of phonemic hearing is only one, the most elementary, form of disturbance of the initial component concerned with the decoding of speech. The second form is that distinctive disorder of speech understanding which can be compared with Lissauer's 'associative mental blindness', in which the phonemic composition of speech remains unimpaired, but recognition of its meaning is grossly disturbed. The nature of this associative form of sensory aphasia, as well as the physiological mechanisms lying at its basis, are still unknown and we can only postulate, as I have done, that the possible basis of this disturbance (for which the pathological focus most commonly lies in the posterior zones of the temporal or temporo-occipital region of the left hemisphere) is impairment of the concerted working of the speech-hearing and visual analysers, as a result of which the articulated word no longer evokes its corresponding image. However, we have insufficient reliable evidence to support this hypothesis, and until new facts are available we can neither accept it nor reject it. I shall try to analyse this problem in future communications (Luria, 1972) and other studies in neuro-linguistics.

The next stage in impressive speech is the understanding of the meaning of a whole phrase or a whole connected speech expression. The cerebral organization of this process is evidently much more complex than that of the simple, direct decoding of word meanings. At the time of writing, it appears that there are three principal mechanisms involved in this process. They rest on the participation of different brain zones and they assume different forms.

The first condition essential for the decoding of narrative speech ①
is retention of all the elements of the expression in the speech memory. If this condition is not satisfied, it is impossible for the patient to understand a long sentence or an expression of narrative speech requiring the comparison of its elements. The patient may retain the beginning of the expression, but because of the increased mutual inhibitory effect of the elements, he loses its end (or the opposite may be the case), and he is therefore unable to understand the meaning of the complete sentence although he still understands the individual words perfectly well. We have seen (part 2, ch. 4) that lesions of the middle zones of the left temporal region or deep lesions of the left temporal lobe, causing dysfunction of the temporal cortex and the phenomena of acoustico-mnestic aphasia, lead to the same result, and the participation of systems of the left temporal region in disturbances of the understanding of narrative speech of this type will be clear. The mechanisms of this kind of defects will be discussed in greater detail elsewhere (Luria, 1973).

The second essential condition for the understanding of narrative ②
speech is the simultaneous synthesis of its elements, and the ability not only to retain all the elements of the narrative speech structure, but also to be able to 'survey' it simultaneously and to form it into a simul-taneously perceived logical scheme. This condition is not equally essential to the understanding of expressions which differ in their structure. It is by no means essential to the understanding of many forms of simple narrative speech, belonging to the category of what Svedelius (1897) called the 'communication of events', which do not incorporate complex grammatical relationships. Conversely, this

simultaneous surveying and formation of simultaneous logical schemes are absolutely essential to the understanding of speech constructions incorporating complex *logical-grammatical relationships*, expressed with the aid of prepositions, case endings, and word order, which Svedelius called 'communications of relationships'.

We have seen that an intimate role in this type of decoding process is played by the *parieto-occipital* (or *temporo-parieto-occipital*) *zones of the left hemisphere*, a pathological lesion of which leads to the disruption of simultaneous spatial schemes, and which, on the symbolic (speech) level, gives rise to such phenomena as a *disturbance of the understanding of logical-grammatical relationships* (*semantic aphasia*) and gross disturbances of constructional activity and arithmetical operations which cannot proceed without these simultaneous (quasi-spatial) syntheses.

It is important to note in this connection that the study of disturbances of speech understanding in patients with lesions of the left parieto-occipital cortex provides a *new and reliable means of distinguishing between two types of linguistic construction*. Some of them can be understood without the simultaneous syntheses described above, and can thus be understood in patients with lesions of these zones (as we have seen, these include the simple forms of communication of events), while others are absolutely dependent on these simultaneous (quasi-spatial) schemes for their understanding, and cannot be decoded by patients with the lesion described. The neuropsychological method of analysis will undoubtedly be of considerable use to linguists when they study the details distinguishing these two forms of grammatical construction and their 'deep structures' from each other.

The third, and most important condition for the understanding of narrative speech and the decoding of its meaning is *active analysis of its most significant elements*. This active analysis is hardly required at all for the decoding of simple phrases and the most elementary forms of narrative speech. However, it becomes an absolutely indispensable condition for decoding the meaning of complex sentences or, more especially, for the understanding of the general meaning and, in particular, the undertone of a complex narrative statement. It will suffice to recall the complex searching movements of the eyes, with their repeated returning to segments of the text already read, made by a person reading a difficult text and attempting to pick out its essential aspects and to grasp the general meaning, in order to realize the importance of this active behaviour in the decoding of complex information. We now know, however, that active searching behaviour, requiring integrity of a stable intention, the formation of a programme or the appropriate actions, and the checking of their course, is achieved with the intimate participation of other brain zones, and that the inclusion of the appropriate zones of the *frontal zones* into the system is an essential condition for the performance of this active searching activity. It is for this reason that in patients with lesions of the frontal lobes (part 2, ch. 7) this goal-directed, programmed, selective activity becomes impossible and the required forms of organized, active behaviour are replaced either by impulsive, fragmentary responses or by inert stereotypes.

Thus it will be readily understood that the participation of the *frontal lobes* in the decoding of complex expressions, requiring active work for their decoding, is absolutely necessary, and that a lesion of the frontal lobes, while not preventing the understanding of words and simple sentences, will completely prevent the understanding of complex forms of narrative speech and, in particular, the understanding of the hidden meaning of a complex expression. I have frequently seen for myself how the planned process of decoding of complex speech constructions is replaced in patients with a marked frontal syndrome either by a series of guesses, not based upon analysis of the text, or by inert semantic stereotypes which the patient has transferred from information received previously.

I shall not dwell in more detail on this phenomena, because we shall need to pay special attention to them later when we examine the cerebral organization of complex forms of intellectual activity and also because these topics will be discussed in a series of special papers dealing with the basic problems in neurolinguistics.

Expressive speech

As we have seen, expressive speech consists of the coding of thought in an expanded expression, and it includes a series of operative components. However, to explain its cerebral organization, we proceed in reverse and begin by examining its most elementary forms in order to elucidate their cerebral mechanisms. The most elementary type of expressive speech is *repetitive* speech.

(1) The simple repetition of a sound, syllable or word naturally requires its accurate auditory perception; clearly, therefore, the systems of the temporal (auditory) cortex which we have discussed must participate in the act of repetition of the elements of speech. Lesions of the secondary zones of the left auditory cortex, leading to disturbance of phonemic hearing, must therefore be accompanied by defects of repetition (substitution of similar phonemes, their incorrect reproduction), which I have already mentioned.

(2) The presence of precise phonemic hearing, however, is only one condition for intact repetitive speech. The second condition is the participation of a sufficiently precise system of articulations, and as I have already stated (part 2, ch. 6), this is dependent on the participation of the inferior zones of the *postcentral* (*kinaesthetic*) cortex of the *left* hemisphere. That is why, as we have already seen, a lesion of these brain zones leads to disintegration of the precise *articulemes*, the substitution of similar 'oppositional' articulemes by one another, and the appearance of literal paraphasias, such as repetition of the word 'khalat' as 'khadat', 'stol' as 'ston' or 'snot' and so on. In patients with more massive lesions of the inferior postcentral zones of the left hemisphere these defects may be much more severe and may give rise to a marked form of afferent motor aphasia, based on disintegration of articulemes. The identification of this form of aphasia and its differentiation from efferent motor aphasia or 'Broca's aphasia' (Luria, 1947; 1970b; Vinarskaya, 1971) are important modern developments in the science of speech disorders.

Afferent Motor Aphasia

(3) The third essential condition for repetitive speech is the ability to *switch from one articuleme to another* or from one word to another. We have already seen that the structures of the *premotor* cortex of the left hemisphere and, in particular, of its inferior zones play an essential role in ensuring the necessary plasticity of the motor processes for this purpose (part 2, ch. 6). That is why lesions of these brain zones lead to the development of pathological inertia in the sphere of speech movements and to the appearance of articulatory perseverations which prevent the switching from one articuleme to another and which constitute the pathophysiological basis of efferent motor aphasia or Broca's aphasia.

314 Synthetic Mental Activities

It remains for us to consider the last condition necessary for normal repetitive speech. Goldstein (1948) was particularly interested in this last condition, but it still requires psychophysiological interpretation.

The repetition of any acoustic structure (and, in particular, of meaningless syllables or their combinations) inevitably comes into conflict with the reproduction of phonetically similar, but meaningful and firmly established words. For such a task to be performed correctly some degree of *abstraction* from these well-established stereotypes, the subordination of articulation to an assigned programme, and the inhibition of irrelevant alternatives are necessary. We have already seen that this programming of selective action and inhibition of all irrelevant connections require the close participation of the *frontal lobes*, and it will thus be perfectly clear that a lesion of these zones of the brain may deprive the programme of its necessary stability, so that the repetition of a given speech structure (particularly if meaningless or complex) will be replaced by the repetition of a similar word, firmly established in the patient's previous experience. All that is required to verify this fact is to instruct such a patient to repeat a phrase which is logically or structurally *incorrect*, when he will immediately reproduce it in the more habitual, *correct* form. It can easily be seen what a complex group of conditions is incorporated into such an apparently simple act as repetition, and what a complex system of zones of the cerebral cortex (each of which provides one of the conditions for this act) is implicated. We shall not dwell here with a psychological analysis of the defects of the repetition of words known in clinical neurology as the phenomenon of 'conduction aphasia'. A special analysis of this phenomenon will be made in a separate study 'Towards the revision of conduction aphasia' (in press).

The next type of expressive speech, the naming of objects, is much more complex. In this case, there is no acoustic model of the required word and the subject must find it himself, starting from the visual image of the object perceived (or imagined) and then coding the image by an appropriate word of spoken speech. The performance of this task is naturally dependent on a series of new conditions and, consequently, on the participation of other cortical zones.

The first condition for adequate naming of objects or their pictures

(1) is a sufficiently clear level of *visual perception*. As soon as visual perception loses its precision (as in cases of disturbance of visual syntheses or optical agnosia), or even acquires certain weakened forms (expressed by difficulty in recognizing stylized drawings or in identifying 'disguised' pictures), or as soon as the weakening of visual ideas appears, the naming of objects becomes severely impaired, having lost its concrete optical basis. This phenomenon is described in classical neurology as 'optical aphasia', and as a rule it arises in lesions of the temporo-occipital zones of the left hemisphere. It can also form the pathophysiological basis of some types of amnestic aphasia arising in lesions of the parieto-occipital zones, and as such it was the subject of a special analysis undertaken recently by Tsvetkova (1972). She showed that the source of the disturbance of the nominative function of speech may be a disturbance of the formation of visual images of objects.

 Optical Aphasia

Patients with this type of amnestic aphasia, for instance, could not form sufficiently clear visual ideas of the objects they were required to name. They could not distinguish the essential features of these objects mentally, and they could not, therefore draw them intelligibly or complete a drawing which had already been started. They could produce only general, vague drawings of the object (but they had no difficulty in copying a drawing shown to them). This showed that the difficulties in naming experienced by these patients were in all probability based on the blurred character, the lack of precise definition of their visual ideas and images and on their inability to pick out in sufficient detail those features of an object essential to its identification and naming (Figure 42).

(2) The second essential, and self-evident condition for normal naming of objects, is integrity of the precise *acoustic structure of speech*, connected with the already familiar function of the speech-hearing systems of the *left temporal region*. A lesion of these zones of the brain, leading directly to a disturbance of the precise phonemic organization of speech structures, thus gives rise to the same difficulties of naming as I have just described in the difficulty of repetition. A feature of this type of disturbance of naming is a superfluity (✗) of *literal paraphasias*, which arise whenever the patient is asked to name an object shown to him. Another is the fact that *prompting* with the initial sounds (or syllables) of the required word in these

acoustico- amnestic aphasia

cases *does not help* the patient, the roots of whose defects lie in the impreciseness of the acoustic composition of words.

③ The third, and by far the most complex condition for the correct naming of objects, is *discovery of the proper, selective meaning and inhibition of all irrelevant alternatives* arising in the course of such attempts. We have already seen that the naming of an object is interwoven into a network or matrix of possible connections, which includes the verbal description of all the various qualities of the object, together with the countless other names describing similar qualities (belonging to the same semantic category), or similar in their acoustic or morphological structure, which spring up. This inhibition of all irrelevant alternatives and the isolation of the required, dominant meaning are easy for the normally working cortex. However, they are severely impaired in pathological (inhibitory) states of the tertiary (parieto-occipital) cortical zones of the left hemisphere when the normal 'law of strength' is not obeyed, and when the transition to a 'phase of equation' permits any irrelevant connection to spring up without adequate restraint. Possibly these pathophysiological mechanisms affecting the work of the tertiary zones of the left hemisphere may lie at the basis of the phenomenon known to the clinician as amnestic aphasia in the narrow sense of this term, and which is accompanied by a flood of uncontrollable verbal paraphasias (the substitution of necessary words by others of similar meaning or structure). An essential feature distinguishing this type of disturbance of expressive speech is that a little *prompting* with the first sound or syllable of the desired word *helps the patient to find it at once*. This sign distinguishes true amnestic aphasia from acoustico-mnestic aphasia, which is based on diffuseness of the acoustic structure of words (Luria, 1972).

④ We are thus left with the fourth condition essential for normal naming of objects, and it is one with which we are already familiar, the mobility of nervous processes. Its essential function is to ensure that, once the name has been found, it is not frozen, it does not become an inert stereotype, so that when the subject has named one object he is unable to switch easily to another name. However, this condition is affected in lesions of the *inferior zones of the left premotor area* (Broca's area), and also, more especially, in lesions of the *left fronto-temporal region*, in which the already familiar pheno-

Amnestic Aphasia

mena of pathological inertia are supplemented by temporal lobe phenomena of 'alienation of word meaning' and in which the patient's critical attitude towards the developing pathological inertia and his ability to correct his mistakes are disturbed. In such cases, although the patient gives the correct name to the picture of, for example, an apple, he is just as likely to call the next picture 'two cherries' as 'two apples'. Having named a pair of pictures correctly as 'a pencil and a key', when another pair of pictures representing 'a cup and a window' are presented he may call them 'a cup and a key' or even 'a pencil and . . . a pencil', without being sufficiently aware of his mistake. Hence, the second – apparently relatively simple – form of expressive speech, i.e. the naming of objects, is just as complex in its structure and requires the combined working of a group of zones of the left cortex for its performance.

Until now we have dealt with the analysis of the psychological structure of relatively simple, effector (operative) forms of expressive speech. It is now the time to turn to the problem of cerebral organization of *expressive speech activity as a whole*.

I shall not dwell in detail on disturbances of narrative expressive speech associated with difficulties in the pronunciation or the finding of individual words, but will turn directly to primary disorders of spontaneous narrative speech activity.

As I stated above, narrative expressive speech or expression begins with an *intention* or *plan*, which subsequently must be recoded into a verbal form and moulded into a speech expression. It is clear (part 2, ch. 7) that both these processes call for the participation of the *frontal lobes*, an apparatus essential for the creation of active intentions or the forming of plans. If this motive of the expression is absent, and no plan is actively formed, naturally there can be no question of spontaneous active speech, although repetitive speech and naming of objects remain intact.

It is these features which characterize patients with a marked frontal syndrome, in whom general aspontaneity and adynamia are accompanied by a well-marked 'aspontaneity of speech'; this is manifested as absence of the subject's own spontaneous expressions and also by the fact that the dialogical speech of such patients consists merely of passive and monotonous (sometimes echolalic) responses to questions. Whereas their responses to questions permitting a simple echolalic response ('Were you drinking tea?' – 'Yes, I was drinking tea') cause little difficulty, questions requiring the introduction of new connections into the answer ('Where have you been today?') give rise to considerable difficulty. The aspontaneity of speech which usually arises in massive frontal lobe lesions (involving the left hemisphere) still cannot be regarded as an 'aphasic' disorder. It is more of a special form of general aspontaneity. By contrast, the type of speech disturbance which I shall now describe occupies a definite, although special, place among the aphasic disorders. This type of speech disturbance I describe as dynamic aphasia (Luria; 1947; 1948; 1962; 1963; 1964; 1965b; 1969a; 1970a; Luria and Tsvetkova, 1968).

The transition from the general plan to narration requires the recoding of the plan into speech, and an important place in this process is played by *internal speech*, with its *predicative structure* (Vygotsky; 1934, 1956), providing what is known in syntax as the 'linear scheme of the sentence'. This process of transition from plan to narration is easily achieved by a normal subject; it remains essentially intact in patients with local lesions of the left temporal or left parieto-temporo-occipital regions, when, although the patient cannot find the necessary words, he retains the general intonational and melodic structure of the sentence, which he may fill with totally inadequate words.

It is this formation of the 'linear scheme of the sentence' which is substantially (sometimes completely) disturbed in patients with lesions of the *inferior postfrontal zones of the left hemisphere*. As a rule these patients have no difficulty whatever in repeating words or in naming objects. They can also repeat relatively simple sentences. However, as soon as they are required to express a thought, or even to produce an elementary verbal expression, they are completely unable to do so.

As a rule they make helpless attempts to find a way of expressing themselves, in such words as: 'well . . . this . . . but how? . . .' and they are completely unable to utter the simplest sentence.

Experience shows that this defect is not due to any absence of plan or to any deficiency of individual words. The patients of this group can easily name objects, but they have the same difficulty even if they are asked to give a fluent description of a thematic picture or, in other words, when the absence of an original plan of expression is ruled out.

The hypothesis that such a disturbance of narration is caused by a disturbance of the *linear scheme of the sentence*, based on a defect of the predicative function of speech, is confirmed by a simple test. If a patient who cannot formulate even a simple sentence such as 'I like walking' is shown three empty cards corresponding to the three elements of the sentence, and if, while he is formulating the sentence, the cards are pointed to in succession:

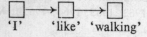

'I'   'like'   'walking'

it is at once apparent that although a short time ago he could not formulate his expression, he can now easily do so; if in a subsequent test we remove this material substitute for the linear scheme of the sentence, he will again be unable to perform the task.

An interesting fact, which Tsvetkova has demonstrated, is that an electromyographic recording from the lips and tongue during direct attempts to formulate expressions revealed no special impulses, whereas as soon as the external support for the scheme of the sentence was suggested, as in the test described, distinct electromyographic impulses from the lips, tongue, and larynx appeared (Figure 74), and the required sentence became ready for articulation.

We still do not know all the physiological mechanisms of this disturbance, but the most probable explanation is that the structures of the inferior frontal (and fronto-temporal) zones of the left hemisphere are intimately connected with the predicative structure of internal speech, for this would provide the complete explanation for this phenomenon.

The symptoms of dynamic aphasia may assume a much more complex form. There is reason to suppose that the physiological mechanisms of this most complex form of dynamic aphasia differ widely from those of the disturbances previously described, and that they require further detailed analysis. The first steps in this analysis have already been made (Ryabova, 1970), but it is still too early to suggest any definite mechanisms for this type of speech inactivity. All that can be said is that this form of disturbance of spontaneous narrative speech (recovery from which does not pass through the

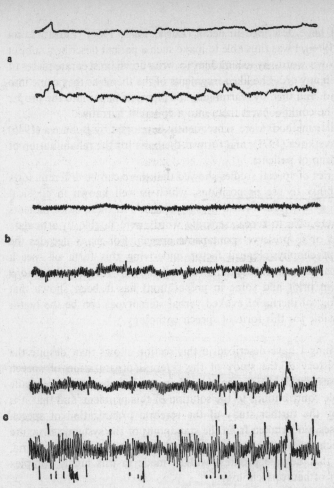

Figure 74 Electromyogram of the speech apparatus in a patient with dynamic aphasia: (a) background; (b) during attempts to formulate a sentence directly; (c) during similar attempts but with the aid of an external scheme of the sentence (after Tsvetkova)

stage of the 'telegraphic style') can be compensated by methods very similar to those I have described, except that the external material supports in this case must stand not for the word elements of the 'linear scheme of the sentence,' but for whole *semantic components of the spoken narrative.*

As I have described in detail (Luria, 1948; 1964; 1969a; Luria *et al.*, 1969), I was thus able to make such a patient describe a subject in his own words by asking him to write down on separate pieces of paper in any order he liked fragments of the theme as they came into his head, and then by rearranging the pieces of paper into the proper order, he could convert them into a coherent narrative.

Similar methods were subsequently developed by Bubnova (1946) and Tsvetkova (1971), and formed the basis for the rehabilitation of this group of patients.

A series of special studies showed that there can be different sorts of inability to use prepositions, which is well known in classical neurology as 'transcortical motor aphasia'. In these cases patients who were able to repeat separate words were unable to articulate phrases or to preserve spontaneous speech. For many decades the basic psychophysiological factor underlying this form of speech disturbances remained unknown, and only in recent publications (some in print and some in preparation) has it been shown that pathological inertia of evoked verbal stereotypes can be the factor responsible for this form of speech pathology.

Everything I have described in this section shows that, despite the long history of the study of the cerebral organization of speech processes, investigations conducted in the last decades have made valuable contributions to the solution of this problem, and that it is only by the further study of the cerebral organization of speech processes, undertaken from the standpoint of the systemic structure of speech activity (which will be the subject of a special book; Luria, 1973), that definite progress will be made in this highly complex chapter of neuropsychology.

Chapter 13
Thinking

Psychological structure

Whereas the history of the cerebral organization of speech extends for a century or more, we should be absolutely justified in saying that the cerebral organization of thinking has no history whatever. From the very beginning of philosophy and psychology, the concept of the 'brain' has always been opposed to the concept of 'thinking', and if an investigator wished to demonstrate that mental processes differ radically from brain processes, he used this opposition. The problem of the cerebral mechanisms of 'abstraction', of 'categorical set', or of 'logical thinking' thus either was not contemplated at all, or it was used simply in relation to such opposites as 'sensory' and 'rational', or 'matter' and 'thought'.

This opposition is seen equally in dualistic philosophy and in psychology, and claims that intellect or 'categorical thinking' cannot be reduced to material brain mechanisms were repeatedly made by almost all brain morphologists, psychiatrists, and neurologists (Monakow, 1914; Goldstein, 1927; 1944; 1948).

In the history of psychology there has been only one group of attempts in the opposite direction; but these attempts, in their various alternative forms, were usually bought very dearly – at the cost of rejection of the intrinsic quality of thinking and its reduction to more elementary mechanisms or associations (nineteenth-century associationism) and structural processes (twentieth-century Gestalt psychology), or by the open refusal to discuss thinking at all and its replacement by the 'formation of conditioned reflexes' or 'learning'. This refusal to undertake the task of discovering the cerebral organization of thinking can be understood if thinking is approached phenomenologically as an indivisible mental act. However, there can be no grounds whatever for this refusal if the solution of this problem is attempted by a scientific analysis of thinking as the form of cognitive activity with the most complex structure, and if the problem considered is not the relation between thinking as a whole (or even more, its product) and the brain, but the relation between this complex form of cognitive activity and its component elements and the brain. This is the approach used by modern neuropsychology, and with it the problem of the cerebral basis of intellectual activity ceases to be purely philosophical and becomes concrete and scientific in character. Let us first examine modern views on thinking, its basic forms and components, before moving on to the problem of its cerebral organization with which we are specially concerned.

Modern psychology regards the process of thinking in a completely different light, as will be apparent from a very brief review, first of the history, and then of the present state of the problem. The dominant views of thinking held by psychologists in the middle of the nineteenth century were very simple: it is a combination of associations of varying complexity; of all these associations, associations by contiguity were rightly regarded as the simplest, while associations by similarity or contrast were regarded as incorporating more complex logical relationships, into which they had to be fitted before these associations could arise. However, these views of the associationists on the psychological nature of thought, which were held for more than a century, had their essential weaknesses which led to its downfall.

The purposive, selective process of thinking could never be understood as the result of mechanical action of individual associations. Whereas Herbart, who made the first attempt to construct something like a mathematical model of thinking, at the beginning of last century attempted to equate the direction of thought with the victory of the strongest and overthrow of the weakest ideas, this remained nothing more than a formal scheme. It failed to explain the factors which would determine the strength of ideas, and at the same time it did not seek to explain the active character of the process which makes thinking such a selective and goal-directed activity, so adaptive to the changing situation.

The simplified associationist views on thinking were not completely rejected until the beginning of the present century when a

number of German psychologists, belonging to the so-called Würzburg school (Külpe, Ach, Bühler, Messer) expressed their doubts
that human thinking in general can be deduced from the association
of ideas. They attempted to show that true thinking consists of the
direct 'perception of relations' and cannot incorporate either images
(concrete), or verbal components, or their associations, so that
the act of thinking is an independent mental 'function', like the acts
of perception or of recollection. The Würzburg school deserves
credit for the fact that for the first time it distinguished thinking as an
independent entity for psychological investigation. However, this
step was made at great cost, for the acceptance of thinking as a
once-and-for-all indivisible act, which can be described by subjective
methods and which cannot be broken down into its components,
was a retrograde step compared with associationism, closing the door
to its scientific investigation.

The story of the attempts to understand thinking as a single structure, based on laws similar to the laws of integral perception, made
by supporters of the Gestalt psychology initially on monkeys
(Kohler, 1917), and later on man (Wertheimer, 1925; 1945; 1957;
Koffka 1925; Duncker, 1935), is very similar. Whereas the basic assumptions for the analysis of thinking as an integral act made by these
investigators undoubtedly deserve attention, their attempts not to
see anything in the construction of this act other than the structural
laws of 'integrity' and 'prägnanz', which were already familiar from
the study of perception, were an impediment to further progress.

Important advances in the psychological analysis of thinking were
made with the transition to the concrete analysis of the basic *methods*
used in thinking and of the fundamental *dynamic structures* which
are revealed on a closer inspection of active thinking and its stochastic structure. In the 1930s, the Soviet psychologist Vygotsky first
demonstrated that the process of analysis and generalization, which
is the basis of the intellectual act, depends on the logical structure of
speech, and that *word-meaning, the basis of ideas, develops in childhood*. Whereas initially it is based on the syncretic unification
of impressions which the child receives from the outside world, later
it is converted into the unification of concrete cues of the whole
practical situation; finally it begins to apply to whole abstract
categories (Vygotsky, 1934; posthumous editions 1956, 1960). This

analysis of the fundamental stages of development of ideas, which Piaget (1926–57) also approached from completely different positions, made it possible to describe the whole complexity of the logical structure of words, the basic tools for the formation of ideas, and to represent with sufficient clarity the wide range of alternatives provided by the logical matrices on which they are based at individual stages of development. It also made it possible to study how these concrete systems of matrices, reflecting the 'situational' character of thinking, are gradually replaced by abstract matrices, incorporating a whole hierarchy of 'community relationships' which consitute the fundamental apparatus of categorical thinking.

The description of this fundamental apparatus of thinking, which has subsequently been developed by many authoritative investigators (Bruner, Goodnow and Austin, 1956; Bruner, 1957), enabled decisive progress to be made in the analysis of thinking as an *integral dynamic act*.

The realization that word meaning is the fundamental tool of thinking was crucial to the approach to the basic problem: the description of the *psychological structure of thinking as a whole*. The investigation of this problem has in fact occupied a whole generation of psychologists and it has received a powerful impetus both from the development of psychological science itself in recent decades and also from the development of high-speed computers, which has necessitated a more detailed description of the structure of real thinking in order that the best possible models of it can be constructed.

Attempts to construct the basic concepts of thinking as an integral process, by breaking it down into its components, have been made in different countries. In the Soviet Union, the problem of the structure of thinking has been investigated on the basis of the general concept of inner structure of *mental activity* formulated by a number of leading Soviet psychologists who are followers of Vygotsky (Leontiev, 1954; 1959; Galperin, 1959, and others). In other countries the psychological analysis of concrete forms of thinking has been associated with the study of chess playing (de Groot, 1964) and, above all, with the development of the heuristic theory of thought, which compares human thinking with the principles of operation of high-speed computers (Newell, Shaw and Simon, 1958; Feigenbaum and Feldman, 1963).

As a result of this series of investigations, we now have a sufficiently clear idea about thinking as a concrete mental activity. We can distinguish those components of it which are exhibited equally in concrete-active and in verbal-logical and discursive thinking, and which enable neuropsychologists to abandon the attempt to seek a cerebral substrate of 'thinking in general' and instead to seek a *system of cerebral mechanisms* responsible for the components of thinking and for its stages. Let us now attempt to summarize very briefly those ideas of human thinking as an integral form of mental activity which are now accepted by all investigators.

Psychologists studying the concrete process of thinking are unanimous in assuming that thinking arises only when the subject has an appropriate motive which makes the task urgent and its solution essential, and when the subject is confronted by a *situation for which he has no ready-made (inborn or habitual) solution*. This basic proposition can be formulated in other words by saying that the origin of thought is always the presence of a task, by which the psychologist understands that the problem which the subject must solve is given under *certain conditions*, which he must first investigate in order to discover the path leading to an adequate solution.

The next stage which follows immediately after the discovery of the task is not, therefore, a direct attempt to respond suitably, but the *restraining* of impulsive responses, the *investigation of the conditions* of the problem, the analysis of its components, recognition of the most essential features, and their correlation with one another. This work of preliminary investigation into the conditions of the problem is a vital and essential step in any concrete process of thought, without which no intellectual act could take place.

The third stage in the process of thinking is the *selection of one from a number of possible alternatives* and the creation of a *general plan (scheme) for the performance* of the task, deciding which alternatives are most likely to succeed, and at the same time rejecting all inadequate alternatives. Many psychologists describe this phase of the intellectual act as the general *strategy* of thinking, and they regard it as its most essential component.

The existence of these multidimensional matrices of word meanings, which I have already mentioned, and which participate in all forms of thought, naturally makes this stochastic structure of the intellectual act understandable and points to the fact that each task inevitably gives rise to a multiple network of alternatives, from which one system can be chosen by the subject on the basis of the predominance of one particular system of associations concealed behind the word meaning.

This analysis of the conditions of the problem and choice of a certain system from many possible alternatives constitutes the psychological essence of the processes of 'heuristics' whose investigation has received special attention in recent years.

The formation of a general scheme for the solution of the problem and the choice of adequate systems of alternatives bring the subject to the next (fourth) phase of thinking, which is choosing the appropriate *methods* and considering which *operations* will be adequate for putting the general scheme of the solution into effect. These operations are most frequently the use of suitable ready-made algorithms (linguistic, logical, numerical) which have evolved in the course of social history and are well fitted to represent such a scheme or hypothesis. Some psychologists describe this stage of the discovery of the essential operations as the *tactics*, distinguishing it from the stage of discovery of the appropriate *strategy* for the solution of the problem.

The process of using the appropriate operations is naturally the *operative* stage of the intellectual act, rather than its creative stage, although it is sometimes one of considerable complexity. As the work of Vygotsky (1934; 1956; 1960), followed by the investigations of Galperin and his collaborators (Galperin, 1959), showed, the process of thinking passes through several stages. It starts with an extended series of successive external actions (trials and errors), progresses to extended internal speech, in which the necessary searches are made, and concludes with the contraction and condensation of these external searches and the transition to a specific *internal process*. In this the subject is able to obtain assistance from ready-made systems of codes (linguistic and logical, in discursive verbal thinking; numerical in the solution of arithmetical problems), which he has learned. The existence of these well assimilated internal codes, which form the operative basis of the 'mental act', thus also forms the basis for performance of required intellectual operations, and in the adult subject, who has mastered the use of these algorithms, it beguins to provide a solid foundation for the operative stage of thinking.

The use of these algorithms leads the subject to the next phase of the intellectual act, regarded for many decades as the last, but in the modern view, still not its final stage. This phase is the actual *solution* to the problem or the discovery of the *answer* to the question embodied in the task.

It is only in the last decade that we have learned that the discovery of this solution does not conclude the intellectual act, but is merely the prelude to the final stage. The fact that the process of thinking does not end with the discovery of the answer has been shown by the work of many investigators (Anokhin, 1955; 1963; 1968b; Miller, Pribram and Galanter, 1960). This stage must be followed by a stage of *comparison of the results obtained with the original conditions* of the task (or as Anokhin called it, the stage of the action acceptor). If the results do agree with the original conditions of the problem the intellectual act is complete, but if, on the other hand, they do not correspond to the original conditions, the search for the necessary strategy must begin again and the process of thinking must continue until an adequate solution, in agreement with the conditions, is found.

These views regarding the psychological structure of thinking and the identification of its principal stages present far better opportunities for the analysis of the cerebral mechanisms of this process than those which were available for earlier investigators. Most neurologists who have attempted to study the cerebral mechanisms of the intellectual act thought that they could confine their attention to the search for the hypothetical cerebral substrate for abstract ideas, the fundamental component of the intellectual act. Such was the character of the attempts made by most psychiatrists. Once they had described the phenomena of the 'dementia' accompanying an organic brain lesion, they considered it sufficient to explain the disturbance of thinking in these cases by the disintegration of abstract ideas and by the transition to concrete forms of reflection of reality. Similar views were also expressed by the eminent neurologist Goldstein (1944; 1948), who considered that intellectual defects arising in local brain lesions can be regarded as the disintegration of 'abstract sets' or of 'abstract behaviour'.

I need hardly say that, considering the great importance of this phenomenon, attempts to reduce disturbances of thinking in patients with local brain lesions to a disintegration of 'abstract sets' can at best shed light on only one possible component of the complex pathology of the intellectual act, and they are quite unable to explain the whole complexity of disturbances of thinking. Nor need I mention that the disturbance of 'categorical behaviour' is the result of a long series of changes taking place in the intellectual activity of the sick person rather than its cause, and that the disturbance may be completely different in character in the different components of this behaviour. Naturally, therefore, despite many years of investigations by neurologists such as Goldstein, who adopted this concept as their starting point, no definite results were obtained which could shed light on the cerebral mechanisms of thinking. According to Goldstein himself, a disturbance of 'abstract behaviour' could arise in patients with lesions in widely different parts of the brain, so that his approach was an assessment of the general result of a complex pathological process rather than a true analysis of its structure. We are therefore fully justified in seeking a new approach, in studying how the *indvidual components of the process of thinking*, as I have described it, *are disturbed in patients with lesions of various parts of the brain*. Only in this way can we improve our prospects of success in the analysis of the cerebral mechanisms of disturbances of speech and use these disturbances for the topical diagnosis of local brain lesions.

Disturbances of motives and goals, which may arise in deep brain lesions and also in lesions of the frontal lobes, must inevitably lead to a different type of disturbance of thinking processes from the disturbance of the traces of short-term audio-verbal memory, associated with lesions of the left temporal region, or cases in which a lesion of the parieto-occipital zones prevents the welding of the individual elements of information into unified, simultaneous schemes. It can easily be imagined that disturbances of the ability to retain a problem, to inhibit impulsive attempts to find an answer to questions and to make a preliminary investigation of the basic conditions of the task, a disturbance of the ability to produce hypotheses, to choose, from the many possible alternatives, the most suitable operations or codes and, finally, the ability to compare results obtained with the original conditions of the task and to assess the adequacy of the solution – all these faculties will suffer to different degrees as the result of lesions in different parts of the brain. Naturally, therefore, destruction of different cerebral zones must inevitably lead to *different disturbances of the structure of thinking*. Accordingly, we can approach the analysis of the brain systems participating in the construction of thinking by a completely different method from that used by classical psychiatry and neurology.

I shall therefore follow the course which is accepted in neuropsychology, and first describe the disturbances of practical or constructive thinking, and then the disturbances of verbal-logical (discursive) thinking in patients with lesions of different parts of the brain. This will give a closer insight into the cerebral organization of intellectual activity along similar lines to those which we followed in our analysis of the cerebral basis of perception and actions, of memory and speech.

Practical or constructive thinking

The simplest form of practical, constructive thinking, which is familiar in clinical medicine, is the *solution of constructive tasks*, and its simplest models are tests with Kohs' blocks or Link's cube. In the first of these tests the subject must build a model from the blocks as indicated by a diagram which he is given; the special feature about this test is that *the blocks as shown on the diagram do not correspond, on direct visual perception, to the actual blocks from which the model must be made*. For instance, if the diagram shows a blue triangle on a yellow background, so that there are three distinct visual units, namely a blue triangle and two yellow background elements (Figure 75a), the actual model must be built from two constructive elements (Figure 75b) each consisting of a yellow and blue square, divided diagonally into two triangles.

The intellectual task which the subject must perform is to overcome the vectors of direct perception and to *convert the elements of impression into elements of construction*. This problem can be solved as soon as the subject can overcome the direct perception of the drawing and recode the structure of this perception into the elements of the building blocks.

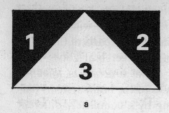 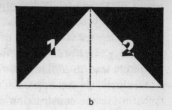

a   b

Figure 75 Scheme of tests using Kohs's blocks (a) structure of
perception of the figure, (b) structure of the required performance

The test known in psychology as Link's cube is similar in its psychological structure. In this test the subject has to construct a large cube of a certain colour (for example, yellow) from twenty-seven smaller cubes, eight of which have three yellow sides, twelve have two yellow sides, six have only one yellow side, and one has no yellow sides.

Direct attempts to construct such a cube obviously will not yield the desired result, for the only possible method of solution of the problem is to investigate its conditions, to form a general strategy (or general plan) of its solution (using the cubes with three yellow sides at the corners) and those with two yellow sides in the middle of the edges, those with one yellow side in the middle of each surface, and the colourless cube in the centre of the model), and after the formation of this plan, to use it in order to find the operations required to perform the task. Other tasks of constructive thinking, large numbers of which are used in modern psychology, all have a similar psychological structure.

The disturbance of spatial syntheses arising in lesions of the *parieto-occipital zones* of the left hemisphere naturally interferes with the performance of such tests of constructive activity. Patients of this group turn the Kohs's blocks over helplessly without knowing how to fit them together, or in what position to put the diagonal so that it will match the outlines of the design.

Both the general principle governing the construction of the model as well as the intention to construct it naturally are completely intact in these cases; this is shown both by the long series of attempts which these patients will make and by their critical attitude towards their defects. The integrity of their activity and the limitation of their defect are shown by the fact that the difficulties experienced by these patients can be compensated by the use of external aids, for example, the spatial coordinates are pointed out to them or their direct attempts to fit the required shape are converted into detailed programmes, incorporating spatial analysis of the direction of the lines ('from the bottom left side to the top right side'). These three-dimensional schemes, as Tsvetkova (Tsvetkova, 1966a; Luria and Tsvetkova, 1968) has shown, enable the patient to get round his difficulties and to solve the problem. The types of defects arising in these patients and the steps which can be taken to overcome them are illustrated in Figure 76a.

The way in which the same tests are performed by patients with *frontal lesions* is completely different in character. These patients have no difficulty in finding the necessary spatial relationships; however, the *activity* of their performance of the test is grossly disturbed. The patients do not analyse the diagram, they make no attempt to convert the 'units of impression' into 'units of construction', and they manipulate the cubes impulsively in accordance with direct impressions. Their mistakes are therefore quite different in character, they work in a quite different manner, they do not proceed by trial and error, they *do not work* actively in order to complete the test, and they do not *evaluate* their mistakes.

The programmes by which these patients can partially compensate their defects are therefore different in nature: in this case the aids are not directed towards the finding of the necessary spatial relationships (they do not need such aids); instead they must direct the *programming of the patient's behaviour*, as in this example: 1. 'Look at the diagram.' 2. 'How many cubes is it made of?' 3. 'Find the first cube.' 4. 'Look and see what colour it must be.' 5. 'Look how the line separating the two colours runs,' and so on. Only by the programming of his behaviour will the subject succeed in his constructive activity; this success will quickly disappear as soon as the detailed programme of behaviour is removed and the patient is forced to perform the constructive activity unaided (Tsvetkova, 1966a; 1972). Types of mistakes made by patients with lesions of the frontal lobe and methods used to compensate the observed defect are illustrated in Figure 76b.

The performance of a test involving the construction of Link's cube can be analysed similarly. Whereas patients with lesions of the

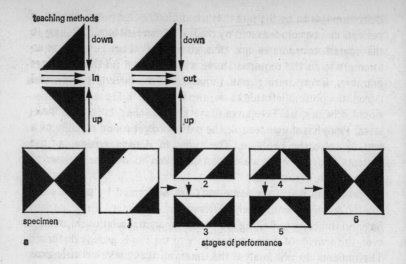

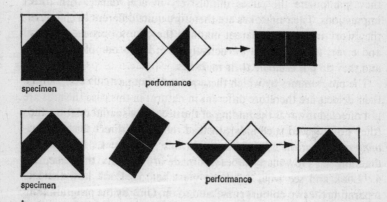

Figure 76 Disturbance of the performance of constructive tasks with Kohs's blocks: (a) by patients with parieto-occipital disturbances and (b) with frontal disturbances (after Tsvetkova)

parieto-occipital zones of the cortex understand the problem perfectly well and start to work diligently at its solution, having difficulty only because of their inability to *picture* the necessary spatial relationships, patients with a marked frontal syndrome can only make direct attempts to perform the test, completely omitting the stage of preliminary investigation of its conditions, and naturally failing to make the intermediate calculations which, in this case, constitute an essential component of normal intellectual activity. All these findings have been analysed in a special publication by Gadzhiev (1966), and no further details of them will be given here.

These facts show that the processes of practical, constructive thinking are complex in structure and take place through the activity of a series of concertedly working brain zones. A careful analysis of the changes taking place in constructive activity in patients with lesions of different parts of the brain will help to identify the role of each of these zones in the structure of these processes.

Verbal-logical (discursive) thinking: the solution of problems

Many different methods are used in psychology to test verbal-logical thinking. They include such methods as the classification of objects or concepts, the finding of logical relationships or analogies, the performance of simple operations of logical deduction, using figures of syllogism, and many others. Some of these have been extensively used in clinical psychiatry (Vygotsky, 1934; Zeigarnik, 1961); some have yielded important results in the investigation of patients with local brain lesions, and I have described them elsewhere (Luria, 1962; 1966a; 1969c).

I do not propose to describe here all the results obtained by the use of these tests for the investigation of patients with local brain lesions, I shall merely examine one of their applications, the neuropsychological analysis of the *solution of arithmetical problems*, as there are good grounds for considering that this test is the most revealing model of discursive thinking. I shall therefore use this test in an attempt to analyse one of the most difficult of problems: the nature of the cerebral systems concerned with the construction of the most complex forms of intellectual activity.

An arithmetical problem always consists of a *goal* (the statement of the problem in the form of a question to which no ready-made answer is available), and the *conditions*, from which a scheme for the solution can be prepared by analysis, alternatively a *strategy* leading to the required solution can be decided. This strategy, expressed in words as a *hypothesis*, initiates searches for the individual *operations* which will be used to obtain the necessary results. The process of solution of the problem ends with a *comparison* between the method used and the result obtained, on the one hand, and the question and the conditions of the problem on the other hand. As we have seen when describing previous cases, depending on whether agreement or disagreement between the solution and the conditions of the problem have been obtained, the intellectual activity will cease, or fresh attempts will be made to find a path leading to an adequate solution.

The fact which lends itself most suitably to investigation is that the different problems have different structures, and it is possible to arrange their structures in the order of increasing complexity. For instance, as I have pointed out elsewhere (Luria and Tsvetkova, 1967), the simplest problems (*Jack has four apples, Jill has three apples. How many apples have they together?*) have a simple algorithm of solution and no special searching is required. More complex forms of this problem (*Jack had four apples, Jill had two apples more. How many apples had they together?*) require the performance of an intermediate operation, which is not expressed in the words in the problem, so that the solution of the task breaks up into two steps: $a+x = y$; $x = (a+b)$; $(2a+b) = y$. The solution of problems with complex algorithms, requiring programmes consisting of a series of successive components, is much more difficult, especially when the components of the programme can be found only after a detailed analysis of the conditions of the problem and the production of a specific strategy. These include the 'prototype tests' requiring *recoding* of the conditions and the introduction of new component elements. (*There were eighteen books on two shelves; there were twice as many books on one shelf as on the other. How many books were there on each shelf?* To solve this problem, in addition to the original condition 'of two shelves' the additional items 'three parts' must be introduced and the number of books on each of these auxiliary 'parts' must first be calculated). Finally, perhaps the most difficult problems are those which I describe as 'conflicting' and in which the correct method of solution involves the inhibition of the impulsive direct method ('*A candle is 15 cm long; the shadow from the candle is 45 cm longer; how many times is the shadow longer than the candle ?*' The tendency here is to perform the direct operation $45 \div 15 = 3$; this must be inhibited and replaced by the more complex programme: $15+45 = 60$; $60 \div 15 = 4$). It will be evident how the solution of problems of each of these types represents a series of increasingly complex psychological actions.

This structural analysis of the demands presented by the solution of problems of different structure provides an approach to the study of the changes in this process of solution when certain conditions connected with the work of particular brain systems are removed. They thus provide a key to the cerebral organization of this complex process.

Lesions of the *left temporal region*, disturbing audio-verbal memory, naturally give rise to difficulty in retention of the conditions of the problem and are accompanied by inability to involve the necessary intermediate speech components in the mechanism of solution. For this reason the solution, even of relatively simple problems, is severely impaired in patients of this group. The process can be facilitated to some extent if the problem is presented *in writing*, but even in these cases the need for intermediate speech components, used as elements for the solution of problems, severely impairs the entire discursive process. Observations on these difficulties, however, are non-specific for intellectual activity. They have been discussed in several publications (Ombrédane, 1951), and I shall not deal with them specially here.

The difficulties in the solution of problems encountered by patients with lesions of the systems of the *left parieto-occipital* region are much more interesting. In these cases (part 2, ch. 5) the lesion causes gross impairment of simultaneous (spatial) syntheses, and this is manifested both in the direct, concrete behaviour and also in the symbolic sphere. As a result of such a disturbance it becomes impossible to operate either with logical-grammatical systems or with systems of numerical operations, so that the normal solution of complex problems is prevented. The general meaning of the problems is often relatively intact in these patients; as a rule they never lose sight of the final question of the problem and they make active attempts to find a method of solution. However, the fact that they cannot understand complex logical-grammatical structures or perform any than the simplest arithmetical operations presents an insuperable obstacle to their problem solving. Even such elements of the conditions as 'A took so many apples from B', or 'A had twice as many apples as B', or again, 'A has two apples more (or less) than B', not to mention more complex logical-grammatical structures, are quite beyond the capacity of such patients. Repetition of the conditions means nothing more to them than the reproduction of their isolated, disconnected fragments, giving rise to a successive series of misunderstandings ('Jack had some apples . . . while Jill . . . two . . . twice . . . what does 'more' mean? and so on), which the patient cannot overcome. Naturally, the system of logical connections embodied in the conditions of more complex problems is completely beyond the grasp of these patients, and despite the fact that the *intention* to solve the problem remains completely intact and the patient continues to make active *attempts* to understand the relationship in the conditions, the solution of the problem remains unattainable.

The disturbance of the process of problem solving differs completely in its structure in patients with lesions of the *frontal zones*. In a special book on this subject (Luria and Tsvetkova, 1967) these peculiarities were analysed in some detail, and I shall now only briefly summarize the facts described there.

The first and principal feature of the disturbance of intellectual activity in patients with massive lesions of the frontal lobes is that, when given a written problem, *they do not perceive it as a problem*, or in other words, as a system of mutually subordinated elements of the condition which must lead to the solution to the problem. If such patients are instructed to repeat the conditions of the problem, they may succeed in reproducing some of the component elements of the condition, *they may be unable to repeat the problem at all*, or *instead of repeating the problem they may repeat only one of its elements*. As an example, let us consider the problem 'There were eighteen books on two shelves, but they were not equally divided; there were twice as many books on one shelf as on the other. How many books were there on each shelf?' The patients of this group will repeat the problem as follows: 'There were eighteen books on two shelves. And on the second shelf there were eighteen books . . .' the task was thus converted into a statement of two facts and no longer had the character of an intellectual problem. In other similar cases (which are very frequent), the patients may repeat the same problem but in a different way: 'There were eighteen books on two shelves; there were twice as many on one shelf as on the other. How many books were there on both shelves?' In this case they do not observe that instead of a problem requiring special solution, they are in fact repeating the first part of the conditions. The patients of this group, as a rule, are unaware of their mistake, and if the problem is presented to them again, they simply repeat their previous mistakes. These facts clearly show that in a patient with a marked frontal syndrome the basic condition, that of the *existence of the problem itself is lacking*, so that there can be no *intention* to 'solve' it.

The second defect characteristic of patients with a frontal lobe lesion, intimately connected with the first, is that these patients *make no attempt at a preliminary investigation of the conditions of the problem*, and as a result, without any preliminary analysis of the conditions and identification of their components, they immediately begin to seek solutions impulsively, usually by combining the numbers specified by the conditions and performing a series of fragmentary observations, totally unconnected with the context of the problems and, consequently, without any plan. A typical example of these fragmentary operations, which replace the true solution of the problem, is given by the course of the answers to the problem of the two shelves with eighteen books: 'There were eighteen books on two shelves ... there were twice as many on the second ... thirty-six ... and there were two shelves ... $18 + 36 = 54! ...$'

This type of 'solution' of a problem is typical of patients with a marked frontal syndrome, and it clearly demonstrates the *disintegration of intellectual activity as a whole* in these patients, so that they cannot solve such problems despite the fact that *their understanding of logical-grammatical structures and of arithmetical operations is intact*. In such cases, patients with a frontal lobe lesion characteristically *do not compare their answer with the original conditions* of the problem and they are *unaware of the meaninglessness of their solution*.

The correct solution to such 'conflicting' problems is clearly quite beyond the capacity of these patients. For example, one such patient, having read out the problem – 'A candle is 15 cm long; the shadow from the candle is 45 cm longer. How many times is the shadow longer than the candle?' – immediately answers 'three times of course!', and even after leading questions he fails to notice anything wrong about his answer.

Neuropsychological analysis thus demonstrates profound differences in the character of disturbance of problem solving by patients with lesions of different parts of the brain. It reveals that whereas the posterior zones of the hemispheres (forming the second functional unit of the brain) are responsible for the *operative conditions* for the performance of intellectual activity, the frontal lobes (forming the third functional unit) are the essential apparatus for *organizing intellectual activity as a whole*, including the *programming* of the intellectual act and the *checking* of its performance.

I am clearly aware that the analysis of the cerebral organization of intellectual activity is only in its infancy, and that much work has still to be done before we have a clear understanding of the cerebral mechanisms of thinking. However, I have no doubt that the method of *systemic analysis* which I have suggested will provide a reliable road to the solution of this complex problem.

Part Four
Conclusion

I have given a brief survey of the basic principles governing the work of the human brain, and I have described the essential features of the new branch of science known as neuropsychology, which has grown up in the last thirty years. The time has now come to draw certain very brief conclusions regarding the role of this new branch of science in theory and practice.

I began this book by stating that until very recently philosophers and psychologists had been quite content to accept the view that the brain is the organ of human mental life rather than to seek and obtain the necessary concrete material from which the fundamental principles governing the functional organization of the brain and the concrete forms of its work could be deduced. This stage is now behind us. We now have a wealth of material to indicate the principles of functional organization of the brain, to identify the principal units of the working brain, and to indicate the role of individual brain systems in the organization of mental processes. The first two parts of this book were devoted to a survey of the data available to modern science when seeking an answer to this problem.

I have used these data to analyse the cerebral organization of complex human mental activity and to show how man, in his perception and action, his memory, speech and thinking, makes use of a highly complex system of concertedly working zones of the cerebral cortex. The third, or synthetic, part of this book deals with this aspect of the problem. I do not suggest for a moment that the material I have described is anything like the complete and final answer to these questions. Neuropsychology is still a very young science, taking its very first step, and a period of thirty years is not a very long time for the development of any science. That is why some very important chapters, such as motives, complex forms of emotions and the structure of personality are not included in this book. Perhaps they will be added in future editions.

I have attempted to describe the ideas which have arisen during this period of forty years of intensive work, using mainly the results of observations made by myself and my collaborators. Naturally, in the years to come many of the ideas I have described will be clarified and developed, while others will prove mistaken and will be revised. This is how any new field of science always develops, and we must be prepared for it.

However, I have no doubt that the stage of the work which is summarized in this book will prove important and useful. The student of the brain will find in it a summary of the data on the functional aspects of the work of the human brain, and this may direct his attention to an aspect of research which until recently has developed much more slowly than the investigation of the intimate electrophysiological mechanisms of brain activity and the study of the functions of single neurons. It is the work of the brain as an apparatus organizing human mental activity which is of the greatest interest, and which must be of the most immediate concern to the philosopher and psychologist, the teacher and physician. I am therefore convinced that the material I have described will stimulate the reader's interest.

There is another aspect of the theoretical significance of the problems discussed in this book. This is of great importance for the development of psychology. Modern psychology has undoubtedly made considerable progress in the study of the genesis of psychological processes, and in their changes in the course of development. It has described the structure of human mental activity. It now has clear ideas on the structure of higher psychological actions and complex conscious activities that cannot in any way be compared with the classical schemes of associationism or with the general ideas of Gestalt psychology, with the simplified phenomenology of behaviourism, or with the pretensions of 'depth psychology'. Despite all these advances, our knowledge of the psychophysiological structure of mental processes and of their internal intimate mechanisms is still grossly inadequate. We still know very little about the internal nature and the neurological structure of complex forms of conscious activity although their course is now reasonably well understood. We know almost nothing about the factors composing the structure of this activity, and how these factors change in the successive stages of mental development and with the acquisition of the complex devices facilitating the course of these processes. It would be wrong to underestimate the important work done in this direction by the various schools of 'factor analysis'. However, it would be equally wrong to suppose that the mathematical methods used by these schools are a natural way of obtaining the solution to the problems which arise.

The purpose of this book was to lay the foundations of another method – of an analysis of the internal structure of psychological processes by the use of neuropsychological methods. These methods begin with a detailed analysis of the changes arising in psychological processes in local brain lesions, after which an attempt is made to show how complexes or systems of psychological processes are disturbed by these lesions. It provides an approach to the analysis of the internal structure of psychological processes and of that inner connection which unites the various psychological processes.

There are thus two aspects to the analysis of changes in psychological processes in local brain lesions. Firstly, it reveals the neurological substrate with which a particular activity is linked, and thus deepens our knowledge of its internal psychophysiological structure. Secondly, it reveals those general structures which exist in different – sometimes apparently completely different – psychological processes, and in this way it can open up yet another path to the factorial analysis of mental activity. This path I describe as the neuropsychological path of syndrome analysis, and the whole of this book is devoted to the attempt to demonstrate the productiveness of this approach.

It is easy to imagine that psychological science, by using this approach, will make new and important advances, and that in another few years new and important additional chapters for example on neuropsychology of emotional life and consciousness will be added and a new branch, neurolinguistics, will be created. As a result we can only predict that in the next fifty years our views on the structure of mental processes will differ substantially from those which we hold today; neuropsychology will deserve much of the credit for this revision and deepening of our knowledge of the internal structure of mental processes.

The field of knowledge to which my book is devoted has another, practical aspect. Every step in the development of neurology, and of its youngest and most active branch – neurosurgery – shows the acute lack of accurate and early methods of local (or at least, regional) diagnosis of focal brain lesions in clinical practice. The classical methods developed by neurology a century ago are absolutely essential, but nevertheless inadequate. The investigation of sensation, movements, reflexes and tone, the basic inventory of neurological investigation, provides only relatively little information on lesions of the most complex, specifically human zones of the brain, and in man these zones occupy nearly two-thirds of the cerebral hemispheres. Naturally, under these conditions neurology and neurosurgery turn hopefully to precise methods: electroencephalography, in all its various forms, contrast methods using arteriography, and various other supporting techniques.

There is another approach which is of decisive importance. This is neuropsychological investigation, capable of obtaining a vast amount of objective information on lesions of the most complex, specifically human parts of the brain and enabling this information to be used for the precise local (or regional) diagnosis of circumscribed brain lesions. In this respect neuropsychology is merely the most complex and newest chapter of neurology, and without this chapter, modern clinical neurology will be unable to exist and develop.

Neuropsychology now has a firm foothold in clinical neurology and neurosurgery. This fact is a source of great satisfaction to the author who, together with his colleagues, has spent a good deal of his life in an effort to make neuropsychology an important practical branch of neurology. It gives him confidence that his scientific life has not been spent in vain, and that new and important prospects lie ahead for neurology, and for those important divisions of neurology – the topical diagnosis of local brain lesions and the rehabilitation of these patients.

To describe the importance of neuropsychology as the science of the working human brain and as a branch of practical medicine, to indicate the contribution which it is making to modern knowledge, and to survey briefly what it has to offer – these are the objects of this book.

References

Adey, W. R., Dunlop, C. W., and Hendrix, C. (1960), 'Hippocampal slow waves: distribution and phase relationships in the course of approach learning', *AMA Arch. Neurol.*, vol. 3.

Adrian, E. D. (1936), 'The spread of activity in the cerebral cortex', *J. Physiol.*, vol. 88.

Adrianov, O. S. (1963), 'Intercortical and thalamocortical relations in conditioned reflex activity', Doctoral Dissertation, Academy of Medical Sciences of the USSR (Russian).

Ajuriaguerra, J., and Hécaen, H. (1960), *Le Cortex Cérébral*, 2nd ed, Masson.

Akbarova, N. A. (1971), 'Neuropsychological analysis of memory disturbances in cranio-cerebral trauma', dissertation, Moscow University (Russian).

Ananev, B. G. (1952), 'Paired working of the cerebral hemispheres', in S. A. Petrushovski (ed.), *I. P. Pavlov and the Philosophical Bases of Psychology*, Izd. Akad. Pedagog, Nauk RSFSR, Moscow (Russian). Pedagog. Nauk RSFSR, Moscow (Russian).

Ananev, B. G. (1954), 'Functional asymmetry in tactile spatial discrimination'. *Uchenye Zapiski Leningradskogo Universiteta*, vol. 189.

Ananev, B. G., Lomov, B. F. *et al.* (ed.) (1959), *Touch*, Izd. Akad. Pedagog. Nauk RSFSR, Moscow (Russian).

Anokhin, P. K. (1935), *Problems of Centre and Periphery in the Physiology of Nervous Activity*, Gosizdat, Gorki (Russian).

Anokhin, P. K. (1940), 'Localization problems from the point of view of systemic ideas of nervous functions', *Nevrologiya i Psikhiatriya* vol. 9, no. 6 (Russian).

Anokhin, P. K. (1949), *Problems in Higher Nervous Activity*, Izd. Akad. Med. Nauk SSSR, Moscow (Russian).

Anokhin, P. K. (1955), 'New data on the afferent apparatus of the conditioned reflex', *Voprosy Psikhologii*, no. 6 (Russian).

Anokhin, P. K. (1959), 'Recent advances in neurophysiology and their importance to the study of higher nervous activity', *Vestnik Akad. Med. Nauk SSSR*, vol. 5. (Russian).

Anokhin, P. K. (1962), 'New data on the character of ascending activation', *Zhurnal Vysshei Nervnoi Deyatel' nosti*, vol. 12 (Russian).

Anokhin, P. K. (1963), 'The theory of the functional system as the basis for the construction of a physiological cybernetics', in *Biological Aspects of Cybernetics*, Izd. Akad. Nauk SSSR, Moscow (Russian).

Anokhin, P. K. (1968a), *Biology and Neurophysiology of the Conditioned Reflex*, Meditsina, Moscow (Russian).

Anokhin, P. K. (1968b), 'Cybernétique, neurophysiologie et psychologie', *Information sur les Sciences Sociales*, vol. 7.

Anokhin, P. K. (1972), *Fundamental Problems in the General Theory of Functional Systems*, Izd. Akad. Nauk SSSR (Russian; special issue on the occasion of a seminar on the general theory of functional systems).

Artemeva, E. Yu. (1965), 'Periodic fluctuations of asymmetry of the EEG waves as criteria of the state of activity', Candidate Dissertation, Moscow University (Russian).

Artemeva, E. Yu., and Homskaya, E. D. (1966), 'Changes in asymmetry of the slow waves in various functional states under normal conditions and in lesions of the frontal lobes', in A. R. Luria and E. D. Homskaya (eds.), *The Frontal Lobes and Regulation of Mental Processes*, Moscow University Press, Moscow (Russian).

Babenkova, S. V. (1954), 'Special features of the interaction between signal systems in the process of restoration of speech in various forms of aphasia', in *Proceedings of the Seventh Session of the Institute of Neurology*, USSR Acad. Med. Sci., Moscow (Russian).

Babkin, B. P. (1910), 'Characteristics of the acoustic analyser in dogs', Trans. *Obshch. Russk. Vrachei v SPb*, vol. 77.

Bálint, R. (1909), 'Seelenlähmung der Schauens', *Monatsckr. f. Psychiat-u. Neurol*, vol. 25.

Balonov, L. Ya. (1950), 'Changes in visual sequential images as a sign of disturbance of cortical dynamics in certain psychopathological syndromes', Candidate Dissertation, Leningrad (Russian).

Baranovskaya, O. P. (1968), 'Effect of the disturbance of attention on frequency characteristics of the EEG under normal conditions and in patients with lesions of the frontal lobes', Candidate Dissertation, Moscow University (Russian).

Baranovskaya, O. P., and Homskaya, E. D. (1966), 'Changes in the frequency spectrum of the EEG during the action of indifferent and signal stimuli in patients with a lesion of the frontal lobes', in A. R. Luria and E. D. Homskaya (eds.), *The Frontal Lobes and Regulation of Psychological Processes*, Moscow University Press, Moscow (Russian).

Baru, A. V., and Karasseva, T. A. (1970), *The Brain and Hearing*, Moscow University Press, Moscow. English translation by N.Y., 1972.

Baruk, H. (1926), 'Les troubles mentaux dans les tumeurs cérébrales', *Thèses de la Faculté de Médecine de Paris*, vol. 4 (Paris).

Bein, E. S. (1947), 'The psychological analysis of temporal aphasia', Doctoral Dissertation (Russian).

Bein, E. S. (1964), *Aphasia and Ways of Overcoming It*, Meditsina, Leningrad (Russian).

Bekhterev, V. M. (1900), 'Demonstration eines Gehirns mit Zerstörung der vorderen und inneren Theile der Hirnrinde beider Schläferlappens', *Z. Neurol.*, vol. 19.

Bekhterev, V. M. (1905–7), *Fundamentals of the Study of Brain Functions*, vols. 1–7 (St Petersburg).

Bekhtereva, N. P. (1971), *Neuropsychological bases of Mental Activity*, Leningrad, Meditsina, Publishing House (Russian).

Benson, D. F., and Geschwind, N. (1969), 'The alexias', in P. J. Vinken and G. W. Bruyn (eds.), *Handbook of Clinical Neurology*, vol. 4, North Holland Publishing Company, Amsterdam.

Benton, A. L. (1961), 'The fiction of the "Gerstmann syndrome"', *J. Neurol. Neurosurg. Psychiat.*, vol. 24.

Benton, A. L. (1965), 'The problem of cerebral dominance', *Canad. Psychol.*, vol. 6.

Benton, A. L. (1967), 'Constructional apraxia and the minor hemisphere', *Confin. Neurol.* (Basel), vol. 27.

Benton, A. L. (1969), 'Disorders of spatial orientation', in P. J. Vinken and G. W. Bruyn (eds.), *Handbook of Clinical Neurology*, vol. 3, North Holland Publishing Company, Amsterdam.

Bergson, H. (1896), *Matière et Mémoire*, Paris.

Bernstein, N. A. (1935), 'The relationship between coordination and localization', *Arkhiv Biol. Nauk*, vol. 38 (Russian).

Bernstein, N. A. (1947), *The Construction of Movements*, Medgiz, Moscow (Russian).

Bernstein, N. A. (1957), 'Some unresolved problems in the regulation of motor acts', *Voprosy Psikhologii*, no. 6 (Russian).

Bernstein, N. A. (1966), *Outlines of the Physiology of Movements and the Physiology of Activity*, Meditsina, Moscow (Russian).

Bernstein, N. A. (1967), *The Coordination and Regulation of Movements*, Pergamon Press, Oxford.

Bianchi, L. (1895), 'The function of the frontal lobes', *Brain*, vol. 18.

Bianchi, L. (1921), *Les mécanismes du cerveau et les fonctions du lobe frontal*, Paris.

Blinkov, S. M. (1955), *Structural Peculiarities of the Human Cerebrum*, Medgiz, Moscow (Russian).

Bodamer, I. (1947), 'Die Prosopagnosie', *Arch. Psychiat. Nervenkr.*, vol. 79.

Bondareva, L. V. (1969), 'Disturbance of the higher forms of memory in certain organic brain lesions', Candidate Dissertation, Moscow University, Moscow (Russian).

Bonin, C. von (1943), 'Architectonics of the precentral motor cortex', in P. C. Bucy (ed.), *The Precentral Motor Cortex*, University of Illinois Press, Urbana.

Bonin, C. von (1948), 'The frontal lobe of primates', *Res. Publ. Assoc. Nerv. Ment. Dis.*, vol. 27.

Bonin, C. von, Garol, H. W., and McCulloch, W. S. (1942), 'The functional organization of the occipital lobe', *Biol. Symp.*, vol. 7.

Bonvicini, H. (1929), 'Die Störungen der Lautsprache bei Temporallappenläsionen', in G. Alexander and O. Marburg (eds.), *Handbuch der Neurologie des Ohres*, vol. 11.

Bornstein, B. (1962), 'Prosopagnosia', in L. Halpern (ed.), *Problems of Dynamic Neurology*, Grune & Stratton.

Bragina, N. N. (1966), 'Clinical syndromes of a lesion of the hippocampus and neighbouring regions', Doctoral Dissertation, USSR Acad. Med. Sci., Moscow (Russian).

Brain, W. R. (1941), 'Visual disorientation with special reference to lesions of the right cerebral hemisphere', *Brain*, vol. 64.

Brazier, M. A. (1960), *The Electrical Activity of the Nervous System*, Macmillan Co

Bremer, F. (1954), 'The neurophysiological problem of sleep', in J. F. Delafresnaye (ed.), *Brain Mechanisms and Consciousness*, Symposium organized by C.I.O.M.S., Blackwell, Oxford.

Bremer, F. (1957), 'Quelques aspects physiologiques des problèmes des relations réciproques de l'écorce cérébrale et des structures sous-corticales', *Acta Neurol. Psychiat. Belg.*, vol. 55.

Brickner, R. M. (1936), *The Intellectual Functions of the Frontal Lobes*, Macmillan Co.

Broadbent, D. E. (1970), 'Recent analysis of short-term memory', in K. Pribram and D. E. Broadbent (eds.), *Biology of Memory*, Academic Press.

Broca, P. (1861a), 'Perte de la parole, etc.', *Bull. Soc. Anthropol.*, vol. 2.

Broca, P. (1861b), 'Remarques sur le siège de la faculté du langage articulé', *Bull. Soc. Anthrop.*, vol. 6.

Brodal, A. (1957), *The Reticular Formation of the Brain Stem*, Oliver & Boyd.

Bronstein, A. I., Itina, N. A., *et al.* (1958), *The Orienting Reflex and Orienting and Investigative Behaviour*, Izd. Akad. Nauk SSSR, Moscow (Russian).

Brown, J. (1958), 'Some tests of the decay theory of immediate memory', *Quart. J. Exp. Psychol*, vol. 10.

Brown, J. (1964), 'Short-term memory', *Brit. Med. Bull.*, vol. 20, no. 1.

Brun, R. (1921), 'Klinische und anatomische Studien über Apraxie', *Schweiz. Arch. Neurol. Psychiat.*, vol. 9.

Bruner, J. (1957), 'On perceptual readiness', *Psychol. Rev.*, vol. 64, no. 2.

Bruner, J., Goodnow, J. J., and Austin, G. A., (1956), *A Study of Thinking*, Wiley.

Brutkowski, S. (1964), 'Prefrontal cortex and drive inhibition', in J. M. Warren and K. Akert (eds.), *Frontal Granular Cortex and Behavior*, McGraw Hill.

Brutkowski, S. (1966), 'Functional peculiarities of the silent zones of the frontal lobes in animals', in A. R. Luria and E. D. Homskaya (eds.), *The Frontal Lobes and Regulation of Psychological Processes*, Moscow University Press, Moscow (Russian).

Brutkowski, S., Konorski, J., Lawicka, W., Stepien, I., and Stepien, L. (1957), 'The effect of the removal of the frontal poles of the cerebral cortex on motor conditioned reflexes', *Acta Biol. Exp.* (Lodz), vol. 17.

Bubnova, V. (1946), 'Disturbance of the understanding of grammatical constructions in brain lesions and its restoration during training', Candidate Dissertation, Institute of Psychology, Moscow (Russian).

Bureš, J., and Burešova, O. (1968), 'The use of spreading depression to study the functional organization of the central nervous system', in *Cortical Regulation of Subcortical Brain Structures*, Tbilisi (Russian).

Buser, P., and Imbert, M. (1961), 'Sensory projections to the motor cortex in cats', in A. Rosenblueth (ed.), *Sensory Communication*, MIT Press.

Butler, R. A., Diamond, I. T., and Neff, W. D. (1957), 'Role of auditory cortex in discrimination of changes in frequency', *J. Neurophysiol.*, vol. 20.

Butters, N., Barton, M., and Brody, B. A. (1970), 'Right parietal lobe and cross-model associations, etc', *Cortex*, vol. 6.

Chlenov, L. G., and Bein, E. S. (1958), 'Agnosias for faces', *Zh. Nevropat. i Psikhiat.*, vol. 58 (Russian).

Conrad, K. (1932), 'Versuch einer psychologischen Analyse des Parietalsyndromes', *Monatsschr. Psychiat. Neurol.*, vol. 84.

Conrad, R. (1960a), 'Very brief delay of immediate recall', *Q. J. Exp. Psychol.*, vol. 12.

Conrad, R. (1960b), 'Serial orders instrusions in immediate memory', *Brit. J. Psychol.*, vol. 51.

Critchley, M. (1953), *The Parietal Lobes*, Arnold.

Danilova, N. N. (1967), 'Neuronal mechanisms of synchronizing and desynchronizing activity of the brain', in E. N. Sokolov (ed.), *Neuronal Mechanisms of the Orienting Reflex*, Moscow University Press, Moscow (Russian).

Danilova, N. N. (1970), 'Neuronal correlates of the EEG activation and inactivation responses', in *Neuronal Mechanisms of Learning*, Moscow University Press, Moscow (Russian).

Dawson, G. D. (1958a), 'Central control of sensory inflow', *Electroenceph. Clin. Neurophysiol.*, vol. 10.

Dawson, G. D. (1958b), 'The effect of cortical stimulation on transmission through the cuneate nucleus in the anaesthetized cat', *J. Physiol.* (London), vol. 412.

Dawson, G. D., Podachin, V. P., and Schatz, S. W. (1959), 'Facilitation of cortical responses by competing stimuli,' *J. Physiol.* (London), vol. 148.

Déjerine, J. (1914), *Sémiologie des affections du système nerveux*, Masson.

Denny-Brown, D. (1951), 'The frontal lobes and their functions', in A. Feiling (ed.), *Modern Trends in Neurology*, Butterworth.

Denny-Brown, D. (1958), 'The nature of apraxia', *J. Nerv. Ment. Dis.*, vol. 176.

Denny-Brown, D., and Chambers (1958), 'The parietal lobe and behaviour', *Res. Publ. Ass. Nerv. Ment. Dis.*, vol. 36.

Denny-Brown, D., Meyer, J., and Hornstein, S. (1952), 'The significance of perceptual rivalry resulting from parietal lesions', *Brain*, vol. 75.

Douglas, R. J., and Pribram, K. H. (1966), 'Learning and limbic lesions', *Neuropsychol.*, no. 4.

Drew, E. A., Ettlinger, G., Milner, B., and Passingham, R. E. (1970), *Cortex*, vol. 6.

Duncker, K. (1935), *Zur Psychologie der produktiven Denken*, Berlin.

Durinyan, R. A., and Rabin, A. G. (1968), 'The projection systems of the brain and problems of the selective mechanisms of the ascending afferent flow', in *Cortical Regulation of Activity of the Subcortical Brain Formations*, Tbilisi (Russian).

Dusser de Barenne, J. G., and McCulloch, W. S. (1941), 'Suppression of motor responses obtained from area 4 by stimulation of area 4s', *J. Neurophysiol.*, vol. 4.

Ebbinghaus, H. (1885), *Über das Gedächtniss: Untersuchungen zur experimentellen Psychologie*, Dunker u. Humbolt, Leipzig.

Eccles, J. C. (1957), *The Physiology of Nerve Cells*, Oxford University Press.

Eccles, J. C. (1961a), 'The mechanisms of synaptic transmission', *Ergebn. Physiol.*, vol. 51.

Eccles, J. C. (1961b), 'The effects of use and disuse on synaptic function', in J. F. Delafresnaye (ed.), *Brain Mechanisms and Learning*, Symposium Organized by C.I.O.M.S., Blackwell.

Eccles, J. C. (1964), *The Physiology of Synapses*, Springer Verlag.

Elkonin, D. B. (1960), *Child Psychology*, Uchpedgiz, Moscow (Russian).

Elyasson, M. I. (1908), 'Investigations of the hearing ability of dogs under normal conditions and after partial bilateral removal of the cortical centre for hearing', Dissertation, St Petersburg, Russian.

Ettlinger, G., Warrington, E., and Zangwill, O. L. (1957), 'A further study of visuo-spatial agnosia', *Brain*, vol. 80.

Farber, D. A. (1969), *Functional Maturation of the Brain in Early Ontogenesis*, Prosveshchenie, Moscow (Russian).

Farber, D. A., and Fried, A. M. (1971), 'Directivity of attention and cortical evoked responses', *Zh. Vysshei Nervnoi Deyatel'nosti im. Pavlova*, vol. 21 (Russian).

Faust, C. (1947), 'Parzielle Seelenblindheit nach occipitalen Hirnverletzung mit besonderer Beeinträchtigung des Physiognomiegedächtnisses', *Nervenartzt*, vol. 18.

Feigenbaum, E. (1970), 'Information processing and memory', in D. A. Norman (ed.), *Models of Human Memory*, Academic Press.

Feigenbaum, E. N., and Feldman, J. (eds.) (1963), *Computers and Thought*, McGraw-Hill.

Feuchtwanger, E. (1923), 'Die Funktionen des Stirnhirns', in O. Foerster and K. Wilmanns (eds.), *Monographien aus dem Gesamtgebiete der Neurologie und Psychiatrie*, vol. 38, Springer, Berlin.

Filimonov, I. N. (1949), *Comparative Anatomy of the Mammalian Cerebral Cortex*, Moscow (Russian).

Filippycheva, N. A., and Faller, T. O. (1970), 'Characteristics of the functional state of the brain in gliomas of midline structures of the cerebral hemispheres', *Zh. Nevropatologii i Psikhiatrii im. Korsakova*, vol. 70 (Russian).

Flourens, M. J. P. (1824), *Recherches expérimentales sur les propriétés et les fonctions du système nerveux dans les animaux vertébrés*, Crevot, Paris.

Foerster, O. (1936), 'Symptomatologie der Erkrankungen des Gehirns. Motorische Felder und Bahnen – Sensible corticale Felder', in O. Bumke and O. Foerster (eds.), *Handbuch der Neurologie*, vol. 6, Springer, Berlin.

Fonarev, A. M. (1969), 'Development of functions of the child's muscular system', Doctoral Dissertation, USSR Acad. Med. Sci., Moscow (Russian).

Frankfurter, W., and Thiele, R. (1912), 'Experimentelle Untersuchungen zur Bezoldschen Sprachsext', *Z. Psychol. u. Physiol. Sinnesorg*, vol. 47.

Franz, S. I. (1907), 'On the function of the cerebrum: The frontal lobes', *Arch. Psychol.*, vol. 1.

French, J. D. (1952), 'Brain lesions associated with prolonged unconsciousness', *A.M.A. Arch. Neurol. Psychiat.*, vol. 68.

French, J. D., Hernández-Peón, R., and Livingston, R. B. (1955), 'Projections from cortex to cephalic brain stem (reticular formation) in monkey', *J. Neurophysiol.*, vol. 18.

French, J. D., and Magoun, H. W. (1952), 'Effects of chronic lesions in central cephalic brain stem of monkeys', *Arch. Neurol. Psychiat.* (Chicago), vol. 68.

Fried, G. M. (1970), 'Effect of the orienting reflex on visual evoked potentials in the EEG of schoolchildren', *Zh. Vysshei Nervnoi Deyatel'nosti*, vol. 10 (Russian).

Fulton, J. F. (1935), 'A note on the definition of the "motor" and "premotor" areas', *Brain*, vol. 58.

Fulton, J. F. (1943), *Physiology of the Nervous System*, 2nd edn, Oxford University Press.

Gadzhiev, S. G. (1966), 'Disturbance of visually-oriented intellectual activity in frontal lobe lesions', in A. R. Luria and E. D. Homskaya (eds.), *The Frontal Lobes and Regulation of Psychological Processes*, Moscow University Press, Moscow (Russian).

Galambos, R. (1956), 'Suppression of auditory nerve activity by stimulation of efferent fibers to the cochleas', *J. Neurophysiol.*, vol. 19.

Galambos, R., and Morgan, C. T. (1960), 'The neural basis of learning', *Handbook of Physiology*, *Amer. Physiol. Soc.*, vol. 3.

Galperin, P. Ya. (1959), 'The development of research into the formation of intellectual actions', in *Psychological Science in the USSR*, Izd. Akad. Pedagog. Nauk RSFSR, Moscow (Russian).

Gastaut, H. (1958), 'Some aspects of the neurophysiological basis of reflexes and behavior', in *Neurological Bases of Behavior*, Little, Brown.

Gelb, A., and Goldstein, K. (1920), *Psychologische Analysen hirnpathologischen Fälle*, Springer, Berlin.

Genkin, A. A. (1962), 'Use of the method of statistical description of the duration of ascending and descending phases of the electrical activity of the brain for the detection of information on processes accompanying intellectual activity', *Doklady Akad. Pedagog. Nauk RSFSR*, no. 6 (Russian).

Genkin, A. A. (1963), 'Asymmetry of the duration of the phases of the encephalogram during intellectual activity', *Doklady Akad. Pedagog. Nauk RSFSR*, no. 6 (Russian).

Genkin, A. A. (1964), 'Duration of the ascending and descending fronts of the EEG as a source of information on neurophysiological processes', Candidate Dissertation, Leningrad (Russian).

Gerbrandt, L. K., Spinelli, D. N., and Pribram, K. H. (1970). 'The interaction of visual attention and temporal cortex stimulation on electrical recording in the striate cortex', *Electroenceph. clin. Neurophysiol.*, vol. 29, pp. 146-55.

Gershuni, G. V. (1949), 'Reflex responses to external stimuli', *Fiziol. Zh. SSSR*, no. 5.

Gershuni, G. V., (ed.) (1968), *Mechanisms of Hearing*, Nauka, Leningrad (Russian).

Geschwind, N. (1965), 'Disconnexion syndromes in animals and man', *Brain*, vol. 88.

Gloning, I., Gloning, K., Jellinger, K., and Tschabitscher, H. (1966), 'Zur Prosopagnosie', *Neuropsychologia*, vol. 4.

Goldberg, J. M., Diamond, I. T., and Neff, W. D. (1957), 'Auditory discrimination after ablation of temporal and insular cortex in cat', *Fed. Proc.*, vol. 16.

Goldstein, K. (1925), 'Das Symptom, seine Entshehung und Bedeutung für unsere Auffassung vom Bau und von der Funktion des Nervensystems', *Arch. Psychiat. Nerven*, vol. 76.

Goldstein, K. (1927), 'Die Lokalisation in der Grosshirnrinde', in A. Bethe *et al.* (eds.), *Handbuch der normalen und pathologischen Physiologie*, vol. 10., Springer, Berlin.

Goldstein, K. (1944), 'The mental changes due to frontal lobe damage', *J. Psychol.*, vol. 17.

Goldstein, K. (1948), *Language and Language Disorders*, Grune & Stratton.

Goldstein, K., and Gelb, A. (1920), 'Psychologische Analysen hirnpathologischen Fälle', *Z. f. Psychol. Physiol. d. Sinnesorg*, vol. 83.

Goltz, F. (1876–84), 'Über die Verrichtungen des Grosshirns', *Pflügers Arch. ges. Physiol.*, vols. 13, 14, 20, 26.

Grastyan, E. (1961), 'The significance of the earliest manifestations of conditioning in the mechanism of learning', in J. F. Delafresnaye (ed.), *Brain Mechanisms and Learning*, Blackwell.

de Groot, A. D. (1964), *Thought and Choice in Chess*, Mouton, The Hague.

Gross, C. G., and Weiskrantz, L. (1964), 'Some changes in behavior produced by lateral frontal lesions in the macaque', in J. M. Warren and K. Akert (eds.), *The Frontal Granular Cortex and Behavior*, McGraw-Hill.

Grünthal, E. (1939), 'Über das Corpus mamillare und den Korsakowschen Symptomencomplex', *Confin. Neurol.*, vol. 2.

Halstead, W. C. (1947), *Brain and Intelligence*, Chicago University Press,

Harlow, J. (1968), 'Recovery from the passage of an iron bar through the head', *Proc. Massachusetts Med. Soc.*, vol. 2.

Head, H. (1926), *Aphasia and Kindred Disorders of Speech*, 2 vols., Cambridge University Press.

Hebb, D. O. (1945), 'Man's frontal lobes', *Arch. Neurol. Psychiat.*, Chicago, vol. 54.

Hebb, D. O. (1955), 'Drives and the CNS', *Psychol. Rev.*, vol. 62, p. 243.

Hebb, D. O., and Penfield, W. (1940), 'Human behavior after extensive bilateral removal from the frontal lobes', *Arch. Neurol. Psychiat.* (Chicago), vol. 44.

Hécaen, H. (1969), 'Aphasic, apraxic and agnostic syndromes in right and left hemisphere lesions', in P. J. Vinken and G. W. Bruyn (eds.), *Handbook of Clinical Neurology*, vol. 4, North Holland Publishing Company, Amsterdam.

Hécaen, H., and Ajuriaguerra, J. (1960), *Le cortex cérébral*, Masson, Paris.

Hécaen, H., and Ajuriaguerra, J. (1963), *Les gauchers. Prévalence manuelle et dominance cérébrale*, Presses Universitaires de France, Paris.

Hécaen, H., Ajuriaguerra, J., and Angelergues, R. (1957), 'Les troubles de la lecture dans le cadre des modifications symboliques', *J. Psychol. Neurol.* (Basel), vol. 134.

Hécaen, H., Ajuriaguerra, J., and Massonet, J. (1951), 'Les troubles visuoconstructifs par lésion pariéto-occipitale droite', *Encéphale*, vol. 40.

Hécaen, H., and Angelergues, R. (1963), *La cécité psychique*, Masson, Paris.

Hécaen, H., and Assal, H. (1970), 'A comparison of constructive deficits following right and left hemisphere lesions', *Neuropsychologia*, vol. 8.

Hécaen, H., Penfield, W., Bertrand, C., and Malmo, R. (1956), 'The syndrome of apractagnosia following lesions of the minor cerebral hemisphere', *Arch. Neurol. Psychiat.* (Chicago), vol. 75.

Hernández-Peón, R. (1961), 'Reticular mechanisms of sensory control', in W. A. Rosenblith (ed.), *Sensory Communication*, MIT Press.

Hernández-Peón, R. (1966), 'Physiological mechanisms of attention', in R. Russell (ed.), *Frontiers in Physiological Psychology*, Academic Press.

Hernández-Peón, R. (1969), 'Neurophysiology of attention', in P. J. Vinken and G. W. Bruyn (eds.), *Handbook of Clinical Neurology*, vol. 3, North Holland Publishing Company, Amsterdam.

Hernández-Peón, R., Charrer, H., and Jouvet, M. (1958), 'Modification of electrical activity in cochlear nuclei during attention in unanesthetized cats', *Science*, vol. 123.

Hernández-Peón, R., Guzman-Flores, C., Alcaraz, M., and Fernandez-Guardiola, A. (1956), 'Sensory transmission in visual pathway during "attention" in unanesthetized cats', *Acta Neurol. Lat.-Amer.*, vol. 3.

Hochheimer, W. (1932), 'Analyse eines "Seelenblinden" von der Sprache aus', *Psychol. Forsch.*, vol. 16.

Hoff, H., Gloning, L., and Gloning, H. (1962), 'Die zentralen Störungen der optischen Wahrnemung', *Wien. med. Wschr.*, vol. 112.

Hoff, H., and Pötzl, O. (1930), 'Über Grosshirnprojektion der Mitte und der Aussengrenzen des Gesichtsfeldes', *Jahrb. d. Psychiat.*, vol. 52.

Hoff, H., and Pötzl, O. (1937), 'Über einer optisch-agnostische Störung des Physiognomiegedächtnisses', *Z. Gesell. Neurol. Psychiat.*, vol. 159.

Holmes, G. (1919), 'Disturbances of vision by cerebral lesions', *Brit. J. Ophthalm.*, vol. 1.

Homskaya, E. D. (1958), 'Investigation of the effect of speech responses on motor responses in children with cerebral asthenia', in A. R. Luria (ed.), *Problems of Higher Nervous Activity of the Normal and Subnormal Child*, vol. 2, Izd. Akad. Pedagog. Nauk RSFSR, Moscow (Russian).

Homskaya, E. D. (1960, 1961), 'Effect of a verbal instruction on vascular and psychogalvanic components of the orienting reflex in local brain lesions', Communications I–III, *Doklady Akad. Pedagog. Nauk RSFSR*, no. 6, (Russian).

Homskaya, E. D. (1965), 'Regulation of autonomic components of the orienting reflex by the aid of verbal instructions in patients with various brain lesions', *Voprosy Psikhologii*, no. 1 (Russian).

Homskaya, E. D. (1966a), 'Autonomic components of the orienting reflex in response to irrelevant and informative stimuli in patients with frontal lobe lesions', in A. R. Luria and E. D. Homskaya (eds.), *The Frontal Lobes and Regulation of Psychological Processes*, Moscow University Press, Moscow (Russian).

Homskaya, E. D. (1966b), 'Regulation of the intensity of voluntary motor responses in frontal lobe lesions', in A. R. Luria and E. D. Homskaya (eds.), *The Frontal Lobes and Regulation of Psychological Processes*, Moscow University Press, Moscow (Russian).

Homskaya, E. D. (1969), 'The role of the frontal lobes of the brain in the regulation of activation processes', *Voprosy Psikhologii*, no. 2.

Homskaya, E. D. (1972), *The Brain and Activation*, Moscow University Press, Moscow (Russian).

Hubel, D. M., and Wiesel, T. N. (1962), 'Receptive fields, binocular interaction and functional interaction and functional architecture of the cat's visual cortex', *J. Physiol.*, vol. 106.

Hubel, D. M., and Wiesel, T. N. (1963), 'Receptive fields of cells in striate cortex of very young, visually inexperienced kittens', *J. Neurophysiol.*, vol. 26.

Hydén, H. (1960), 'The neuron', in J. Brachet and A. E. Mirsky (eds.), *The Cell*, Academic Press.

Hydén, H. (1962), 'A molecular basis of neuron–glia interaction', in F. O. Schmitt (ed.), *Macromolecular Specificity and Biological Memory*, MIT Press.

Hydén, H. (1964), 'RNA: a functional characteristic of neuron and glia in learning', in M. Brazier (ed.), *RNA and Brain Function in Learning*, Berkeley and Los Angeles.

Ioshpa, A. Ya., and Homskaya, E. D. (1966), 'Regulation of the temporal parameters of voluntary motor responses under normal conditions and in frontal lobe lesions', in A. R. Luria and E. D. Homskaya (eds.), *The Frontal Lobes and Regulation of Psychological Processes*, Moscow University Press, Moscow (Russian).

Isserlin, M. (1929–32), 'Die pathologische Physiologie der Sprache', *Ergebn. Physiol.*, vols. 29, 33, 34.

Jackson, J. H. (1874), 'On the nature of the duality of the brain', in *Selected Writings of John Hughlings Jackson*, vol. 2, Hodder & Stoughton, 1932.

Jacobsen, C. F. (1935), 'Function of frontal association area in primates', *Arch. Neurol. Psychiat.* (Chicago), vol. 33.

Jakobson, R., and Halle, M. (1956), *Fundamentals of Language*, Mouton, The Hague.

Jasper, H. H. (1954), 'Functional properties of the thalamic reticular system', in J. L. Delafresnaye (ed.), *Brain Mechanisms and Consciousness*, Blackwell.

Jasper, H. H. (1957), 'Recent advances in our understanding of ascending activities of the reticular system', in H. H. Jasper (ed.), *Reticular Formation of the Brain*, Churchill.

Jasper, H. H. (1963), 'Studies in non-specific effects upon electrical responses in sensory systems', in *Brain Mechanisms, Progress in Brain Research*, vol. 1, Elsevier, Amsterdam.

Jasper, H. H. (1964), 'Transformation of cortical sensory responses by attention and conditioning', *IBRO Bulletin*, no. 3.

Jouvet, M. (1956), 'Analyse encéphalographique de quelques aspects du conditionnement chez le chat', *Acta Neurol. Lat.-Amer.*, vol. 2.

Jouvet, M. (1961), 'Recherches sur les mécanismes neurophysiologiques du sommeil et de l'apprentissage négatif', in J. F. Delafresnaye (ed.), *Brain Mechanisms and Learning*, Blackwell.

Jouvet, M., and Courrion, E. J. (1958), 'Variations of the subcortical responses during attention in man', *Electroenceph. Clin. Neurophysiol.*, vol. 10.

Jouvet, M., and Hernández-Peón, R. (1957), 'Mécanismes neurophysiologiques concernant l'attention et le conditionnement', *Electroenceph. Clin. Neurophysiol*, Suppl. 6.

Jouvet, M., and Michel, F. (1959), 'Aspects électroencéphalographiques de l'habituation de la réaction de l'éveil', *J. Physiol.* (Paris), vol. 51.

Kabelyanskaya, L. G. (1957), 'The state of the auditory analyser in sensory aphasia', *Zh. Nevropat. i Psikhiat. im. Korsakova*, vol. 57 (Russian).

Kaidanova, S. I. (1954), 'Features of the auditory analyser in children with impaired development of sensory speech', in *Abstracts of Proceedings of a Scientific Session of the Lesgaft State Scientific Institute*, Leningrad (Russian).

Kaidanova, S. I. (1967), 'Character of the auditory analyser in adults with sensory alalia and aphasia', Candidate Dissertation, Leningrad University, Leningrad (Russian).

Kaplan, A. K. (1949), 'Visual after-images in cases of disturbance of the normal activity of the central nervous system', Dissertation, Institute of Physiology, USSR Academy of Sciences, Leningrad (Russian).

Karasseva, T. A. (1967), 'Diagnosis of temporal lobe lesions with the aid of quantitative methods of investigation of hearing', Candidate Dissertation, USSR Academy of Medical Sciences, Moscow (Russian).

Karpov, B. A., Luria, A. R., and Yarbus, A. L. (1968), 'Disturbances of the structure of the posterior and anterior regions of the brain', *Neuropsychologia*, vol. 6.

Katz, F. G. (1930), 'Die Bezoldsche Sprachsexte und das Sprachverständniss', *Passow-Schaeffers Beitr.*, vol. 28.

Keppel, G. (1968), 'Retroactive and proactive inhibition', in T. R. Dixon and D. L. Horton (eds.), *Verbal Behavior and General Behavior Theory*, Prentice-Hall.

Khoroshko, V. K. (1912), *Relation of the Frontal Lobes of the Brain to Psychology and Psychopathology*, Moscow (Russian).

Khoroshko, V. K. (1921), 'Personal investigations of the frontal lobes of the brain', *Med. Zh.*, nos. 5–6 and 6–7 (Russian).

Kimura, D. (1963), 'Right temporal lobe damage, perception of unfamiliar stimuli after damage', *Arch. Neurol.* (Chicago), vol. 8.

Kintsch, W. (1970a), 'Models for free recall and recognition', in D. A. Norman (ed.), *Models of Human Memory*, Academic Press.

Kintsch, W. (1970b), *Memory and Conceptual Processes*, Wiley.

Kiyashchenko, N. K. (1969), 'Structure of memory disturbances in local brain lesions', Candidate Dissertation, Moscow University, Moscow (Russian).

Kleist, K. (1907), 'Corticale (innervatorische) Apraxie', *J. Psychiat.*, vol. 28.

Kleist, K. (1911), 'Der Gang und der gegenwärtige Stand der Apraxieforschung', *Ergebn. Neurol.*, vol. 1.

Kleist, K. (1934), *Gehirnpathologie*, Barth, Leipzig.

Klimkovsky, M. (1966), 'Disturbance of audio-verbal memory in lesions of the left temporal lobe', Candidate Dissertation, Moscow University, Moscow (Russian).

Klüver, H. (1952), 'Brain mechanisms and behaviour with special reference to the rhinencephalon', *Lancet*.

Klüver, H., and Bucy, P. C. (1938), 'An analysis of certain effects of bilateral temporal lobectomy in the rhesus monkey', *J. Psychol.*, vol. 5.

Koffka, K. (1925), *Grundlagen der psychischen Entwicklung*, Berlin.

Köhler, W. (1917), *Intelligenzprüfungen an Anthropoiden*, Berlin.

Kok, E. P. (1967), *The Visual Agnosias*, Meditsina, Leningrad (Russian).

Konorski, J. (1961), 'The physiological approach to the problem of recent memory', in J. F. Delafresnaye (ed.), *Brain Mechanisms and Learning*, Blackwell.

Konorski, J., and Lawicka, W. (1964), 'Analysis of errors by prefrontal animals in the delayed response test', in J. W. Warren and K. Akert (eds.), *The Frontal Granular Cortex and Behavior*, McGraw-Hill.

Konorski, J., Stepien, L., Brutkowski, S., Lawicka, W., and Stepien, I. (1952), 'The effect of the removal of interoceptive fields of the cerebral cortex on the higher nervous activity of animals', *Bull. Soc. Sci. Lett.* (*Lodz*), vol. 3.

Korchazhinskaya, V. I. (1971), 'Unilateral spatial agnosia in local brain lesions', Candidate Dissertation, USSR Acad. Med. Sci., Moscow (Russian).

Kryzhanovsky, I. I. (1909), 'Conditioned reflexes after ablation of the temporal regions of the brain in dogs', Candidate Dissertation, Military Medical Academy, St Petersburg (Russian).

Kubie, L. S. (1969), 'Preconscious factors in the process of remembering', in G. Talland and N. Waugh (eds.), *The Pathology of Memory*, Acadamic Press.

Kudrin, A. I. (1910), 'Conditioned reflexes in dogs after extirpation of the posterior halves of the cerebral hemispheres', Candidate Dissertation, Military Medical Academy, St Petersburg (Russian).

Lashley, K. S. (1929), *Brain Mechanisms and Intelligence*, University of Chicago Press, Chicago.

Lashley, K. S. (1950), 'In search of the engram', in *Physiological Mechanisms in Animal Behavior*, Academic Press.

Latash, L. P. (1968), *The Hypothalamus, Adaptive Activity and the Electroencephalogram*, Meditsina, Moscow (Russian).

Lebedinsky, V. V. (1966), 'Performance of symmetrical and asymmetrical programmes by patients with frontal lobe lesions', in A. R. Luria and E. D. Homskaya (eds.), *The Frontal Lobes and Regulation of Psychological Processes*, Moscow University Press, Moscow (Russian).

Leontiev, A. N. (1931), *Development of the Memory*, Krupskaya Acad. of Communist Education Press, Moscow (Russian).

Leontiev, A. N. (1954), 'The experimental investigation of thought', *Proceedings of a Conference on Psychology*, Izv. Akad. Pedagog. Nauk RSFSR, Moscow (Russian).

Leontiev, A. N. (1959), *Problems in Mental Development*, Izd. Akad. Pedagog. Nauk RSFSR, Moscow (Russian).

Liepmann, H. (1905), *Über Störungen des Handelns bei Gehirnkranken*, Karger, Berlin.

Liepmann, H. (1920), *Apraxie. Brugsch's Ergebn. Ges. Med.*, Berlin and Vienna.

Lindsley, D. B. (1951), 'Emotion', in S. S. Stevens (ed.), *Handbook of Experimental Psychology*, Wiley.

Lindsley, D. B. (1958), 'The reticular system and perceptual discrimination', in *Reticular Formation of the Brain*, Little, Brown.

Lindsley, D. B. (1960), 'Attention, consciousness, sleep and wakefulness', in J. Field (ed.), *Handbook of Physiology. Section: Neurophysiology*, vol. 3, Thomas.

Lindsley, D. B. (1961), 'The reticular activating system and perceptual integration', in F. Sheer (ed.), *Electrical Stimulation of the Brain*, Austin.

Lindsley, D. B., Bowden, J., and Magoun, H. W. (1949), 'Effect upon the EEG of acute injury to the brain-stem activating system', *Electroenceph. Clin. Neurophysiol.*, vol. 1.

Lissauer, H. (1898), 'Ein Fall von Seelenblindheit etc.', *Arch. Psychiat. Neurol.*, vol. 21.

Livanov, M. N. (1962), 'Spatial analysis of bioelectrical activity of the brain', *Zh. Vyssh. Nervn. Deyat.*, vol. 12 (Russian).

Livanov, M. N., Gavrilova, N. A., and Aslanov, A. S. (1964), 'Cross correlation between different areas of the human brain during mental work', *Zh. Vyssh. Nervn. Deyat.*, vol. 14, no. 2 (Russian).

Livanov, M. N., Gavrilova, N. A., and Aslanov, A. S. (1967), 'Intercorrelation between different cortical regions of the human brain during mental activity', *Neuropsychologia*, no. 3.

Lorenz, K. (1950), 'The comparative method in studying innate behaviour patterns', *Physiological Mechanisms in Animal Behaviour. Symposia Soc. Exp. Biol.*, vol. 4.

Lotmar, F. (1919), 'Zur Kenntnis der erschwerten Wortfindung und ihre Bedeutung für das Denken des Aphasischen', *Schweiz. Arch. Neurol. Psychiat.*, vol. 15.

Lotmar, F. (1935), 'Zur Pathophysiologie der erschwerten Wortfindung bei Aphasischer', *Schweiz. Arch. Neurol. Psychiat.*, vol. 30.

Luria, A. R. (1946), 'Disturbance of grammatical operations in brain lesions', *Izvest. Akad. Pedagog. Nauk RSFSR*, no. 3.

Luria, A. R. (1947), '*Traumatic Aphasia*', Izd. Akad. Med. Nauk SSSR, Moscow (Russian; English translation, Mouton, The Hague, 1970).

Luria, A. R. (1948), *Restoration of Function after Brain Injury*, Medgiz, Moscow (Russian; English translation by B. Haigh: Pergamon Press, 1963).

Luria, A. R. (ed.), (1956, 1958a), *Problems in the Higher Nervous Activity of the Normal and Abnormal Child*, vols. 1 and 2, Izd. Akad. Pedagog. Nauk RSFSR, Moscow (Russian).

Luria, A. R. (1957), 'The genesis of voluntary movements', *Voprosy Psikhologii*, no. 2.

Luria, A. R. (1958a), see Luria, A. R. (1956).

Luria, A. R. (1958b), 'Brain disorders and language analysis', *Language and Speech*, vol. 1.

Luria, A. R. (1959a), 'Disorders of simultaneous perception in a case of bilateral occipito-parietal brain injury', *Brain*, vol. 82.

Luria, A. R. (1959b), 'The directive role of speech in development and dissolution', *Word* (New York), vol. 15.

Luria, A. R. (1959c), 'The development of speech and formation of mental processes', in *Psychological Science in the USSR*, Vol. 1, Izd. Akad. Pedagog. Nauk RSFSR, Moscow (Russian).

Luria, A. R. (1960), 'Verbal regulation of behavior', in M. Brazier (ed.), *The Central Nervous System and Behavior*, Third Macy Conference, National Institutes of Health, Bethesda, Md.

Luria, A. R. (1961), *The Role of Speech in Regulation of Normal and Abnormal Behaviour*, Pergamon Press, Oxford.

Luria, A. R. (1962, 1966a, 1969c), *Higher Cortical Functions in Man*, 1st edn, 1962; 2nd edn, 1969, Moscow University Press, Moscow (Russian). English translation of 1st edn, by B. Haigh, Basic Books and Plenum Press, New York, 1966.

Luria, A. R. (1963, 1966b, 1970c), *Human Brain and Psychological Processes*, vol. 1, Izd. Akad. Pedagog. Nauk RSFSR, Moscow, 1963 (Russian). English translation by B. Haigh: Harper & Row, New York, 1966). Vol. 2, Izd. Akad. Pedagog. Nauk RSFSR, Moscow, 1970 (Russian).

Luria, A. R. (1964); 'Factors and forms of aphasia', in *Disorders of Language*, Ciba Foundation Symposium.

Luria, A. R. (1965a), 'Aspects of aphasia', *J. Neurol. Sci.*, vol. 2.

Luria, A. R. (1965b), 'Two kinds of motor perseverations in massive injury of the frontal lobes', *Brain*, vol. 88.

Luria, A. R. (1966a), see Luria, A. R. (1962).

Luria, A. R. (1966b), see Luria, A. R. (1963).

Luria, A. R. (1969a), 'The frontal syndrome', in P. J. Vinken and G. W. Bruyn (eds.), *Handbook of Clinical Neurology*, vol. 2, North Holland Publishing Company, Amsterdam.

Luria, A. R. (1969b), 'The origin and cerebral organization of man's conscious action', An Evening Lecture to the 19th International Congress of Psychology, London.

Luria, A. R. (1969c), see Luria, A. R. (1962).

Luria, A. R. (1969d), 'Conscious action, its origin and cerebral organization', *Voprosy Psikhologii*, no. 5.

Luria, A. R. (1970a), see Luria, A. R. (1947).

Luria, A. R. (1970b), 'The functional organization of the brain', *Scientific American*, vol. 222 (3).

Luria, A. R. (1970c), see Luria, A. R. (1963).

Luria, A. R. (1970d), 'Brain and mind', *Priroda*, no. 3.

Luria, A. R. (1971), 'Memory disturbances in local brain lesions', *Neuropsychologia*, vol. 9.

Luria, A. R. (1972), 'Aphasia reconsidered', *Cortex*, vol. 81, no. 1.

Luria, A. R. (1973), *Neuropsychology of Memory*, vol. 1, Moscow, Pedagogika Publishing House (Russian).

Luria, A. R., and Homskaya, E. D. (1962), 'An objective study of ocular movements and their control', *Psychol. Beitr.*, vol. 6.

Luria, A. R., and Homskaya, E. D. (1963), 'Le trouble du role régulateur de langage au cours des lésions du lobe frontal', *Neuropsychologia*, vol. 1.

Luria, A. R., and Homskaya, E. D. (eds.) (1966), *The Frontal Lobes and Regulation of Psychological Processes*, Moscow University Press, Moscow (Russian)

Luria, A. R., and Homskaya, E. D. (1970), 'Frontal lobes and the regulation of activation processes', in D. Mostofsky (ed.), *Attention: Contemporary Theory and Analysis*, Appleton, Century, Crofts.

Luria, A. R., Homskaya, E. D., Blinkov, S. M., and Critchley, M. (1967), 'Impairment of selectivity of mental processes in association with lesions of the frontal lobe', *Neuropsychologia*, vol. 5.

Luria, A. R., Karpov, E. A., and Yarbus, A. L. (1965), 'Disturbance of perception of complex objects in lesions of the frontal lobes', *Voprosy Psikhologii*, no. 5.

Luria, A. R., Konovalov, A. N., and Podgornaya, A. Ya. (1970), *Memory Disturbances in the Syndrome of Aneurysm of the Anterior Communicating Artery*, Moscow University Press, Moscow (Russian).

Luria, A. R., Pravdina-Vinarskaya, E. N., and Yarbus, A. L. (1961), 'The mechanism of fixation movements and their pathology', *Voprosy Psikhologii*, no. 6 (Russian).

Luria, A. R., Pribram, K. H., and Homskaya, E. D. (1964), 'An experimental analysis of the behavior disturbances produced by a left frontal arachnoidal endothelioma (meningioma)', *Neuropsychologia*, vol. 2.

Luria, A. R., and Rapoport, M. Yu. (1962), 'Regional symptoms of disturbance of the higher cortical functions in intracerebral tumours of the left temporal lobe', *Voprosy Neirokhirurgii*, no. 4 (Russian).

Luria, A. R., Simernitskaya, E. G., and Tubylevich, B. (1970), 'The structure of psychological processes in relation to cerebral organization', *Neuropsychologia*, vol. 8.

Luria, A. R., and Skorodumova, A. V. (1950), 'The phenomenon of fixed hemianopia', in *Collection in Memory of S. V. Kravkov*, Moscow (Russian).

Luria, A. R., Sokolov, E. N., and Klimkovsky, M. (1967a), 'Some neurodynamic mechanisms of memory', *Zh. Vysshei Nervnoi Deyatel'nosti*, vol. 17 (Russian).

Luria, A. R., Sokolov, E. N., and Klimkovsky, M. (1967b), 'Towards a neurodynamic analysis of memory disturbances with lesions of the left temporal lobe', *Neuropsychologia*, vol. 5.

Luria, A. R., and Tsvetkova, L. S. (1965a), 'The programming of constructive activity in local brain lesions', *Voprosy Psikhologii*, no. 2 (Russian).

Luria, A. R., and Tsvetkova, L. S. (1965b), 'Rehabilitative training and its importance to psychology and education', *Sovetskaya Pedagogika*, no. 2 (Russian).

Luria, A. R., and Tsvetkova, L. S. (1967), *Les troubles de la résolution des problèmes analyse neuropsychologie*, Gautier Villar, Paris.

Luria, A. R., and Tsvetkova, L. S. (1968), 'Towards the mechanisms of "dynamic aphasia"', *Foundation of Language* (Amsterdam), vol. 4.

Luria, A. R., Tsvetkova, L. S., and Futer, J. C. (1965), 'Aphasia in a composer', *J. Neurol. Sci.*, vol. 2.

Luria, A. R., and Vinogradova, O. S. (1959), 'An objective investigation of the dynamics of semantic systems', *Brit. J. Psychol.*, vol. 50.

Luria, A. R., and Vinogradova, O. S. (1971), 'An objective investigation of the dynamics of semantic systems', in *Semantic Structure of the Word*, Nauka, Moscow (Russian).

Lyublinskaya, A. A. (1959), *Outlines of the Mental Development of the Child*, Izd. Akad. Pedagog. Nauk RSFSR, Moscow (Russian).

McConnell, J. V., Jacobson, A. L., and Kimble, D. P. (1970), 'The effect of regeneration on retention of a conditioned response in the planarian', *J. Comp. Physiol. Psychol.*, vol. 52.

McCulloch, W. S. (1943), 'Inter-areal interactions of the cerebral cortex', in P. C. Bucy (ed.), *The Precentral Motor Cortex*, University of Illinois Press.

McFie, J., Piercy, M., and Zangwill, O. L. (1950), 'Visual spatial agnosia associated with lesions of the right hemisphere', *Brain*, vol. 73.

McGeoch, J. A. (1932), 'Forgetting and the law of disuse', *Psychol. Rev.*, vol. 39.

MacLean, P. D. (1952), 'Some psychiatric implications of psychophysiological studies of the fronto-temporal portion of the limbic system', *Electroenceph. Clin. Neurophysiol.*, vol. 4.

MacLean, P. D. (1958), 'The limbic system with respect to self preservation and preservation of the species', *J. Nerv. Ment. Dis.*, vol. 127.

MacLean, P. D. (1959), 'The limbic system in respect to two basic life principles', in M. Brazier (ed.), *The Central Nervous System and Behavior*, Transactions of the 2nd Conference of the Josiah Macy, Jr Foundation.

Magoun, H. W. (1963), *The Waking Brain*, 2nd edn., Thomas, Springfield.

Malmo, R. B. (1942), 'Interference factors in delayed response in monkeys after removal of the frontal lobe', *J. Neurophysiol.*, vol. 5.

Maruszewski, M. (1966), 'Disturbance of the simplest forms of voluntary action in focal lesions of the frontal lobes', in A. R. Luria and E. D. Homskaya (eds.), *The Frontal Lobes and Regulation of Psychological Processes*, Moscow University Press, Moscow (Russian).

Melton, A. W. (1963), 'Implication of short term memory for a general theory of memory', *J. Verbal Learning*, vol. 2.

Melton, A. W. (1970), 'Short-term and long-term postperceptual memory', in K. H. Pribram and D. E. Broadbent (eds.), *The Biology of Memory*, Academic Press.

Melton, A. W., and Irvin, I. M. (1940), 'The influence of degree of interpolated learning on retroactive inhibition', *Amer. J. Psychol.*, vol. 53.

Melton, A. W., and von Lackum, W. L. E. (1941), 'Retroactive and proactive inhibition in retention', *Amer. J. Psychol.*, vol. 54.

Miller, N. E. (1966), 'Experiments relevant to learning theory and perception', evening lecture for the XVIII International Congress of Psychology, Moscow (see also Proceedings of the Congress, Moscow, 1969).

Miller, G. (1969), 'The organization of lexical memory: are associations sufficient?', in G. Talland and N. Waugh (eds.), *The Pathology of Memory*, Academic Press.

Miller, G., Galanter, E., and Pribram, K. (1960), *Plans and the Organization of Behavior*, Holt, Rinehart & Winston.

Milner, B. (1954), 'The intellectual functions of the temporal lobe', *Psychol. Bull.*, vol. 51.

Milner, B. (1958), 'Psychological defects produced by temporal lobe excision', *Res. Pub. Assoc. Nerv. Ment. Dis.*, vol. 36.

Milner, B. (1962), 'Les troubles de la mémoire accompagnant des lésions hippocampiques bilatérales', in *Physiologie de l'hippocampe*, Paris.

Milner, B. (1966), 'Amnesia following operation on the temporal lobes', in C. W. M. Witty and O. L. Zangwill (eds.), *Amnesia*, Butterworth.

Milner, B. (1968), 'Visual recognition and recall after right temporal lobe excision in man', *Neuropsychologia*, vol. 6.

Milner, B. (1969), 'Residual intellectual and memory deficits after head injury', in A. E. Walker, W. F. Caverners and M. Critchley (eds.), *The Late Effects of Head Injury*, Thomas.

Milner, B. (1970), 'Memory and the mesial temporal region of the brain', in K. H. Pribram and D. E. Broadbent (eds.), *The Biology of Memory*, Academic Press.

Mishkin, M. (1954), 'Visual discrimination performance following partial ablation of the temporal lobe', *J. Comp. Physiol. Psychol.*, vol. 48.

Mishkin, M. (1957), 'Effects of small frontal lesions in delayed alternation in monkey', *J. Neurophysiol.*, vol. 20.

Mishkin, M., and Pribram, K. H. (1955, 1956), 'Analysis of the effects of frontal lesions in monkeys', I, II, *J. Comp. Physiol. Psychol.*, vols. 48, 49.

Mishkin, M., and Weiskrantz, L. (1958), 'Effects of delaying reward on visual discrimination performance in monkeys with frontal lesions', *J. Comp. Physiol. Psychol.*, vol. 51.

Monakow, C. (1910), *Über Lokalisation der Hirnfunktionen*, Wiesbaden.

Monakow, C. (1914), *Die Lokalisation im Grosshirn und der Abbau der Funktionen durch corticale Herde*, Bergmann, Wiesbaden.

Monakow, C., and Mourgue, R. (1928), 'Introduction biologique à l'étude de la neurologie et de la psychopathologie', Alcan, Paris.

Money, J. (1962), *Reading Disabilities*, Johns Hopkins Press.

Monnier, M. (1956), 'Reticular cortical and motor responses to photic stimuli in man', *Science*, vol. 123.

Morrell, F. (1967), *Electrical Signs of Sensory Coding. The Neurosciences*, Rockefeller University Press.

Morton, J. (1969), 'The interaction of information in word recognition', *Psychol. Rev.*, vol. 76.

Morton, J. (1970), 'A functional model for memory', in D. A. Norman (ed.), *Models of Human Memory*, Academic Press.

Moruzzi, G., and Magoun, H. W. (1949), 'Brain stem reticular formation and activation of the EEG', *Electroenceph. Clin. Neurophysiol.*, vol. 1.

Müller, G. E. (1873), *Zur Theorie der sinnlichen Aufmerksamkeit*, Edelmann, Leipzig.

Müller, G., and Pilzecker, A. (1900), 'Experimentelle Beiträge zur Lehre vom Gedächtniss', *Z. f. Psychol.*, vol. 1.

Narikashvili, S. P. (1961), 'Cortical regulation of the function of the reticular formations of the brain', *Uspekhi Sovrem. Biol.*, vol. 52.

Narikashvili, S. P. (1962), *Non-specific Brain Structures and the Perceptual Function of the Cerebral Cortex*, Izd. Gruzinsk. Akad. Sci., Tbilisi. (Russian)

Narikashvili, S. P. (1963), 'Cortico-subcortical interaction in analyser activity', *Fiziol. Zh. SSSR*, vol. 49, no. 11.

Narikashvili, S. P. (1968), 'Cortical influence on the thalamic nuclei and reticular formation of the brain stem', in *Cortical Regulation of Activity of Subcortical Brain Structures*, Tbilisi (Russian).

Narikashvili, S. P., and Kadzhaya, D. V. (1963), 'Cortical regulation of response activity of the relay nucleus', *Fiziol. Zh. SSSR*, vol. 49.

Nauta, W. J. (1964), 'Some efferent connections of the prefrontal cortex in the monkey', in J. M. Warren and K. Akert (eds.), *Frontal Granular Cortex and Behavior*, McGraw-Hill.

Nauta, W. J. (1968), 'A survey of the anatomical connections of the prefrontal cortex', in *Problems in Dynamic Localization of Brain Functions*, Meditsina, Moscow (Russian).

Nauta, W. J. (1971), 'The problem of the frontal lobe: A reinterpretation', manuscript.

Newell, A., Shaw, I. C., and Simon, H. A. (1958), 'Elements of a theory of human problem solving', *Psychol. Rev.*, vol. 65.

Nielsen, J. M. (1946), *Agnosia, Aphraxia and Aphasia*, Los Angeles.

Norman, D. A. (1966), 'Acquisition and retention in short-term memory', *J. Exp. Psychol.*, vol. 72.

Norman, D. A. (1968), 'Towards a theory of memory and attention', *Psychol. Rev.*, vol. 75.

Norman, D. A., and Rumelhart, D. I. (1970), 'A system for perception and memory', in D. A. Norman (ed.), *Models of Human Memory*, Academic Press.

Olds, J. (1955), 'Physiological mechanisms of reward', in *Nebraska Symposium on Motivation*, University of Nebraska Press.

Olds, J. (1958), 'Selective effects of drives and drugs on "reward" system of the brain', in G. E. W. Wolstenholme and C. M. O'Connor (eds.), *Neurological Basis of Behaviour*, Ciba Foundation Symposium, Churchill.

Olds, J. (1959), 'Higher functions of the nervous system', *Ann. Rev. Physiol.*, vol. 21.

Ombrédane, A. (1951), *L'aphasie et l'élaboration de la pensée explicite*, Presses Universitaires de France.

Paterson, A., and Zangwill, O. L. (1944), 'Disorders of visual space perception associated with lesions of the right cerebral hemisphere', *Brain*, vol. 67.

Paterson, A., and Zangwill, O. L. (1945), 'A case of topographical disorientation associated with an unilateral cerebral lesion', *Brain*, vol. 68.

Pavlov, I. P. (1949a), *Complete Collected Works*, vols. 1–6, Izd. Akad. Nauk SSSR, Moscow and Leningrad (Russian).

Pavlov, I. P. (1949b), *Pavlov's Wednesday Clinics*, vols. 1–3, Izd. Akad. Nauk SSSR, Moscow and Leningrad (Russian).

Peimer, I. A. (1958), 'Local bioelectrical responses of the human cortex and their correlation with generalized responses during conditioned-reflex activity', *Fiziol. Zh. SSSR*, no. 9 (Russian).

Peimer, I. A. (1966), 'Correlations between local and generalized responses during the transmission of information in the human central nervous system', in *Problems in Neurocybernetics*, Rostov-on-Don (Russian).

Penfield, W., and Jasper, H. (1959), *Epilepsy and the Functional Anatomy of the Human Brain*, Little, Brown.

Penfield, W., and Milner, B. (1958), 'Memory deficit produced by bilateral lesions of the hippocampal zone', *Arch. Neurol. Psychiat.* (Chicago), vol. 74.

Pham Ming Hac (1971), 'Modes of memory disturbances in lesions of the convexital parts of the left hemisphere', Dissertation, Moscow University.

Pick, A. (1905), *Studien über motorische Aphasie*, Vienna.

Piercy, M. F., Hécaen, H., and Ajuriaguerra, J. (1960), 'Constructional apraxia associated with unilateral cerebral lesions', *Brain*, vol. 83.

Piercy, M. S., and Smith, V. (1962), 'Right hemisphere dominance for certain non-verbal intellectual skills', *Brain*, vol. 85.

Polikanina, R. M. (1966), *Development of Higher Nervous Activity in Premature Infants in the Early Period of Life*, Meditsina, Moscow (Russian).

Polyakov, G. I. (1965), *Principles of Neuronal Organization of the Brain*, Moscow University Press, Moscow (Russian).

Polyakov, G. I. (1966), 'Structural organization of the frontal cortex in relation to its functional role', in A. R. Luria and E. D. Homskaya (eds.), *The Frontal Lobes and Regulation of Psychological Processes*, Moscow University Press, Moscow (Russian).

Popova, L. T. (1964), 'Disturbance of mnestic processes in patients with some local brain lesions', Candidate Dissertation, First Moscow Medical Institute (Russian)

Posner, M. I. (1963), 'Immediate memory in sequential tasks', *Psychol. Bull.*, vol. 60.

Posner, M. I. (1967), 'Short-term memory systems in human information processing', *Acta Psychol.*, vol. 27.

Posner, M. I. (1969), 'Representational systems for storing information in memory', in G. Talland and N. Waugh (eds.), *The Pathology of Memory*, Academic Press.

Postman, L. (1954), 'Learning principles of organization of the memory', *Psychol. Monogr.*, no. 68.

Postman, L. (1961a), 'Extra-experimental interference and the retention of words', *J. Exp. Psychol.*, vol. 61.

Postman, L. (1961b), 'The present state of interference theory', in C. N. Cofer (ed.), *Verbal Learning and Verbal Behavior*, McGraw-Hill.

Postman, L. (1963), 'Does interference theory predict much forgetting?' *J. Verbal Learning Verb. Behav.*, vol. 2.

Postman, L. (1967), 'The effect of inter-item associative strength on the acquisition and retention of serial lists', *J. Verbal Learning Verb. Behav.*, vol. 6.

Postman, L. (1969), 'Mechanisms of interfering in forgetting', in G. Talland and N. Waugh (eds.), *The Pathology of Memory*, Academic Press.

Pötzl, O. (1928), *Die Aphasi lehre vom Standpunkt der klinischen Psychiatrie. Die optisch-agnostischen Störungen*, Deutike, Leipzig.

Pötzl, O. (1937), 'Zum Apraxieproblem', *J. Neurol. Psychol.*, vol. 54.

Pribram, K. H. (1954), 'Towards a science of neuropsychology', in R. A. Patton (ed.), *Current Trends in Psychology and the Biological Sciences*, University of Pittsburgh Press.

Pribram, K. H. (1958a), 'Neocortical functions in behavior', in *Symposium on Interdisciplinary Research in the Behavioral Sciences*, University of Wisconsin Press, Madison.

Pribram, K. H. (1958b), 'Comparative neurology and evolution of behavior', in *Behavior and Evolution*, Yale University Press.

Pribram, K. H. (1959a), *On the Neurology of Thinking*, Behavioral Sciences Series, vol. 4., Harper & Row.

Pribram, K. H. (1959b), 'The intrinsic systems of the forebrain', in J. Field and H. W. Magoun (eds.), *Handbook of Physiology*, McGraw-Hill.

Pribram, K. H. (1960), 'A review of the theory in physiological psychology', *Ann. Rev. Psychol.*, vol. 11.

Pribram, K. H. (1961), 'A further analysis of the behavior deficit that follows injury to the primate frontal cortex', *J. Exp. Neurol.*, vol. 3.

Pribram, K. H. (1963a), 'The new neurology: memory, novelty, thought and choice', in G. H. Glaser (ed.), *The Electroencephalogram and Behavior*, Basic Books.

Pribram, K. H. (1963b), 'Reinforcement revisited', in M. Jones (ed.), *Nebraska Symposium on Motivation*, University of Nebraska Press.

Pribram, K. H. (1966a), 'Contemporary investigations of the function of the frontal lobes in the monkey and man', in A. R. Luria and E. D. Homskaya (eds.), *The Frontal Lobes and Regulation of Psychological Processes*', Moscow University Press (Russian).

Pribram, K. H. (1966b), 'The limbic system, efferent control of inhibition of behavior', in T. Tokizane and J. P. Schadé (eds.), *Progress in Brain Research*, Elsevier, Amsterdam.

Pribram, K. H. (1967), 'Steps towards a neuropsychological theory', in D. C. Glass (ed.), *Neurophysiology and Emotion*, Rockefeller University Press.

Pribram, K. H. (1971), *Languages of the Brain: Experimental Paradoxes and Principles of Neuropsychology*, Prentice-Hall.

Ramon-y-Cajal, S. (1909–11), *Histologie du système nerveux de l'homme et des vertébrés*, 2 vols., Maloine.

Reitman, W. (1970), 'What does it take to remember?' in D. A. Norman (ed.), *Models of Human Memory*, Academic Press.

de Renzi, E., and Spinnler, H. (1966a), 'Facial recognition in brain-damaged patients', *Neurology* (Minneapolis), vol. 16.

de Renzi, E., and Spinnler, H. (1966b), 'Visual recognition in patients with unilateral cerebral disease', *J. Nerv. Ment. Dis.*, vol. 142.

Revault d'Allones, G. (1923), 'La schématisation. L'attention', in Dumas, *Traité de psychologie*, Paris.

de Robertis, E. D. P. (1964), *Histopathology of Synapses and Neurosecretion*, Pergamon Press, Oxford.

Robinson, E. (1920), 'Some factors determining the degree of retroaction', *Psychol. Monogr.*, vol. 28, no. 128.

Rose, J. E., and Woolsey, C. N. (1949), 'Organization of the mammalian thalamus and its relationship to the cerebral cortex', *Electroenceph. Clin. Neurophysiol.*, vol. 1.

Rosvold, H. E. (1959), 'Physiological psychology', *Ann. Rev. Psychol.*, vol. 10.

Rosvold, H. E., and Delgado, J. M. R. (1956), 'The effect on delayed alternation test performance of stimulating and destroying electrical structures within the frontal lobes', *J. Comp. Physiol. Psychol.*, vol. 51.

Ryabova, R. V. (1970), 'Psycholinguistic and neuropsychological analysis of dynamic aphasia', Candidate Dissertation, Moscow University, Moscow (Russian).

Rylander, G. (1939), *Personality Changes after Operations on the Frontal Lobes*, London.

Sager, O. (1962), *The Diencephalon*, Romanian Acad. Sci. Press, Bucharest (Russian).

Sager, O. (1965), 'Mechanisms of self-regulation of cortico-subcortical relationships', in *Reflexes of the Brain*, Nauka, Moscow (Russian).

Sager, O. (1968), 'The study of functions of the cerebral cortex in regulating subcortical centres', in *Cortical Regulation of Activity of Subcortical Brain Structures*, Tbilisi (Russian).

Sapir, I. D. (1929), 'Die Neurodynamik des Sprachapparates bei Aphasikern', *J. Psychol. Neurol*, vol. 38, no. 1.

Scheibel, M. E., and Scheibel, A. B. (1958), 'Structural substrates for integrative patterns in the brain stem reticular core', in *Reticular Formation of the Brain*, Little, Brown.

Scoville, W. B. (1954), 'The limbic system in man', *J. Neurosurg.*, vol. 11.

Scoville, W. B., and Milner, B. (1957), 'Loss of recent memory after bilateral hippocampal lesions', *J. Neurol. Neurosurg. Psychiat.*, vol. 20.

Segundo, J. P., Arana-Ingues, R., and French, J. D. (1955), 'Behavioral arousal by stimulation of the brain in the monkey', *J. Neurosurg.*, vol. 12.

Segundo, J. P., Naquet, R., and Buser, P. (1955), 'Effects of cortical stimulation on electrocortical activity in monkeys', *J. Neurophysiol.*, vol. 18.

Semernitskaya, F. M. (1945), 'Rhythm and its disturbance in various brain lesions', Candidate Dissertation, Institute of Psychology, Acad. Pedagogic Sci. RSFSR, Moscow (Russian).

Semmes, J. (1965), 'Hemispheric specialization: a possible clue mechanism', *Neuropsycholgia*, vol. 3.

Semmes, J., Weinstein, S., Ghent, L., Teuber, H. L. (1955), 'Spatial orientation in man after cerebral injury', *J. Physchol.*, vol. 39.

Sharples, F., and Jasper, H. H. (1956), 'Habituation of the arousal reaction', *Brain*, vol. 79.

Sherrington, C. S. (1934), *The Brain and Its Mechanisms*, Cambridge University Press.

Sherrington, C. S. (1942), *Man on his Nature*, Cambridge University Press, London.

Shiffrin, R. M. (1970), 'Memory search', in D. A. Norman (ed.), *Models of Human Memory*, Academic Press.

Shmar'yan, A. S. (1949), *Cerebral Pathology and Psychiatry*, Medgiz, Moscow (Russian).

Simernitskaya, E. G. (1970), *The Study of the Regulation of Activity by the Evoked Potentials Method*, Moscow University Press (Russian).

Simernitskaya, E. G., and Homskaya, E. D. (1966), 'Changes in the parameters of evoked responses depending on differences in informative value of stimuli under normal conditions and in frontal lobe lesions', in A. R. Luria and E. D. Homskaya (eds.), *The Frontal Lobes and Regulation of Psychological Processes*, Moscow University Press, Moscow (Russian).

Sittig, O. (1931), *Apraxie*, Karger, Berlin.

Skaggs, E. (1925), 'Further studies in retroactive inhibition', *Psychol. Monogr.*, vol. 34, no. 161.

Smirnov, A. A. (1948), *The psychology of remembering*, Izd Akad. Pedagog. Nauk, Moscow (Russian).

Smirnov, A. A. (1966), *The Psychology of Memory*, Prosveshchenie Press, Moscow (Russian).

Smirnov, L. I. (1946), *The Pathological Anatomy of Brain Trauma*, Medgiz, Moscow (Russian).

Smirnov, L. I. (1948), *The Topography, Anatomy and Histology of Brain Tumours*, Medgiz, Moscow (Russian).

Smith, A. (1966), 'Speech and other functions after left (dominant) hemispherectomy', *J. Neurol. Neurosurg. Psychiat.*, vol. 29.

Smith, A. (1969), 'Nondominant hemisphere', *Neurology*, vol. 19.

Smith, A., and Burkland, C. W. (1966), 'Dominant hemispherectomy', *Science*, vol. 135.

Sokolov, E. N. (1958), *Perception and the Conditioned Reflex*, Macmillan.

Sokolov, E. N. (1960), 'Neuronal model of the orienting reflex', in M. Brazier (ed.), *The Central Nervous System and Behavior*, J. Macy Jr Foundation, New York.

Sokolov, E. N., *et al.* (eds.) (1959), *The Orienting Reflex and Problems of Higher Nervous Activity*, Izd. Akad. Pedagog. Nauk RSFSR, Moscow (Russian).

Sokolov, E. N., *et al.* (eds.) (1964), *The Orienting Reflex and Problems of Perception under Normal and Pathological Conditions*, Prosveshchenie Press, Moscow (Russian).

Soloviev, I. M. (1966), *The Psychology of the Gnostic Activity of Normal and Abnormal Children*, Prosveshchenie Press, Moscow (Russian).

Sperling, G. (1960), 'The information available in brief visual perception', *Psychol. Monogr.*, vol. 74, no. 11.

Sperling, G. (1963), 'A model for visual memory tasks', *Human Factors*, vol. 5.

Sperling, G., and Spellman, R. G. (1970), 'Acoustic similarity and auditory short term memory: experiments and a model', in D. A. Norman (ed.), *Models of Human Memory*, Academic Press.

Sperry, R. W. (1959), 'Preservation of high-ordered functions in isolated somatic cortex in callosum-sectioned cat', *J. Neurophysiol.*, vol. 22.

Sperry, R. W. (1966), 'Brain dissection and mechanisms of consciousness', in J. C. Eccles (ed.), *Brain and Conscious Experience*, Springer.

Sperry, R. W. (1967a), *Mental Unity Following Surgical Disconnections of the Hemispheres*, Academic Press.

Sperry, R. W. (1967b), 'Split-brain approach to learning problems', in G. C. Quarton *et al.* (eds.), *The Neurosciences*, Rockefeller University Press.

Sperry, R. W. (1968), 'Hemisphere disconnection and unity of conscious awareness', *Amer. Psychologist*, vol. 23.

Sperry, R. W., and Gazzaniga, M. S. (1967), 'Language following surgical disconnection of the hemispheres', in C. H. Millikan and F. L. Darley (eds.), *Brain Mechanisms Underlying Speech and Language*, Grune & Stratton.

Sperry, R. W., Gazzaniga, M. S., and Bogen, J. E. (1969), 'Interhemispheric relationships: the neocortical commissures; syndromes of hemisphere disconnection', in P. J. Vinken and G. W. Bruyn (eds.), *Handbook of Clinical Neurology*, vol. 4, North Holland Publishing Co.

Spinelli, D. N., and Pribram, K. H. (1967), 'Changes in visual recovery function and unit activity produced by frontal and temporal cortex stimulation', *Electroenceph. clin. Neurophysiol.*, vol. 22, pp. 143-9.

Subirana, A. (1952), 'La droiterie', *Schweiz. Arch. Neurol. Psychiat.*, vol. 69.

Subirana, A. (1964), 'The relationship between handedness and language function', *Internat. J. Neurol.*, vol. 4.

Subirana, A. (1969), 'Handedness and cerebral dominance', in P. J. Vinken and G. W. Bruyn (eds.), *Handbook of Clinical Neurology*, vol. 4, North Holland Publishing Co.

Sugar, O., French, J. D., and Ghusid, J. G. (1948), 'Cortico-cortical connections of the superior surface of temporal operculum in monkey', *J. Neurophysiol.*, vol. 11.

Sugar, O., Petr, R., Amador, L. V., and Criponissiotu, B. (1950), 'Cortico-cortical connections of the cortex buried in intraparietal and principal sulci of monkey', *J. Neuropath. Exp. Neurol.*, vol. 9.

Svedelius, C. (1897), *L'analyse du langage*, Uppsala.

Tecce, J. I. (1970), 'Attention and evoked potentials in man', in D. Mostofsky (ed.), *Attention*, Appleton, Century, Crofts.

Teuber, H. L., *et al.* (1960), *Somatic Sensory Changes after Penetrating Brain Wounds in Man*, Harvard University Press.

Teuber, H. L. (1962), 'Effects of brain wounds implicating right or left hemispheres in man', in V. B. Mountcastle (ed.), *Interhemispheric Reactions and Cerebral Dominance*, Johns Hopkins Press.

Tinbergen, N. (1957), *The Study of Instincts*, Oxford University Press.

Titchener, E. B. (1908), *Lectures of the Elementary Psychology of Feeling and Attention*, New York.

Traugott, N. N. (1947), *Sensory alalia and aphasia in childhood*. *Medico-Biological Science*, no. 1, Izd. Akad. Med. Nauk SSSR, Moscow (Russian).

Troubezkoi, N. (1939), *Grundriss der Phonologie*, Prague.

Tsvetkova, L. S. (1966a), 'Disturbance of constructive activity in frontal lobe lesions', in A. R. Luria and E. D. Homskaya (eds.), *The Frontal Lobes and Regulation of Psychological Processes*, Moscow University Press, Moscow (Russian).

Tsvetkova, L. S. (1966b), 'Disturbance of analysis of a written text in patients with frontal lobe lesions', in A. R. Luria and E. D. Homskaya (eds.), *The Frontal Lobes and Regulation of Psychological Processes*, Moscow University Press, Moscow (Russian).

Tsvetkova, L. S. (1966c), 'Disturbance of the solution of arithmetical problems in patients with lesions of the parieto-occipital and frontal zones of the brain', in A. R. Luria and E. D. Homskaya (eds.), *The Frontal Lobes and Regulation o Psychological Processes*. Moscow University Press, Moscow (Russian).

Tsvetkova, L. S. (1969), 'Disturbance of active forms of speech in dynamic aphasia', *Voprosy Psikhologii*, no. 1.

Tsvetkova, L. S. (1970), 'Rehabilitative training in local brain lesions', Doctoral Dissertation, Moscow University (Russian).

Tsvetkova, L. S. (1972), *Rehabilitative training in local brain lesions*, Pedagogika, Publishing House Moscow (Russian).

Underwood, B. J. (1945), 'The effect of successive interpolation on retroactive and proactive inhibition', *Psychol. Monogr.*, vol. 59, no. 3.

Underwood, B. J. (1957), 'Interference and forgetting', *Psychol. Rev.*, vol. 64.

Underwood, B. J., and Ekstrand, B. R. (1966), 'An analysis of some shortcomings in the interference theory of forgetting', *Psychol. Rev.*, vol. 73.

Underwood, B. J., and Postman, L. (1960), 'Extraexperimental sources of interference in forgetting', *Psychol. Rev.*, vol. 67.

Underwood, B. J., and Postman, L. (1962), 'Extraexperimental sources of interference and forgetting', *Amer. J. Psychol.*, vol. 75.

Uznadze, D. N. (1966), *Experimental Psychological Investigations*, Nauka, Moscow (Russian).

Vinarskaya, E. N. (1971), Clinical problems of aphasia', *Neurolinguistic Analysis*, Meditsina Publishers, Moscow.

Vinogradova, O. S. (1958), 'Dynamics of the orienting reflex during conditioning', in *The Orienting Reflex and Orienting and Investigative Activity*, Izd. Akad. Pedagog. Nauk RSFSR, Moscow (Russian).

Vinogradova, O. S. (1959a), 'Role of the orienting reflex in conditioning in man', in *The Orienting Reflex and Problems in Higher Nervous Activity*, Izd. Akad. Pedagog. Nauk SSSR, Moscow (Russian).

Vinogradova, O. S. (1959b), 'Investigation of the orienting reflex in children by a plethysmographic method', in *The Orienting Reflex and Problems in Higher Nervous Activitiy*, Izd. Akad. Pedagog. Nauk RSFSR, Moscow (Russian).

Vinogradova, O. S. (1961), *The Orienting Reflex and Its Neurophysiological Mechanisms*, Izd. Akad. Pedagog. Nauk RSFSR, Moscow (Russian).

Vinogradova, O. S. (1969), 'Functional properties of cortical neurons', in A. R. Luria, *Higher Cortical Functions in Man*, 2nd edn, Moscow University Press, Moscow (Russian).

Vinogradova, O. S. (1970a), 'The hippocampus and the orienting reflex', in *Neuronal Mechanisms of the Orienting Reflex*, Moscow University Press, Moscow (Russian).

Vinogradova, O. S. (1970b), 'The limbic system and registration of information', in R. Hinde and G. Korn (eds.), *Short-term Processes in Nervous Activity and Behaviour*, Cambridge University Press.

Vladimirov, A. D. (1972), *Methods of Eye Movement Studies*, Moscow University Press.

Vladimirov, A. D., and Homskaya, E. D. (1962), 'A photo-electric method of recording eye movements during the examination of objects', *Voprosy Psikhologii*, no. 5 (Russian) (English translation, *American Psychologist*, 1969, vol. 24.)

Vygotsky, L. S. (1934), *Thought and Speech*, Sotsekgiz (Russian).

Vygotsky, L. S. (1956), *Selected Psychological Investigations*, Izd. Akad. Pedagog. Nauk RSFSR, Moscow (Russian).

Vygotsky, L. S. (1960), *Development of the Higher Mental Functions*, Izd. Akad. Pedagog. Nauk RSFSR, Moscow (Russian).

Vygotsky, L. S., and Luria, A. R. (1930), *Studies in the History of Behaviour*, OGIZ, Moscow (Russian).

Wada, J. (1949), 'A new method for determination of the side of cerebral speech dominance', *Med. Biol.*, vol. 14.

Wada, J., and Rasmussen, T. (1960), 'Intracarotid injection of sodium amytal for the lateralization of cerebral speech dominance', *J. Neurosurg.*, vol. 17.

Walter, W. Grey (1966), 'Role of the human frontal lobes in the regulation of activity', in A. R. Luria and E. D. Homskaya (eds.), *The Frontal Lobes and Regulation of Psychological Processes*, Moscow University Press, Moscow (Russian).

Walter, W. Grey, Cooper, R., Aldridge, V. J., McCallum, W. C., and Winter, A. L. (1964), 'Contingent negative variation, etc.', *Nature*, vol. 203.

Warrington, E. K. (1971), 'Neurological disorders of memory', *Brit. Med. Bull.*, vol. 27, no. 3.

Warrington, E., and James, M. (1967), 'Disorders of visual perception in patients with localized brain lesions', *Neuropsychologia*, vol. 5.

Warrington, E., James, S., and Kinsbourne, M. (1966), 'Drawing disability in relation to laterality of cerebral lesion', *Brain*, vol. 89.

Weigl, E. (1964), 'Some critical remarks concerning the problem of so called simultanagnosia', *Neuropsychologia*, vol. 2.

Weinstein, E. A., Cole, M., Mitchell, M. S., and Lyerly, O. G. (1964), 'Anosognosia and aphasia', *Arch. Neurol. Psychiat.* (Chicago), vol. 10.

Weiskrantz, L. (1964), 'Neurological studies and animal behaviour', *Brit. Med. Bulletin*, vol. 20, no. 1.

Weiskrantz, L. (ed.) (1968), *Analysis of Behavioral Change*, Harper & Row.

Welt, L. (1888), 'Über Charakterveränderungen des Menschen in Folge der Läsionen des Stirnhirns', *Dtsch. Arch. klin. Med.*, vol., 42.

Wernicke, C. (1894), 'Grundriss der Psychiatrie', *Psychophysiologische Einleitung*, Wiesbaden.

Wertheimer, M. (1925), *Drei Abhandlungen zur Gestalttheorie*, Erlangen.

Wertheimer, M. (1945), *Produktives Denken*, Frankfurt-am-Main.

Wertheimer, M. (1957), *Productive Thinking*, New York.

Wickelgren, W. A. (1970), 'Multitrace strength theory', in D. A. Norman (ed.), *Models of Human Memory*, Academic Press.

Woerkom, W. van (1925), 'Über Störungen im Denken bei aphasischen Patienten', *Monatsschr. Psychol. Neurol.*, vol. 59.

Woolsey, C. N. (1958), 'Organization of the somatic sensory and motor areas of the cerebral cortex', in *Biological and Biochemical Bases of Behavior*, University of Wisconsin Press, pp. 63–81.

Yarbus, A. L. (1965), *Eye Movements and Vision*, Nauka (Russian; English translation by B. Haigh: Plenum Press, New York, 1967).

Yoshii, N., Miyamoto, K., Shimokoti, M., and Halse, S. (1969), 'The study of the EEG changes specific for a certain type of behaviour and the neurophysiological mechanism of the conditioned reflex', in *Systemic Organization of Physiological Functions*, Meditsina, Moscow (Russian).

Zangwill, O. L. (1960), *Cerebral Dominance and Its Relation to Psychological Function*, Oliver & Boyd.

Zaporozhets, A. V. (1960), *Development of the Child's Voluntary Movements*, Izd. Akad. Pedagog. Nauk RSFSR, Moscow (Russian).

Zaporozhets, A. V. (ed.) (1967), *Perception and Action*, Prosveshchenie Press, Moscow (Russian).

Zaporozhets, A. V. (1968), *Formation of Perception in the Preschool Child*, Prosveshchenie Press, Moscow (Russian).

Zeigarnik, B. V. (1961), *The Pathology of Thinking*, Moscow University Press, Moscow (Russian; English translation by B. Haigh: Consultants Bureau, New York, 1965).

Zeigarnik, B. V. (1968), *Introduction to Psychopathology*, Moscow University Press, Moscow (Russian).

Zimkin, N. V., and Zimkina, A. M. (1953), 'The role of various zones of the nervous system in the course of trace processes in the tactile, temperature and taste analysers', in *Problems in Physiological Optics*, vol. 8, Izd. Akad. Med. Nauk SSSR, Moscow (Russian).

Zimkina, A. M. (1957), 'Some special features of tactile trace processes (after images) in man', *Material on Evolutionary Physiology*, vol. 2, Izd. Akad. Nauk SSSR, Moscow (Russian).

Zinchenko, P. J. (1961), *Involuntary Recall*, Izd. Akad. Pedagog. Nauk, Moscow (Russian).

Zinchenko, V. P., Wang Chih-ts'ing, and Tarakanov, V. V. (1962), 'The formation and development of perceptive actions', *Voprosy Psikhologii*, no. 3 (Russian).

Zinchenko, V. P., and Vergiler, N. Yu., (1972), *Formation of Visual Images*, N.Y. Consultants Bureau.

Zislina, N. N. (1955), 'Disturbance of visual after images in lesions of the cerebral cortex', *Problems in Physiological Optics*, vol. 11, Izd. Akad. Med. Nauk SSSR, Moscow (Russian).

Zucker, R. (1934), 'An analysis of disturbed function in aphasia', *Brain*, vol. 57.

Zurif, E. B., and Carson, G. (1970), 'Dyslexia in relation to cerebral dominance and temporal analysis', *Neuropsychologia*, vol. 8.

Author Index

Drew, E. A., 78, 236
Duncker, K., 325
Durinyan, R. A., 58, 86
Dusser de Barenne, J. G., 88

Eccles, J. C., 281, 282
Elkonin, D. B., 29
Elyasson, M. I., 131
Ettlinger, G., 78, 236, 239

Faller, T. O., 273
Farber, D. A., 259, 261, 268, 269
Faust, C., 126, 239
Feigenbaum, E., 284, 326
Feldman, J., 326
Feuchtwanger, E., 188, 223
Filimonov, I. N., 60, 113
Filippycheva, N. A., 273
Flechsig, P., 73, 81
Flourens, M. J. P., 25
Foerster, O., 114–15, 172, 173, 179
Fonarev, A. M., 258
Frankfurter, W., 135
Franz, S. I., 89, 188
French, J. D., 47, 49, 50, 58, 86, 88
Fried, A. M., 259, 261, 268, 269, 270
Fulton, J. F., 179
Futer, J. C., 41, 143

Gadzhiev, S. G., 335
Galambos, R., 58
Galanter, E., 92, 250, 329
Gall, F. J., 20, 21, 22
Galperin, P. Ya., 29, 30, 94, 326, 328
Gastaut, H., 55, 56
Gavrilova, N. A., 98, 265
Gazzaniga, M. S., 162, 163
Gelb, A., 110, 230, 235, 236
Genkin, A. A., 193, 265
Gershuni, G. V., 55, 129
Geschwind, N., 148, 237, 239
Ghent, L., 148
Ghusid, J. G., 88
Gloning, I., 237
Gloning, K., 237
Goldberg, J. M., 131

Goldstein, K., 24–5, 110, 156, 230,
  235, 236, 305, 315, 323, 330
Goltz, F., 25
Grastyan, E., 272
Groot, A. D. de, 326
Gross, C. G., 93
Grünthal, E., 64, 288

Haigh, B., 12
Halle, M., 134
Halstead, W. C., 188
Harlow, J., 188
Head, H., 24–5, 154, 305
Hebb, D. O., 55, 188, 221
Hécaen, H., 111, 121, 126, 160, 162,
  164, 165, 166, 167, 231, 235, 237,
  238, 239
Hering, K. E., 280
Hernández-Peón, R., 49, 58, 86, 265–7
Hochheimer, W., 236
Hoff, H., 166, 237, 239
Holmes, G., 109, 110–11, 121, 165,
  231
Homskaya, E. D., 37, 58, 63, 86, 180,
  189–92, 194, 195, 201–2, 210, 211,
  216, 222, 224, 243, 264, 272, 276,
  277, 279
Hornstein, S., 125
Hubel, D. M., 68, 231
Hunter, W. S., 28
Hydén, H., 281

Ioshpa, A. Ya., 180
Isserlin, M., 156
Itina, N. A., 258
Irvin, I. M., 285

Jackson, J. H., 24, 165, 221, 238
Jacobsen, C. F., 89, 90, 188, 274
Jacobson, A. L., 281
Jakobson, R., 134
James, S., 165, 235, 239
Janet, P., 123
Jasper, H. H., 15, 47, 55, 56, 131, 270
Jellinger, K., 237
Jouvet, M., 47, 49, 58, 194, 265

Subject Index